W9-CLJ-871

BARRON'S

CCRN®

EXAM

Pat Juarez, APN, CCNS

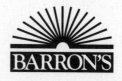

BARRON'S

ABOUT THE AUTHOR

Pat Juarez, MS, APN, CCNS has over 30 years of critical care nursing experience as a Clinical Nurse Specialist, staff nurse, and educator. As the Clinical Development Specialist for Critical Care, Pat developed and provided oversight for the critical care nursing curriculum for Advocate Health Care for over 10 years. She is currently the Clinical Practice Specialist for Advocate Health Care and continues to teach the CCRN Certification course on a consulting basis.

ACKNOWLEDGMENTS

For critical care nurses, I remain in awe of your knowledge, skills and caring after all these years ... the learning and caring are an unending journey.

And for Alicia, my daughter, and Wayne, my best friend, for their love and support.

© Copyright 2015 by Barron's Educational Series, Inc.

All rights reserved.
No part of this publication may be reproduced or distributed in any form or by any means without the written permission of the copyright owner.

All inquiries should be addressed to:
Barron's Educational Series, Inc.
250 Wireless Boulevard
Hauppauge, NY 11788
www.barronseduc.com

ISBN-13: 978-1-4380-0458-7

Library of Congress Catalog Card No. 2015931164

PRINTED IN THE UNITED STATES OF AMERICA
9 8 7 6 5 4 3 2 1

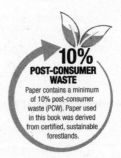

10%
POST-CONSUMER WASTE
Paper contains a minimum of 10% post-consumer waste (PCW). Paper used in this book was derived from certified, sustainable forestlands.

CONTENTS

PRACTICE TESTS

Introduction

1

The purpose of this book is to identify the key concepts you need to master in order to successfully pass the adult critical care nursing certification exam (CCRN®). The exam is developed and administered by the AACN Certification Corporation, an organization separately incorporated from the American Association of Critical Care Nurses (AACN). Certification is a process by which a nongovernmental agency validates, based upon predetermined standards, an individual nurse's qualifications and knowledge for practicing in a defined functional or clinical area of nursing. Achieving certification in your specialty nursing practice is a major professional achievement.

This book is a succinct review. It focuses on the key concepts included in the test blueprint. It does not provide a comprehensive critical care nursing curriculum review, nor does it provide detailed information about every aspect of the test blueprint. You do not need to spend your time studying material that is not covered on the exam. You should spend time understanding and studying the concepts included in the test blueprint. Nurses who have successfully passed the test have reported that self-testing and retesting themselves by using practice questions is one of the best strategies for test preparation. With this in mind, this book provides more than 450 practice questions for you to answer as you study.

For detailed information on the qualifications needed to take the exam and to register for the exam online, go to the AACN website, *www.aacn.org*.

> Throughout this book you will see certain subjects or sections marked with a star icon (☆). Pay special attention to these concepts, as they are very likely to appear on the CCRN test!

Test-Taking Tips

2

A journey of a thousand miles begins with a single step.

—Lao Tzu

Congratulations on taking the first step in your certification journey by acquiring *Barron's CCRN Exam*. This section will provide you with strategies that have worked for others who have successfully completed their certification journey by passing the CCRN exam. Although everyone learns at a different pace, one thing's for sure—you will not pass the test if you do not study or if you rely solely on your clinical experience.

You must understand some facts about the CCRN test:

- The test is a computerized 150-question test, of which 125 will count.
    - 25 questions (you will not know which ones) are in the process of validation by AACN for future tests.
- The test is designed to measure your command of the common body of knowledge needed to function effectively in an acute/critical care setting.
- The test blueprint is based on studies done by AACN of acute/critical care nursing practice.
- The **AACN Synergy Model for Patient Care** serves as the organizing framework of the exam. Although no questions refer directly to the Synergy Model, you must understand it, especially to prepare for the 30 questions (20% of the exam) that cover professional caring and ethical practice.
- You will have 3 hours to complete the exam. I have never met anyone who did not have enough time to complete the test. However, it's a good idea to pace yourself and remain aware of the time.

PASSING SCORE

- In order to pass, you need to answer 88 of 125 questions correctly, which is 70% of the 125 questions counted.
- The passing score is evaluated in total, NOT by each category. For example, you can get all 6 endocrine questions wrong and still be able to pass the test if you do well on the other topics.

Knowledge of the test blueprint is important to guide your study time. For instance, you will probably see only three hematology questions, so you should not spend 30 hours studying hematology. On the other hand, there are about 30 cardiovascular questions. Therefore, you should definitely plan on more study time for this topic. Clinical judgment accounts for 80% of the test, and professional caring and ethical practice accounts for 20% of the test. See the specific breakdown of test topics that follows (Table 2-1).

Table 2-1. Adult CCRN Test Blueprint

Clinical Judgment	# of Questions	% of Test
Topic	**120 Questions**	**80%**
Cardiovascular	30 questions	20%
Pulmonary	27 questions	18%
Neurology	18 questions	12%
Multisystem	12 questions	8%
GI	9 questions	6%
Renal	9 questions	6%
Endocrine	6 questions	4%
Behavioral	6 questions	4%
Hematology/immunology	3 questions	2%
Professional Caring and Ethical Practice	**30 questions**	**20%**
Advocacy/moral agency	4 questions	3%
Caring practices	6 questions	4%
Collaboration	6 questions	4%
Systems thinking	3 questions	2%
Response to diversity	3 questions	2%
Clinical inquiry	4 questions	2%
Facilitation of learning	4 questions	3%

TEST QUESTIONS

You will need to memorize many facts. However, most questions require you to go a step further and apply or evaluate the facts. For instance, you are expected to know normal hemodynamic parameters. The questions on hemodynamics, though, will test your ability to apply a plan of care for abnormal values. Overall question types include:

- Knowledge/comprehension questions (36%)
  - Require memory of previously learned information and an understanding of the information
- Application/analysis questions (39%)
  - Require an ability to use information appropriately and to recognize commonalities, differences, interrelationships
- Synthesis/evaluation questions (25%)
  - Require the ability to put parts together to form a new conclusion and judge the value of the information
- All phases of the nursing process are included on the exam, with intervention being the phase with the greatest percentage:
  - Assessment   32%
  - Planning   15%
  - Intervention   40%
  - Evaluation   13%

The CCRN exam is NOT an easy test. The pass rate has been about the same for years. These are the test statistics as of December 30, 2013:

Candidates Tested (2014)	First-Time Pass Rate	Total Certificants
11,824	72%	65,081

This data should not scare you but, instead, serve as a reality check. You need to STUDY. You also need to study the material covered on the test—not the entire core curriculum for critical care! As T. Boone Pickens said:

A fool with a plan can outsmart a genius with no plan.

Smart critical care nurses without a good study plan have failed this test. So ask yourself, how do you, as an adult learner, learn best? Most nurses would rather study on their own according to a schedule based on the test blueprint. But others do better by participating in a study group. Even if you attend an instructor-led course, you cannot walk out of a course and successfully pass the test without studying what was covered in the class.

The following strategies are recommended to pass the CCRN exam:

- Before studying, take the brief pretest in this book. The pretest questions are primarily knowledge-based questions to provide you with a baseline snapshot of where you are.
- Review the test blueprint, and determine how much time you will spend studying each topic, e.g., 30 hours to study cardiovascular, 6 hours to study hematology, etc.
- Plan your study time by the number of hours, not by the number of days or weeks. The phrase "weeks of study" is rather vague. Instead, determine how many hours per day/ days of the week you are capable of studying.
- You MUST include practice questions when studying.
- Review, study each section of the book, and then do the practice questions at the end of each section.
- **IMPORTANT:** As you complete the practice questions, answer them without looking back into the section material. You need to test your knowledge, not your ability to look up information. After you score yourself, then go back into the section material and review.
- Look over the material for the questions you missed. Make sure you understand where you went wrong when you first answered the question. Then retake the section test until you get at least 80% correct. As you retake the questions and improve your score, you will build the confidence that you need to succeed!
- After completing each section of the book and doing the section questions until you score at least 80%, take the first 150-question practice exam. Review the questions you missed, and retake these questions until you score at least 80%.
- At least one or two weeks before you are scheduled to take the exam, proceed to the second 150-question practice test and do the same. By now, your confidence should be increasing.
- The week before the test date, answer 100–150 questions in one sitting at least once. This is your mental training. You would not attempt to complete a marathon without training first. Similarly, you should not attempt to sit and answer 150 test questions without practicing at least 100 questions in one sitting. If you don't do this, you may find your attention wavering during the actual exam.

- Do not plan on cramming the night before. This usually results in decreased self-confidence and increased anxiety.
- Your clinical experience will be an advantage. However, you should not rely totally on your unit practice patterns, which may sometimes vary from correct AACN answers.

EXAM APPLICATION

Understanding the process for exam application is important for creating your study plan. Once you get approval to take the exam, you have **90 days** to schedule and take the exam at an H&R Block testing site (or paper/pencil exam at the annual AACN National Teaching Institute (NTI)). Consider the time of year and the overall personal commitments in your life before developing your plan for studying. For example, if you are getting married on July 1, you probably should not plan on taking the certification exam on June 21! In order to apply to take the exam, you must do the following.

- Go to *www.aacn.org* and have the following available: your RN license, a credit card, and the name, address, and phone number of an RN coworker or supervisor who can verify your eligibility. You will need to enter your member/customer number or e-mail address and password to sign in.
  - Initial exam candidates not already in AACN's database must register to create a new customer account.
  - Candidates who are not current AACN members will be given the opportunity to purchase membership and pay member pricing upon certification.
- You will need to provide your current mailing address and e-mail address in order to receive an e-mail confirmation of your registration and facilitate AACN communication with you in case AACN has questions regarding your registration.
  - Approval to register for the exam will arrive via e-mail several days after you complete the online application.
  - The approval number you receive will be good for 90 days. The clock starts ticking immediately!
- You will use the AACN approval number to schedule online the date and time of the exam at an H&R Block testing site.
- You can choose either a morning or an afternoon time. Choose the time when you tend to be most alert.

Test-Taking Pearls

- Get plenty of rest the night before the test . . . no alcohol, sedating drugs, or overtime shifts! You need to be on your game.
- Plan on taking a watch, sweater, and glasses (if you need them) to the testing site.
- Eat a healthy meal before the test, include protein and carbs. Avoid eating sugar.
- Remember to bring two pieces of ID, and make sure that one is a photo ID.
- Plan to arrive early, at least 15 minutes before the scheduled time.

- Control your anxiety:
  - Some anxiety increases performance, but panic does not.
  - Adequate preparation decreases anxiety.
  - Use deep breathing/progressive muscle relaxation.
  - Visualize yourself receiving your passing score.
  - No negative self-talk!
- Performance during exam:
  - Read each question thoroughly.
  - Look for key words such as *except, least, most, never, always, initially, first, last, early, late, indicated, contraindicated, priority,* and *best.*
  - Read all options as well as the question stem.
  - After you read the question stem, answer the question without looking at the options. Then look at the answer choices. If your answer is there, it is most likely right, BUT still go ahead and read all options. A different choice may be one better than your answer.
  - Do not assume information that is not given.
  - Do not leave any question blank.
  - If you don't know the answer, don't dwell after reading it over a couple of times. Go to the next question. Come back to the difficult question later since the answer may become more apparent to you.
- You will be given one blank sheet of paper and a pen at the test site to make notations. You will be able to go back and forth among the questions.
- Guessing:
  - Use this only as a last resort.
  - First, eliminate any choices that you can.
  - If you still do not know the answer, look for the option that is different than the others.
  - If the content has nothing to do with what you have studied, you can rationalize that perhaps this is one of the 25 questions that will not be counted!
- Changing answers:
  - If you tend to miss answers due to not reading thoroughly and you realize that you misread a question, change your answer.
  - If you tend to miss questions even though you read them thoroughly, don't change your initial answer—your first selection is most likely correct.
- If any questions ask you what to do first in a situation, look at the options and see if any of them address airway, breathing, circulation (ABCs). Let that guide you.
- When in doubt, fall back on your ABCs!

EXAM RESULTS

After you complete the exam, you will get a printout of the results (see the following example).

> Congratulations! You have passed the CCRN® Examination. Your score is 111 correct answers.
> The passing score is 87 correct answers.
>
> **Note:** The scores below are PERCENT OF ITEMS ANSWERED CORRECTLY in each major content category. The examination you took included pretest items for future tests that were not included in your score. For more information about interpreting the score report, please refer to your *Exam Handbook*.

Content Area	Your % Score
1. Cardiovascular	90%
2. Pulmonary	81%
3. Endocrine	100%
4. Hematology Immunology	100%
5. Neurology	100%
6. Gastrointestinal	100%
7. Renal	100%
8. Multisystem	70%
9. Professional/Synergy Model	88%

> **Congratulations!**
>
> **You have passed the CCRN® Certification Examination.**

During the minutes while you are waiting for your scores, you might be nervous. When you pass, though, the feeling is exhilarating!

BENEFITS OF CERTIFICATION

What are the benefits of critical care certification? Why bother to undertake this professional challenge? Research has demonstrated that certification has the following benefits:

- Validates specialized knowledge
- Indicates a level of competence
- Enhances professional credibility
- Provides access to higher job levels and higher salaries
- Promotes recognition of nurses by other professionals and patients
- Improves nurses' confidence and personal satisfaction
- Increases nurse retention and, in some facilities, garners financial benefits

Value of certification to patients and their families:

- Certified nurses make decisions with more confidence.
- Certification has been linked to better patient safety.
- Certification has been linked to increased patient satisfaction.

More simply expressed…

When you know better, you do better.

—Maya Angelou

1. Ⓐ Ⓑ Ⓒ Ⓓ 6. Ⓐ Ⓑ Ⓒ Ⓓ 11. Ⓐ Ⓑ Ⓒ Ⓓ 16. Ⓐ Ⓑ Ⓒ Ⓓ 21. Ⓐ Ⓑ Ⓒ Ⓓ

2. Ⓐ Ⓑ Ⓒ Ⓓ 7. Ⓐ Ⓑ Ⓒ Ⓓ 12. Ⓐ Ⓑ Ⓒ Ⓓ 17. Ⓐ Ⓑ Ⓒ Ⓓ 22. Ⓐ Ⓑ Ⓒ Ⓓ

3. Ⓐ Ⓑ Ⓒ Ⓓ 8. Ⓐ Ⓑ Ⓒ Ⓓ 13. Ⓐ Ⓑ Ⓒ Ⓓ 18. Ⓐ Ⓑ Ⓒ Ⓓ 23. Ⓐ Ⓑ Ⓒ Ⓓ

4. Ⓐ Ⓑ Ⓒ Ⓓ 9. Ⓐ Ⓑ Ⓒ Ⓓ 14. Ⓐ Ⓑ Ⓒ Ⓓ 19. Ⓐ Ⓑ Ⓒ Ⓓ 24. Ⓐ Ⓑ Ⓒ Ⓓ

5. Ⓐ Ⓑ Ⓒ Ⓓ 10. Ⓐ Ⓑ Ⓒ Ⓓ 15. Ⓐ Ⓑ Ⓒ Ⓓ 20. Ⓐ Ⓑ Ⓒ Ⓓ 25. Ⓐ Ⓑ Ⓒ Ⓓ

PRETEST

ANSWER SHEET

Pretest

Directions: The purpose of this pretest is to get a quick baseline assessment of your knowledge and understanding before you begin studying. The questions cover all topics on the CCRN exam. However, most are knowledge-based questions and do not cover application, evaluation, and analysis of knowledge. After you complete all sections of the book and study each section's practice questions but before you take one of the comprehensive practice tests, revisit this pretest. You should notice an improvement! Read each question and choose the one best response. The answers can be found at the end of the test.

1. Which of the following are symptoms of hypoglycemia?

   (A) Tachycardia and trembling
   (B) Bradycardia and diaphoresis
   (C) Anxiety and flushed dry skin
   (D) Flushed dry skin and tachycardia

2. Which of the following is TRUE for a patient with a right-sided stroke who develops increased intracranial pressure?

   (A) Pupils will change before level of consciousness, right-sided paralysis, eyes deviated to the left, left pupil change
   (B) Pupils will change before level of consciousness, left-sided paralysis, eyes deviated to the right, right pupil change
   (C) Level of consciousness will change before pupils, right-sided paralysis, eyes deviated to the left, left pupil change
   (D) Level of consciousness will change before pupils, left-sided paralysis, eyes deviated to the right, right pupil change

3. Which of the following interventions would the nurse consider to be inappropriate for the patient with increased intracranial pressure?

   (A) Maintaining oxygenation and normal $PaCO_2$
   (B) Feeding the patient via an NGT
   (C) Administering 5% dextrose in water (D5W) at 75 mL/hour
   (D) Log roll when turning the patient

4. Which of the following is associated with mitral regurgitation?

   (A) Systolic murmur, sinus bradycardia
   (B) Diastolic murmur, heart failure
   (C) Systolic murmur, inferior wall myocardial infarction
   (D) Diastolic murmur, complete heart block

5. You know that research supports unrestricted access of a designated support person to the patient, but your unit restricts all patient visitors to set times. Your best response would be to:

   (A) gather the facts and propose a policy change to your manager for the unit.
   (B) tell patients/visitors that the unit's policy is outdated but there is nothing you can do about it.
   (C) continue to follow the unit policy.
   (D) complain to colleagues about the unit's outdated policy.

6. Nitrate therapy is indicated for the treatment of unstable angina and acute heart failure because it:

   (A) decreases preload and increases myocardial O_2 demand
   (B) increases preload and increases myocardial O_2 demand
   (C) increases preload and decreases myocardial O_2 demand
   (D) decreases preload and decreases myocardial O_2 demand

7. All of the following support the diagnosis of cardiac tamponade EXCEPT:

   (A) widening pulse pressure.
   (B) equalization of right and left heart pressures.
   (C) pulsus paradoxus.
   (D) enlarged heart on chest X-ray (CXR).

8. Your patient has just consented to a bedside chest tube insertion and requests that his wife be allowed to be present during the procedure. You should:

   (A) explain to the patient that this is against infection control practice.
   (B) tell the patient he will be able to see his wife as soon as the procedure is completed.
   (C) tell the patient it would be too much for his wife to handle.
   (D) prepare the wife for what to expect and allow her to be present.

9. ECG changes associated with ST-elevation myocardial infarction (STEMI) affecting the lateral wall would include changes in which of the following leads?

   (A) II, III, aVf
   (B) V1, V2, V3
   (C) V2, V3, V4
   (D) V5, V6, I, aVl

10. Which of the following laboratory findings are most specifically indicative of disseminated intravascular coagulation (DIC) as the cause of bleeding?

    (A) elevated fibrin split products and d-dimer
    (B) prolonged PT, PTT, and bleeding time
    (C) decreased platelet count
    (D) decreased hemoglobin and hematocrit

11. A 29-year-old female has been in the critical care unit for 2 days after a motor vehicle crash and has developed acute tubular necrosis (ATN). She was normotensive on admission. What would be the most likely cause of her ATN?

    (A) hemorrhage
    (B) rhabdomyolysis
    (C) creatinine release
    (D) cardiac dysrhythmias

12. A patient with acute tubular necrosis (intrarenal failure) is differentiated from a patient with decreased renal perfusion (prerenal failure) because in ONLY decreased renal perfusion (prerenal failure):

    (A) the urine specific gravity is low.
    (B) the urine osmolality is greatly reduced.
    (C) the BUN to creatinine ratio is at least 20:1.
    (D) the urinary sodium is 40 to 100 mEq/L.

13. A patient with a history of heroin and alcohol abuse is admitted for treatment of cellulitis. The patient has flushed, slightly moist skin and is slow to respond to verbal stimuli. The affected arm is edematous and hard to the touch with yellow exudates noted from puncture wounds on the skin. Vital signs are:

    Temperature 102°F (38.9°C); B/P 88/50; heart rate 120/minute; respiratory rate 26/minute. The nurse should anticipate orders for:

    (A) antibiotic and crystalloid administration.
    (B) antipyretic and dopamine administration.
    (C) CT scan of the head and a drug screen.
    (D) colloid followed by norepinephrine administration.

14. A patient with a history of hyperlipidemia and alcohol abuse reports left upper-quadrant abdominal pain. Vital signs are: Temperature 101°F (38.3°C); B/P 85/50; heart rate 110/minute; respiratory rate 24/minute. Which of the following lab values should the nurse anticipate?

    (A) decreased serum amylase level and increased WBC count
    (B) decreased hematocrit (HCT) and increased lipase level
    (C) decreased sedimentation rate and elevated calcium level
    (D) increased LDH and increased SGOT (AST)

15. Your patient is admitted with diabetic ketoacidosis (DKA). Arterial blood gases (ABGs) on room air show:

pH	7.22
$PaCO_2$	21
pO_2	94
HCO_3	11

    The ABG demonstrates:

    (A) compensated metabolic alkalosis.
    (B) compensated respiratory acidosis.
    (C) partially compensated metabolic acidosis.
    (D) uncompensated metabolic acidosis.

16. What is the recommended initial position to improve oxygenation for a patient with unilateral pneumonia?

    (A) Trendelenburg's
    (B) supine
    (C) side lying on affected side
    (D) side lying on unaffected side

17. A patient is admitted with a respiratory infection. The patient has shortness of breath with a frequent productive cough and is expectorating light-green sputum. Vital signs are stable except for temperature, which is 39°C, and increased respiratory rate. The nurse should anticipate which of the following ABG results?

    (A) respiratory acidosis
    (B) respiratory alkalosis
    (C) metabolic acidosis
    (D) metabolic alkalosis

18. Your patient has been receiving mechanical ventilation for 2 days, but you note there is no order for nutrition. Your best response would be to:

    (A) insert a feeding tube and begin enteral nutritional therapy.
    (B) complain about the practice patterns of the physicians to your colleagues.
    (C) ask the physician for an order for enteral feeding for the patient.
    (D) assume it is the physician's responsibility for the nutritional plan of care.

19. A patient with status asthmaticus is admitted. His breath sounds are diminished throughout his lung fields, respiratory rate is 38/minute. After giving the patient an aerosol bronchodilator, the patient now has bilateral wheezes. This indicates:

    (A) the patient is getting better.
    (B) the patient has gotten worse.
    (C) the need for anesthesia to be present STAT.
    (D) the patient does not have asthma.

20. In a patient with acute lung injury (ALI), which of the following contribute to the development of atelectasis?

    (A) loss of surfactant and interstitial fluid accumulation
    (B) increased pulmonary vascular resistance and hypoxemia
    (C) increased pulmonary compliance and hypoxemia
    (D) mucosal edema and mucus plugging

21. The following are TRUE related to acute subarachnoid hemorrhage EXCEPT for:

    (A) sudden explosive headache.
    (B) nuchal rigidity.
    (C) decreased level of consciousness.
    (D) pinpoint pupils.

22. The patient with an inferior wall ST-elevation myocardial infarction (STEMI) also has a right ventricular (RV) infarction. He soon develops right ventricular failure. Which of the following data obtained would correlate with this patient's condition if PAP = pulmonary artery pressure, PAOP = pulmonary artery occlusive pressure, and CVP = central venous pressure?

    (A) PAP 38/22; PAOP 20; CVP 6; ST elevation in II, III, aVF; crackles bilaterally
    (B) PAP 54/28; PAOP 14; CVP 14; ST elevation in V_2–V_6; clear lungs
    (C) PAP 28/10; PAOP 10; CVP 18; ST elevation in II, III, aVF; clear lungs
    (D) PAP 23/8; PAOP 19; CVP 20; ST elevation in V_2–V_6; crackles bilaterally

23. Which of the following hemodynamic profiles would best exemplify that seen in septic shock if PAP = pulmonary artery pressure, PAOP = pulmonary artery occlusive pressure, and CVP = central venous pressure?

    (A) PAP 20/4; PAOP 3; CVP 0; SVR 1,400
    (B) PAP 22/6; PAOP 5; CVP 1; SVR 600
    (C) PAP 45/22; PAOP 21; CVP 8; SVR 1,800
    (D) PAP 55/25; PAOP 15; CVP 10; SVR 1,200

24. Which of the following patients is least likely to return to a normal level of functioning after discharge?

    (A) the 70-year-old admitted with septic shock who is receiving chemotherapy
    (B) the 75-year-old admitted for a scheduled coronary artery bypass graft procedure
    (C) the 21-year-old trauma patient admitted with a pneumothorax and fractured pelvis
    (D) the 65-year-old admitted with acute MI and history of diabetes

25. Which of the following statements is TRUE?

    (A) Delirium is a permanent condition.
    (B) The patient who develops delirium has an increased risk of mortality.
    (C) Most patients with delirium are agitated.
    (D) The patient with dementia cannot develop delirium.

ANSWER KEY
Pretest

1. **A**	6. **D**	11. **B**	16. **D**	21. **D**
2. **D**	7. **A**	12. **C**	17. **B**	22. **C**
3. **C**	8. **D**	13. **A**	18. **C**	23. **B**
4. **C**	9. **D**	14. **B**	19. **A**	24. **A**
5. **A**	10. **A**	15. **C**	20. **A**	25. **B**

ANSWERS EXPLAINED

1. **(A)** When the blood glucose drops, sympathetic stimulation occurs. (Symptoms are masked for the patient receiving beta-adrenergic blocker drugs.) Flushed, dry skin is a sign of hyperglycemia.

2. **(D)** Higher brain centers (cerebral cortex) are the first to be affected by increased intracranial pressure. Therefore, level of consciousness is the first sign (one exception, epidural hematoma). Pupil changes are ipsilateral (same side as the injury) due to compression of cranial nerve III against the transtentorial notch. Motor changes are contralateral (opposite the side of injury) due to motor fiber crossing in the brain stem.

3. **(C)** 5% dextrose in water is a hypotonic solution. When administered, it will cause movement of the D5W into the brain cells, causing swelling and increased intracranial pressure. The other 3 choices are acceptable interventions for the patient with increased ICP.

4. **(C)** Inferior wall MI may result in ischemia and dysfunction (regurgitation) of the mitral valve. The mitral valve is closed during systole (left ventricular ejection). A murmur is produced when the mitral valve is not fully closed during systole.

5. **(A)** The AACN Synergy Model supports patient advocacy. Unrestricted access of a designated support person is evidence-based practice included in the Patient Visitation AACN Practice Alert. Choice (A) is an effective strategy for change.

6. **(D)** Nitrates cause venodilation, which results in a decrease in venous return to the heart (left ventricular preload reduction). The decrease in preload decreases the work of the left ventricle and myocardial oxygen demand.

7. **(A)** The pulse pressure **narrows** with cardiac tamponade. The other 3 choices ARE seen with cardiac tamponade.

8. **(D)** The AACN Synergy Model supports caring practice and family presence. An AACN practice alert indicates family presence may improve patient outcome.

9. **(D)** V5, V6 represents the lower lateral wall of the left ventricle and I, aVL represents the high lateral wall of the left ventricle, supplied by the left circumflex artery in most of the population.

10. **(A)** DIC is a clotting problem, with massive coagulation. As clots break down, fibrin split products are produced. Therefore with DIC, FSPs will be high. In fact, this is the most specific test result for DIC. D-dimer is present due to the presence of clots. While not specific for DIC, it is a good rule-out test.

11. **(B)** The motor vehicle crash most likely resulted in a crush injury with destruction of skeletal muscle cells (rhabdomyolysis). This results in the release of massive amounts of creatinine kinase (CK) that, in turn, may "clog" renal tubules and lead to acute tubular necrosis (ATN). Choice (A) is not correct as there is no history of bleeding. Choice (C), creatinine release, is too vague, could be minor, and does not cause ATN. Arrhythmias, choice (D), are not included in the scenario.

12. **(C)** A BUN with a 10:1 ratio is seen in acute intrarenal renal failure; the 20:1 ratio is typical of prerenal renal failure. The other 3 choices are typically seen in acute intrarenal failure because they are evidence of damage to the basement membrane of renal tubules with the inability to concentrate urine or "hold on" to sodium.

13. **(A)** The scenario is one of septic shock. The patient emergently needs antibiotics and crystalloid administration. The other 3 choices are not as effective as choice (A) for septic shock.

14. **(B)** The scenario describes acute pancreatitis, which may be hemorrhagic and cause the hematocrit to drop. Serum lipase increases with acute pancreatitis.

15. **(C)** The pH is low; there is an acidosis. The low bicarbonate indicates the acidosis is metabolic. Bicarbonate drops as it is attempting to buffer the excess ketoacids. The low $PaCO_2$ is evidence that the lungs are attempting to compensate with hyperventilation, or "blowing off acid." However, compensation is only partial, not complete. (The pH would need to be normal, 7.35, for full compensation.)

16. **(D)** It is best to place the "good" lung down and have the patient on the side that does not have the problem. This is because more blood perfusion is greater to the "down" side due to gravity. If more blood goes to the "bad" side, hypoxemia may occur.

17. **(B)** The increased respiratory rate generally causes hyperventilation, "blowing off," decrease in the $PaCO_2$, and a rise in pH. Tachypnea does not guarantee hyperventilation. However, nothing in the history of this scenario indicates acidosis or metabolic alkalosis.

18. **(C)** Early nutritional therapy for the patient receiving mechanical ventilation improves patient outcomes. Knowledge of evidence-based practice, however, is not enough. The critical care nurse needs to advocate for the patient using strategies that work. Collaboration (AACN Synergy Model of practice) with the physician would be most likely to provide the patient with what he/she needs.

19. **(A)** Diminished or absent breath sounds in the patient with an asthma exacerbation are an ominous sign of lack of air movement through the airways. Development of wheezing is a sign of the patient improving with air now moving, although bronchospasm is still present.

20. **(A)** The pathophysiology of acute lung injury includes damage to Type II alveolar cells (which results in alveolar collapse) and capillary leak (which results in interstitial fluid accumulation). Both alveolar collapse and interstitial fluid lead to atelectasis. Although mucus plugging and mucosal edema may lead to atelectasis, these problems are not associated with acute lung injury.

21. **(D)** All of the other 3 choices **are** features of subarachnoid hemorrhage. Pinpoint pupils are associated with pontine infarct.

22. **(C)** When the right ventricle (RV) fails, the pressure proximal to the RV (CVP) increases, whereas pressures distal to the RV (pulmonary artery pressure and pulmonary arterial occlusive pressure) are normal or even low. This results in clear lungs. ECG changes indicative of an inferior wall MI are found in leads II, III, and aVF.

23. **(B)** The pathophysiology of septic shock includes capillary leak, which decreases intravascular volume (low CVP and relative hypovolemia), and massive vasodilatation, which decreases systemic vascular resistance (low SVR).

24. **(A)** The AACN believes the critical care nurse should assess not only the patient's physiologic status but the patient's resiliency, which has been shown to affect outcome. In addition to acute problems, extremes of age and chronic conditions also need to be considered.

25. **(B)** Studies have shown delirium produces long-term effects. They also indicate that the more severe the delirium, the worse the long-term outcome. The other 3 choices are NOT true regarding delirium.

Cardiovascular Concepts

4

*I'm a great believer in luck, and I find the harder I work,
the more I have of it.*

—Thomas Jefferson

CARDIOVASCULAR BLUEPRINT

Cardiovascular (20%)   **30 Questions**

→ Acute coronary syndromes (including unstable angina)

→ Acute myocardial infarction/ischemia (including papillary muscle rupture)

→ Acute peripheral vascular insufficiency (e.g., acute arterial occlusion, carotid artery stenosis, endarterectomy, peripheral stents, fem-pop bypass)

→ Acute pulmonary edema

→ Cardiac surgery (e.g., valve replacement, CABG)

→ Cardiac trauma

→ Cardiogenic shock

→ Cardiomyopathies (e.g., hypertrophic, dilated, restrictive, idiopathic)

→ Dysrhythmias

→ Heart failure

→ Hypertensive crisis

→ Hypovolemic shock

→ Interventional cardiology (e.g., catheterization)

→ Myocardial conduction system defects

→ Ruptured or dissecting aneurysm (e.g., thoracic, abdominal, thoracoabdominal)

→ Structural heart defects (e.g., acquired and congenital, including valvular disease)

Note: Hypovolemic shock is included in the cardiovascular blueprint but is covered in the multisystem section.

CARDIOVASCULAR TESTABLE NURSING ACTIONS

- ☐ Identify/monitor normal and abnormal physical assessment findings
- ☐ Apply leads for cardiac monitoring
- ☐ Identify, interpret, and monitor cardiac rhythms
- ☐ Monitor hemodynamic status, and recognize signs and symptoms of hemodynamic instability
- ☐ Recognize indications for and manage patients requiring:
  - ○ 12-lead ECG
  - ○ Arterial line
  - ○ Cardiac catheterization
  - ○ Cardiocentesis
  - ○ Cardioversion
  - ○ Central venous access
  - ○ Central venous pressure monitoring
  - ○ Defibrillation
  - ○ PA catheter
  - ○ SvO_2 monitoring
  - ○ Transthoracic pacing
  - ○ Transvenous pacing
- ☐ Manage patients receiving cardiovascular medications (e.g., thrombolytics, vasoactive agents, platelet inhibitors, anti-arrhythmic medications)
- ☐ Monitor patients and follow protocols for cardiac surgery
- ☐ Recognize signs and symptoms of cardiovascular emergencies, initiate interventions, and seek assistance as needed
- ☐ Recognize indications for and manage patients requiring:
  - ○ IABP
  - ○ Percutaneous coronary interventions

Cardiovascular (CV) questions outnumber all of the other clinical topics included on the adult CCRN exam. Plan on spending the most time studying CV. The 30-question total for CV includes hemodynamic monitoring. Plan to spend about 30 hours reviewing the CV and hemodynamics sections of the book and practicing test questions related to CV and hemodynamics. Because hemodynamic monitoring also includes pulmonary and multisystem concepts, hemodynamics is covered after the first 8 clinical judgment topics.

Select assessment concepts are included on the adult CCRN exam. These concepts may be covered in assessment questions or be incorporated in the cardiovascular disorder questions.

Normal Heart Sounds

S1

- "Lub"
- Caused by closure of AV (mitral, tricuspid) valves
- Loudest at **apex** of the heart (midclavicular, 5th intercostal space)
- Marks end of diastole, beginning of **systole**

S2

- "Dub"
- Caused by closure of semilunar (aortic, pulmonic) valves
- Loudest at the **base** (right sternal border, 2nd intercostal space)
- Marks end of systole, beginning of **diastole**
- S2 splits on inspiration; wide, fixed splitting of S2 caused by RBBB
- S2 **louder with pulmonary embolism**

➤ Each of the 4 valves has an auscultatory point on the chest wall. You need to know these points (Figure 4-1).

➤ The "base" of the heart is the aortic area, where S2 ("dub") is loudest. Anatomically, it is at the 2nd intercostal space (ICS), right sternal border.

➤ The "apex" of the heart is the mitral area, where S1 ("lub") is loudest. Anatomically, it is at the 5th ICS, midclavicular.

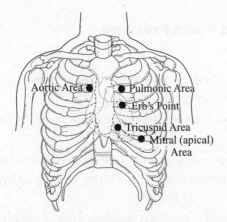

Figure 4-1. Heart auscultatory points on the chest wall and associated valves

Abnormal Heart Sounds in Adults

S3

- Caused by rapid rush of blood into a dilated ventricle
- Occurs early in diastole, right after S2
- Heard best at the apex with the bell of the stethoscope
- ☆ Associated with heart failure, may occur before crackles
- Abnormal in adults
- Ventricular gallop, "Kentucky"
- ☆ S3 is also caused by:
  - ➤ Pulmonary hypertension and cor pulmonale
  - ➤ Mitral, aortic, or tricuspid insufficiency

TIP

S4 is not heard in the presence of atrial fibrillation . . . why??

No atrial contraction!

S4

- Caused by atrial contraction of blood into a noncompliant ventricle
- Occurs right before S1
- Best heard at apex with the bell of the stethoscope
- Associated with myocardial ischemia, infarction, hypertension, ventricular hypertrophy, and **aortic stenosis**
- Atrial gallop, "Tennessee"

PERICARDIAL FRICTION RUB

- Due to pericarditis, associated with pain on deep inspiration
- May be positional

MURMURS

- Valvular disease; see below for a detailed discussion of this topic
- Septal defects (atrial or ventricular)

Blood Pressure and Pulse Pressure

- Pulse pressure:

Systolic – Diastolic = Pulse Pressure

- Normal pulse pressure is 40–60 mmHg, i.e., 120/80.
- Systolic blood pressure is an indirect measurement of the cardiac output and stroke volume.
  - ○ A decrease in systolic pressure with little change or increase in diastolic pressure is narrowing of pulse pressure, seen most often with severe hypovolemia or severe drop in cardiac output (CO), i.e., 100/78
- Diastolic blood pressure is an indirect measurement of the systemic vascular resistance (SVR).
  - ○ A decrease in diastolic pressure that widens pulse pressure may indicate vasodilation, drop in SVR, often seen in severe sepsis, septic shock, i.e., 100/38.
- Diastole is normally one-third longer than systole.
- ☆ Coronary arteries are perfused during diastole.

You will most likely see several questions related to valvular heart disease and/or heart sound assessment. Since there are 4 heart valves and each valve may be diseased with either **stenosis** or **insufficiency**, it would be next to impossible to memorize whether each problem is a systolic or diastolic murmur. If you can picture which valves are open and which are closed during each phase of the cardiac cycle (systole and diastole), you will be able to decide what problem is being described in each question. First, let's review some heart sound basics.

- Normal heart sounds, S1 and S2 in adults, are due to valve closure.
- Valves open and close based on the pressure changes in the chamber above the valve and below the valve. When the pressure in the chamber above a valve is higher than that below the valve, the valve opens. When the pressure drops in the chamber above the valve and the pressure is greater below the valve, the valve closes.
- SYSTOLE . . . ejection, high pressure
- DIASTOLE . . . filling, low pressure
- Which is longer, systole or diastole? DIASTOLE is one-third longer than systole, need time for filling.
- When are coronary arteries perfused, during systole or diastole? DIASTOLE!
- Why does the cardiac output and blood pressure drop with extreme tachyarrhythmias? No time for filling, therefore less output.

Causes of Valvular Heart Disease

- Coronary artery disease, ischemia, and acute MI
- Dilated cardiomyopathy
- Degeneration
- Bicuspid aortic valve . . . genetic
- Rheumatic fever
- Infection
- Connective tissue diseases

MURMURS

- Murmurs of **INSUFFICIENCY** (regurgitation) occur when the valve is **closed**
  - Acute or chronic
- Murmurs of **STENOSIS** occur when the valve is **open**
  - Chronic problem, develops over time
  - NOT acute

Systolic Murmurs (Figure 4-2)

Lub . . . shhhb . . . Dub

- Semilunar valves are OPEN during systole
  - Aortic stenosis
  - Pulmonic stenosis

- AV valves are CLOSED during systole
  - Mitral insufficiency
    - Mitral insufficiency (will cause large, giant V-waves on the pulmonary artery occlusive pressure tracing if patient has a pulmonary artery catheter)
  - Tricuspid insufficiency
- Ventricular septal defect (VSD), which is most common with acute MI, may result in systolic murmur. It is heard at the left sternal border, 5th intercostal space (ICS).

Diastolic Murmurs (Figure 4-3)

Lub . . . Dub . . . shhhb

- Semilunar valves are CLOSED during diastole
  - Aortic insufficiency (AI)
  - Pulmonic insufficiency (PI)
- AV valves . . . OPEN during diastole
  - Mitral stenosis is associated with atrial fibrillation due to atrial enlargement that occurs over time
  - Tricuspid stenosis

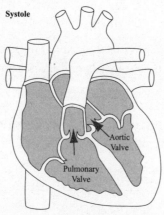

Figure 4-2. Systole, closure of AV valves, S1 "Lub"

→ The semilunar valves (pulmonic, aortic) are OPEN during systole.
→ The AV valves (tricuspid, mitral) are CLOSED during systole.

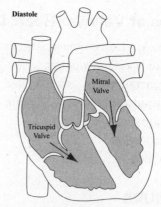

Figure 4-3. Diastole, closure of semilunar valves, S2 "Dub"

→ The semilunar valves (pulmonic, aortic) are CLOSED during diastole.
→ The AV valves (tricuspid, mitral) are OPEN during diastole.

- **Mitral insufficiency** occurs when the mitral valve is closed (murmur occurs). When is the mitral valve closed?

  ➤ Systole!

- **Mitral stenosis** occurs when the mitral valve is open (murmur occurs). When is the mitral valve open?

  ➤ Diastole!

- **Aortic insufficiency** occurs when the aortic valve is closed. When is the aortic valve closed?

  ➤ Diastole!

- **Aortic stenosis** occurs when the aortic valve is **open**. When is the aortic valve open?

  ➤ Systole!

Note: If you can picture what the aortic valve is doing, the pulmonic is doing the same (opening or closing). If you can picture what the mitral valve is doing, the tricuspid valve is doing the same (opening or closing).

Does a murmur due to a VSD occur during systole or diastole?

  ➤ During ejection or systole!

MURMURS ASSOCIATED WITH ACUTE MI

- The mitral valve is attached to the left ventricular wall by the papillary muscles and chordae tendinae. Myocardial ischemia or infarction can affect mitral valve function and lead to acute mitral valve regurgitation.
- Papillary muscle **dysfunction** (Grade I or II), loudest at **apex**
- Papillary muscle **rupture** (Grade V or VI), loudest at **apex** . . . surgical emergency!
- Ventricular septal defect
  - **Sternal border**, 5th ICS

☆ Several questions on the exam always cover this topic. The questions may describe ECG findings and clinical picture and then ask about what type of ACS the patient has. Alternatively, the questions may tell you what type of ACS the patient has, e.g., anterior MI, and expect you to know what the typical clinical picture would be for this type of MI. You do not need to have taken a 12-lead ECG class to do well. However, you DO need to understand which leads are associated with which wall of the heart (Table 4-1). If you master the content below, you should do well!

Table 4-1. Risk Factors for Coronary Artery Disease

Category	Risk Factors
Non-modifiable risk factors	Age, sex, family history, genetics
Modifiable risk factors	Smoking, atherogenic diet, alcohol intake, physical activity, dyslipidemias, hypertension, obesity, diabetes, metabolic syndrome

Spectrum of Ischemic Heart Disease

- Asymptomatic coronary artery disease (CAD)
- Stable angina…Chest pain with activity, predictable, lesions usually fixed and calcified lesions

Acute Coronary Syndromes

NOTE

Patients may not have chest pain with MI, especially women and diabetics.

- Due to platelet-mediated thrombosis, may result in sudden cardiac death.
    1. **UNSTABLE ANGINA:** Chest pain at rest, unpredictable, may be relieved with nitroglycerin, troponin negative, ST depression, or T-wave inversion on the ECG.
    2. **NON-ST ELEVATION MYOCARDIAL INFARCTION (NSTEMI):** Troponin positive, ST depression, T-wave inversion on the ECG, unrelenting chest pain.
    3. **ST ELEVATION MYOCARDIAL INFARCTION (STEMI):** Troponin positive. ST elevation in 2 or more contiguous leads, unrelenting chest pain.

☆ **Variant or Prinzmetal's Angina**

- A type of unstable angina associated with transient ST segment elevation
- Due to coronary artery spasm with or without atherosclerotic lesions
- Occurs at rest, may be cyclic (same time each day)
- May be precipitated by nicotine, ETOH, cocaine ingestion
- Troponin negative
- Nitroglycerin (NTG) administration results in relief of chest pain, STs return to normal

Management of Acute Chest Pain

- Stat ECG, done and read within 10 minutes
    - Allows categorization to STEMI or NSTEMI/unstable angina
    - Allows risk stratification to high, medium, low

ECG Results (3 possibilities)

ST elevation...	ST depression,	No acute change
STEMI	T wave inversion...	
	NSTEMI/UA	

- Aspirin
  - Chew, give **ASAP**, improves morbidity/mortality
- ANTICOAGULANT: heparin or enoxaparin
- Antiplatelet agents
  - Clopidogrel (Plavix)
  - Abciximab (Reopro)
  - Eptifibatide (Integrilin)
  - Tirofiban (Aggrastat)
- Beta blocker
  - Unless ACS due to **cocaine**
  - Use cardioselective such as metoprolol, do not use non-cardioselective such as propranolol
  - Contraindications include hypotension, bradycardia, use of phosphodiesterase-inhibitor drugs such as sildenafil (Viagra)
- Treat pain
  - Nitroglycerin
  - Morphine
- History, risk factor assessment
  - Lab assessment
  - Cardiac biomarkers, lipid profile, CBC, electrolytes, BUN, creatinine, magnesium, PT, PTT

☆ **ECG Lead Changes and Location of Coronary Artery Disease**

  - Changes in II, III, aVF → right coronary artery (RCA), inferior LV
  - Changes in V1, V2, V3, V4 → left anterior descending (LAD), anterior LV
  - Changes in V5, V6, I, aVL → circumflex, lateral LV
  - V5, V6, low lateral LV
  - I, aVL, high lateral LV
  - Changes in V1, V2 → RCA, posterior LV
  - Changes in V3R, V4R → RCA, right ventricular (RV) infarct

Treatment of STEMI

- Determine onset of infarct, if symptoms < 12 hours → **REPERFUSION**
  - Percutaneous coronary intervention, PCI (door to balloon 90 min)
  - Fibrinolytic drug therapy (door to drug < 30 min)
- Eligibility criteria
  - **ST elevation in 2 or > contiguous leads, or** new onset left bundle branch block (LBBB)
  - Onset of chest pain < 12 hours
  - Chest pain of 30 minutes in duration
  - Chest pain unresponsive to sublingual (SL) nitroglycerin (NTG)

PATIENT CARE FOLLOWING REPERFUSION FOR STEMI

PCI (90 minutes, door to balloon inflation in coronary artery at point of lesion)

- Monitor for signs of re-occlusion: chest pain, ST elevation → contact physician
- Monitor for vasovagal reaction during sheath removal → give fluids, atropine
  - Hypotension < 90 systolic with or without bradycardia, absence of compensatory tachycardia
  - Associated symptoms of pallor, nausea, yawning, diaphoresis
- Monitor for bleeding: sheath site
  - Immediately apply manual pressure 2 finger breadths above the puncture site
  - Continue manual pressure for minimum of 20 min (30 min if still on GP IIb/IIIa inhibitors) to achieve hemostasis
- Monitor for bleeding: retroperitoneal → fluids, blood products
  - Sudden hypotension
  - Severe low back pain
- Monitor for vascular complications → pulse assessments

Fibrinolytic Therapy (30 minutes door to drug administration)

- Absolute contraindications
  - Any prior intracranial hemorrhage
  - Known structural cerebral vascular lesion (e.g., arteriovenous malformation)
  - Known malignant intracranial neoplasm (primary or metastatic)
  - Ischemic stroke within 3 months EXCEPT acute ischemic stroke within 3 hours
  - Suspected aortic dissection
  - Active bleeding or bleeding diathesis (excluding menses)
  - Significant closed-head or facial trauma within 3 months
- ☆ **Evidence of reperfusion**
  - Chest pain relief: due to fibrinolysis of clot
  - Resolution of ST segment deviations: due to return of blood flow
  - Marked elevation of troponin/CK-MB: due to myocardial "stunning" when vessel opens
  - Reperfusion arrhythmias (VT, VF, accelerated idioventricular rhythm (AIVR)): due to myocardial "stunning" when vessel opens
- Nursing management
  - Assess for major and minor bleeding
    - Major bleed, change in LOC, brain bleed
  - Institute bleeding precautions
  - Assess for reperfusion (see above)
  - Assess for re-occlusion as evidenced by recurring chest pain, ST deviation

Treatment of NSTEMI

- **No** emergent reperfusion
- Same meds as STEMI
- If high risk score **or** continued chest pain, signs of instability, start GP IIb/IIIa inhibitors (Integrilin, Reopro) and prepare for diagnostic cardiac catheterization within 24 hours

☆ **Inferior MI**

- ○ Associated with right coronary artery (RCA) occlusion
- ○ ST elevation in II, III, aVF (Figure 4-4)
- ○ Reciprocal changes in lateral wall (I, aVL)
- ○ Associated with AV conduction disturbances: 2nd-degree Type I, 3rd-degree heart block, sick sinus syndrome (SSS), and sinus bradycardia
- ○ Development of systolic murmur: mitral valve regurgitation (MVR) secondary to papillary muscle rupture (Posterior papillary muscle-tethering distance is significantly greater in inferior compared with anterior myocardial infarction.)
- ○ Tachycardia associated with inferior MI → higher mortality
- ○ Also associated with RV infarct and posterior MI
- ○ Use beta blockers and NTG with CAUTION

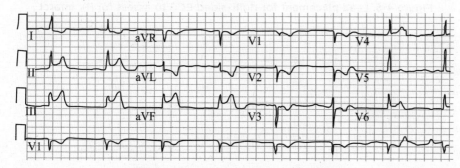

Figure 4-4. Acute inferior wall STEMI

☆ **Right Ventricular Infarct**

- ○ The right coronary artery, which supplies the inferior wall of the left ventricle, also supplies the right ventricle. Therefore, about 30% of inferior wall MI patients also have a right ventricular (RV) infarct.
- ○ Size of the infarct will determine symptoms.
- ○ A right-sided ECG (Figure 4-5) may demonstrate the ST changes.
- ○ Signs/symptoms
    - JVD at 45°, high CVP, hypotension, usually clear lungs, bradyarrhythmias
    - ECG with ST elevation in V_{4R} (Figure 4-6)
- ○ Treatment
    - Fluids
    - Positive inotropes
- ○ Avoid
    - Preload reducers → nitrates, diuretics
    - Caution with beta blockers, often cannot give initially due to hypotension

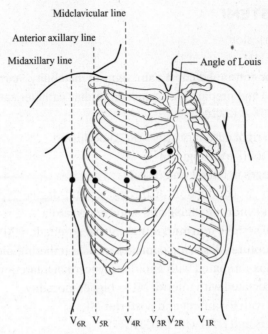

Figure 4-5. Lead placement for right-sided ECG to assess for RV infarct

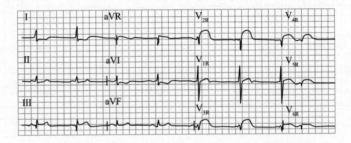

Figure 4-6. Right-sided ECG results with evidence of RV infarct

⭐ Anterior MI

- ○ Associated with left anterior descending (LAD) occlusion
- ○ ST elevation in V1–V4: precordial leads, V leads (Figure 4-7)
- ○ Reciprocal changes (ST depression) in inferior wall (II, III, aVF)
- ○ May develop second degree Type II heart block or RBBB (the LAD supplies the common bundle of HIS)... **ominous** sign
- ○ Development of systolic murmur: possible ventricular septal defect
- ○ Higher mortality than inferior: **HEART FAILURE**

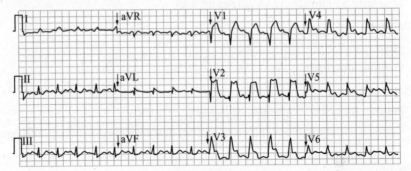

Figure 4-7. Anterior STEMI

LATERAL MI

- ST elevation in V5, V6 (low lateral)
- ST elevation in I, aVL (high lateral)
- Generally involves left circumflex artery.

Complications of Acute MI

ARRHYTHMIAS . . . MOST COMMON!

- Ventricular
  - Defibrillate VF
  - Drug therapy for stable, sustained VT and to prevent recurrent VF
  - Synchronized cardioversion for unstable, sustained VT
- Bradycardia, heart blocks, sick sinus syndrome (SSS)
- Atrial fibrillation
  - 10% to 15% of all MIs, have increased mortality, even when returned to NSR
- Heart failure
- Cardiogenic shock
- Re-infarction
- Thromboembolic events
- Pericarditis
- Ventricular aneurysm
- Ventricular septal defect
- Papillary muscle rupture
- Cardiac wall rupture

INTERVENTIONAL CARDIOLOGY

Cardiac Catheterization Lab Procedures

- Diagnostic cardiac catheterization
- Percutaneous Coronary Interventions (PCI)
  - Intracoronary stenting: most common PCI procedure
  - Balloon angioplasty without stent (PTCA): seldom used, high re-occlusion rates
- Percutaneous balloon valvotomy
- Pacemaker implantation
- Electrophysiology Studies (EP)
  - Intracardiac defibrillator (ICD)
  - Cardiac ablation therapy

GOAL OF PCI WITH STENT

- Restoration of blood flow distal to a coronary artery lesion with partial or total occlusion

COMPLICATIONS OF PCI

- In hospital death is rare, ~0.71%
- In-hospital MI 0.4%
- Coronary artery perforation
- Distal coronary artery embolization
- Intramural hematoma
- Failure of stent deployment
- ☆ **Stent thrombosis is most likely to be on the test**

  ○ Most incidents occur acutely (within 24 hours of stent placement) or subacutely (within the first 30 days)

- Stroke or TIA: greater risk if with aortic stenosis
- Arrhythmias
- Renal failure
- ☆ **Retroperitoneal bleed is most likely to be on the test**

PATIENT CARE DURING SHEATH REMOVAL

- Record baseline peripheral pulses and vitals
- Provide comfort, i.e., morphine 2–4 mg IV before removal
- Monitor B/P q 5–10 min during sheath removal
- Monitor for **vasovagal response** (hypotension < 90 systolic with or without bradycardia, absence of compensatory tachycardia and associated symptoms of pallor, nausea, yawning, diaphoresis)
- Vasovagal management

  ○ Hold nitrates

  ○ Atropine 0.5 mg IV (even in absence of bradycardia if other signs occur)

  ○ IV bolus of 250 mL 0.9 NS if not immediately responsive to atropine

  ○ Assess for anxiety/pain as contributing factors

- Achieve hemostasis

  ○ Manual pressure for 20 to 30 minutes

  ○ Mechanical clamp compression using Femostop or C-clamp

  ○ Closure device

MANAGE COMPLICATIONS OF PCI

- Monitor for signs of coronary artery re-occlusion: chest pain, ST elevation → contact physician
- Monitor for vasovagal reaction during sheath removal → give fluids, atropine
- Monitor for bleeding: sheath site

  ○ Immediately apply manual pressure 2 finger breadths above the puncture site

  ○ Continue manual pressure for minimum of 20 min (30 min if still on GP IIb/IIIa inhibitors) to achieve hemostasis

- Monitor for bleeding: retroperitoneal → fluids, blood products

  ○ Sudden hypotension

  ○ Severe low back pain

- Monitor for vascular complications: pulse assessments
- Monitor for hematoma at sheath insertion site: assess sheath insertion site for swelling

HYPERTENSIVE CRISIS, EMERGENCY

One question may be on this topic. The question is usually related to how the topic differs from hypertensive urgency or what drugs are used for treatment.

- Hypertensive **emergency or CRISIS** is elevated B/P with evidence of end-organ damage (brain, heart, kidney, retina) that can be related to acute hypertension → need critical care admission
- Hypertensive **urgency** is elevated B/P without evidence of acute end-organ damage → usually no need for critical care admission
- Treatment of hypertensive crisis or emergency → emergent lowering of B/P needed
  - **Nitroprusside**
    - Preload **and** afterload reducer
    - Assess for cyanide toxicity secondary to drug metabolite (Thiocyanate): mental status change (restlessness, lethargy), tachycardia, seizure, a need for ↑ in dose, unexplained metabolic acidosis, especially in those with renal impairment or when drug is used > 24 hrs
  - **Labetalol**
    - Intermittent IV doses preferred to continuous infusion due to possibility of continuing of drug beyond maximum dose of 300 mg
    - Duration of effect persists 4–6 hrs after IV dose is discontinued
- Biggest risk is STROKE

ACUTE PERIPHERAL VASCULAR INSUFFICIENCY

One question about this topic may appear. It generally covers ACUTE issues.

- Peripheral arterial disease signs and symptoms (the 6 "Ps")
  - **Pain** (activity, rest)
  - **Pallor**
  - **Pulse** absent or diminished
  - **Paresthesia**
  - **Paralysis**
  - **Poikilothermia**: chronic, not acute sign, but could have acute on chronic; loss of hair on toes or lower legs; glossy, thin, cool, dry skin
  - Additionally, cool to touch, minimal edema
- Ankle-brachial Index (ABI)
  - Test to assess for PAD
  - Used to assess adequacy of lower extremity perfusion
  - Normal is > 1
    - Divide the ankle pressure by the brachial pressure on the same side
  - **Need to remember only what normal is**
- Additional diagnostic testing
  - Doppler ultrasound testing
  - Arteriography

- ■ Patient care management for PAD
  - ○ Embolectomy, bypass graft, angioplasty
- ☆ Bed in reverse Trendelenburg
- ☆ **Do NOT elevate the affected extremity**—will decrease perfusion
  - ○ Medications
    - – Thrombolytics (tPA)
    - – Anticoagulants (heparin)
    - – Antiplatelet agents (ASA, clopidogrel)
    - – Vasodilators

ARRHYTHMIA INTERPRETATION, ARRHYTHMIA EMERGENCIES, PACEMAKER THERAPY

Test candidates are expected to have mastered arrhythmia interpretation and have an understanding of ACLS principles. So look these over. However, do not spend a great deal of time on this part of the test blueprint because there is not always an arrhythmia strip, and when there is, it is usually not complex.

☆ **For test questions that include development of an arrhythmia, pay close attention to the clinical response of the patient to the arrhythmia. Is the patient stable or unstable? If the clinical description is NOT provided, consider this fact and do NOT assume patient response!**

☆ **Prolongation of the QT interval** (causes, treatment) is often addressed on the CCRN test. QT prolongation may lead to torsades de pointes. Causes of prolonged QT include:

- ○ Drugs—amiodarone, quinidine, haloperidol, procainamide
- ○ Electrolyte problems—hypokalemia, hypocalcemia, hypomagnesemia
- ○ Treatment for torsades VT—magnesium

For pacemaker therapy, which includes some knowledge of implantable cardiac defibrillator (ICD) devices, review the following information.

Pacemaker Code

A = atria   V = ventricle   D = dual (both)

- ■ First initial = Chamber **paced;** this was "invented" first
- ■ Second initial = Chamber **sensed;** this function came along second
- ■ Third initial = Response to sensing; last to be developed
  - ○ I = inhibits (pacer detects intrinsic cardiac activity and withholds its pacing stimuli) . . . demand
  - ○ D = inhibits **and** triggers (pacer detects intrinsic cardiac activity and fires a pacing stimulus in response)
  - ○ O = None

On the CCRN test, you may see a question that asks how a "VVI" or a "DDD" pacemaker works. If you remember the code, you should be able to figure out the answer.

Sample questions:

a. Which pacemaker paces both the atria and ventricles, senses both the atria and ventricles, and in response to sensing can inhibit and trigger in response?

b. Which pacemaker paces the ventricle, senses the ventricle, and inhibits pacing in response to sensing?

Answers: a. DDD   b. VVI

Review the 3 basic pacer malfunctions:

1. Failure to pace (no spike at all when expected)
2. Failure to capture (spikes without a QRS for ventricular pacing)
3. Failure to sense (pacing in native beats)

ICDs can provide "tiered" therapy:

- Programmed to **shock** (defibrillate or synchronized cardioversion)
- Programmed to **burst pace** (sense tachyarrhythmia, provide a series of beats faster than the tachyarrhythmia, then stop suddenly with hopefully the SA node recovering)
- Programmed to provide pacing for **bradyarrhythmias**

If the ICD does not correct the sudden death arrhythmia, shock as usual; do not place shocking pads directly over the ICD.

- The patient will require special education related to the device and emotional support as many patients experience FEAR of being shocked.

HEART FAILURE

Heart failure (HF) is a broad topic. For the test, if you focus on the following, you will be ready!

Heart failure may be acute, chronic, acute exacerbation of chronic HF, systolic or diastolic failure, or right or left HF. The most extreme HF occurs when all compensatory mechanisms have failed and the result is cardiogenic shock. An understanding of these concepts and the management of each as well as an understanding of heart failure classifications is needed in order to answer the CCRN test questions on this topic successfully.

- **Heart failure** is a clinical syndrome characterized by signs and symptoms associated with high intracardiac pressures and decreased cardiac output.
- **Acute decompensated heart failure** is the abrupt onset of symptoms severe enough to merit hospitalization.
  - ~ 75% have history of chronic heart failure
- Heart failure with **systolic dysfunction** (left ventricular systolic dysfunction, LVSD): EF 40% or less, problem with ejection
- Heart failure with **diastolic dysfunction:** EF > 50%, problem with filling, ejection is OK

TIP

When studying, compare and contrast systolic and diastolic heart failure and differentiate clinical signs of left-sided vs. right-sided heart failure.

What Is BNP?

- Beta natriuretic peptide (BNP) is released by the ventricle when under wall stress in attempts to dilate and decrease ventricular pressure.
- High with heart failure, indicator of a ventricle (left or right) under stress.

Pathophysiology of Acute Decompensated Systolic Dysfunction

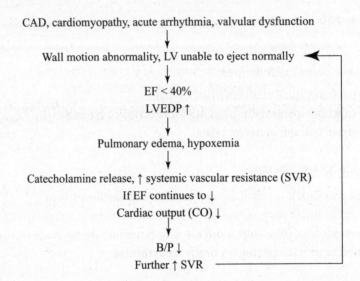

CAD, cardiomyopathy, acute arrhythmia, valvular dysfunction

↓

Wall motion abnormality, LV unable to eject normally

↓

EF < 40%
LVEDP ↑

↓

Pulmonary edema, hypoxemia

Catecholamine release, ↑ systemic vascular resistance (SVR)
If EF continues to ↓
Cardiac output (CO) ↓

↓

B/P ↓
Further ↑ SVR

- When systolic dysfunction is prolonged and becomes chronic, compensatory **hormones** lead to ventricular remodeling over time.
- Drugs are used to decrease neurohormonal effects.

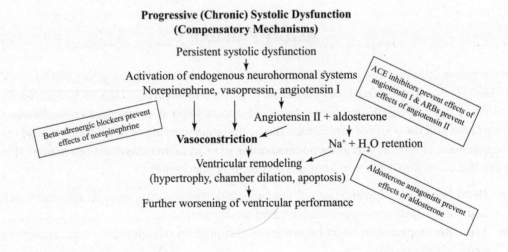

**Progressive (Chronic) Systolic Dysfunction
(Compensatory Mechanisms)**

Persistent systolic dysfunction

↓

Activation of endogenous neurohormonal systems
Norepinephrine, vasopressin, angiotensin I

ACE inhibitors prevent effects of angiotensin I & ARBs prevent effects of angiotensin II

Angiotensin II + aldosterone

Beta-adrenergic blockers prevent effects of norepinephrine

Vasoconstriction

$Na^+ + H_2O$ retention

Ventricular remodeling
(hypertrophy, chamber dilation, apoptosis)

Aldosterone antagonists prevent effects of aldosterone

Further worsening of ventricular performance

Pathophysiology of HF with Diastolic Dysfunction

Chronic hypertension, valvular disease,
restrictive or hypertrophic cardiomyopathy

↓

Stiff LV due to inability of myofibrils to relax
Impaired LV filling (empties OK, EF normal)
↑ LVEDP

↓

Pulmonary edema

See Table 4-2 for a summary of differences between systolic and diastolic heart failure.

☆ **Table 4-2. Summary of Differences Between Systolic and Diastolic Heart Failure**

	Systolic	Diastolic
Primary problem	Ejection problem, dilated chamber • Can fill OK	Filling problem, hypertrophied chamber or septum • Can eject OK
Signs	Dilated left ventricle PMI shifted to left Valvular insufficiency (dilation causes mitral v. insufficiency) EF ≤ 40% Pulmonary edema due to poor ventricular emptying S3 B/P normal or low (usually) BNP elevated	Normal ventricular size Thick ventricular walls and/or thick septum Normal contractile function Normal EF Pulmonary edema due to high ventricular pressure S4 with hypertension B/P often high BNP elevated
Treatment	Beta blockers ACEI/ARB Diuretics Dilators Aldosterone antagonists Positive inotropes	Beta blockers ACEI/ARB Calcium channel blockers Diuretics (low dose) Aldosterone antagonists
Contraindicated	Negative inotropes (calcium-channel blockers and, in acute phase, beta blockers)	Positive inotropes Dehydration further worsens filling Tachyarrhythmias decrease filling time and worsen symptoms
Cardiomyopathy Types	Dilated results in systolic HF Dilated may result in mitral insufficiency as left ventricular wall enlarges	Cardiomyopathies resulting in diastolic HF: • Idiopathic hypertrophic subaortic stenosis (IHSS) • Hypertrophic cardiomyopathy (HCM) • Hypertrophic obstructive cardiomyopathy (HOCM)

☆ Chest X-Ray Findings: Systolic vs. Diastolic HF

- Systolic HF may be evidenced by a large, dilated heart **or** by normal heart size on chest film.

  - An enlarged heart is often associated with a shift of the point of maximal impulse (PMI) from midclavicular to the **left** (Figure 4-8).

- Diastolic HF generally is evidenced by a normal heart size on the chest film. However, on the 12-lead ECG, there **may** be left ventricular hypertrophy pattern, especially when the patient has a history of uncontrolled hypertension.

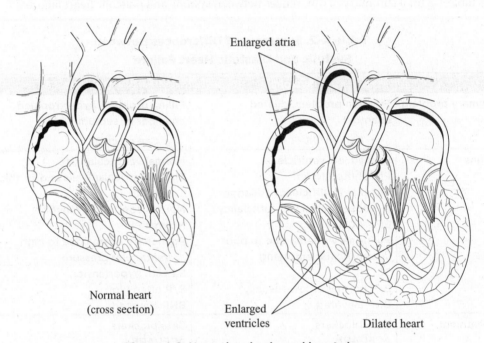

Enlarged atria

Normal heart
(cross section)

Enlarged
ventricles

Dilated heart

Figure 4-8. Normal and enlarged heart size

Heart failure may also be categorized according to which ventricle is failing, the right or the left (Tables 4-3 and 4-4). The etiologies and treatment are different. The test may describe a case scenario with background information, signs and symptoms, and whether the HF is right or left. Then you will be asked to identify the correct treatment.

Table 4-3. Causes of Right and Left Heart Failure

Right Sided	Left Sided
Acute RV infarct	Coronary artery disease, ischemia
Pulmonary embolism (massive)	Myocardial infarction
Septal defects	Cardiomyopathy
Pulmonary stenosis/insufficiency	Fluid overload
COPD	Chronic, uncontrolled hypertension
Pulmonary hypertension	Aortic stenosis/insufficiency
Left ventricular failure	Mitral stenosis/Insufficiency
	Cardiac tamponade

Table 4-4 Signs and Symptoms of Right vs. Left Heart Failure

Right Sided	Left Sided
Hepatomegaly	Orthopnea, dyspnea, tachypnea
Splenomegaly	Hypoxemia
Dependent edema	Tachycardia
Venous distention	Crackles
Elevated CVP/JVD	Cough with pink, frothy sputum
Tricuspid insufficiency	Elevated PA diastolic/PAOP
Abdominal pain	Diaphoresis
	Anxiety, confusion

The CCRN test may include a question related to heart failure classifications. The New York Heart Association (NYHA) classification is based on patient report of symptoms, not objective findings. The patient should be classified only **after** optimal drug therapy has been achieved, not during an acute exacerbation.

NYHA Heart Failure Classes

- **Class 1**—Ordinary activity does not cause fatigue, dyspnea, palpitation, or anginal pain. There is no limitation of physical activity. **EXTRAORDINARY ACTIVITY** results in heart failure symptoms.
- **Class 2**—Comfortable at rest, but ordinary physical activity results in heart failure symptoms. There is some limitation of physical activity. **ORDINARY ACTIVITY** results in heart failure symptoms.
- **Class 3**—Comfortable at rest, but less than ordinary activity causes heart failure symptoms. There is marked limitation of physical activity. **MINIMAL ACTIVITY** results in heart failure symptoms.
- **Class 4**—Symptoms of heart failure occur at rest. If any physical activity is attempted, discomfort is increased. There is severe limitation of physical activity. Remaining **AT REST** results in heart failure symptoms.
- The main cause of death for heart failure patients is sudden arrhythmia. Select patients with Class 2 to 4 heart failure are candidates for an implantable cardiac defibrillator (ICD).

CARDIOMYOPATHY

If the test includes a question on cardiomyopathy, it will most likely be on either **dilated** or **hypertrophic** cardiomyopathy (Table 4-5).

Table 4-5. Differences Between Dilated and Hypertrophic Cardiomyopathy

Dilated	Hypertrophic
SYSTOLIC dysfunction, problem ejecting Classical sign • Thinning, dilation, enlargement of LV chamber • Mitral valve regurgitation (MVR) common due to ventricular dilation Symptoms similar to **SYSTOLIC** heart failure Treatment • Similar to systolic heart failure • Heart failure may progress through stages, classes • May need ventricular assist device (VAD), heart transplant	**DIASTOLIC** dysfunction, problem filling Classical sign • Increased thickening of the heart muscle and septum inwardly at the expense of the LV chamber Symptoms similar to **DIASTOLIC** heart failure • Fatigue • Dyspnea • Chest pain • Palpitations • S3, S4 • Presyncope or syncope Treatment as for diastolic heart failure **Increased risk of sudden cardiac death!**

CARDIOGENIC SHOCK

When compensatory mechanisms fail to maintain the cardiac output, the most extreme end on the continuum of heart failure occurs—cardiogenic shock (Table 4-6). Cardiogenic shock has several causes. Most commonly, it is due to an extreme drop in stroke volume secondary to systolic dysfunction, which results in . . .

■ Elevated left ventricular preload (PAOP) with associated pulmonary symptoms
■ Elevated left ventricular afterload (SVR) due to vasoconstrictive compensatory mechanisms
■ A resultant drop in cardiac output to the point where perfusion to organs is no longer adequate

Etiologies of Cardiogenic Shock

■ Acute MI
■ Chronic heart failure
■ Cardiomyopathy
■ Dysrhythmias
■ Cardiac tamponade
■ Papillary muscle rupture

　　○ Obliterates the mitral valve
　　○ Life-threatening emergency
　　○ Requires immediate surgical intervention

Table 4-6. Clinical Presentation of Cardiogenic Shock

Compensatory Stage	Progressive Stage
Tachycardia	Hypotension
Tachypnea	Worsening tachycardia, tachypnea, oliguria
Crackles, mild hypoxemia	Metabolic acidosis
ABG with respiratory alkalosis or early metabolic acidosis	Worsening crackles and hypoxemia
Anxiety, irritability	Skin clammy, mottled
Neck vein distention	Worsening anxiety, or lethargy
S3 (S4 if also acute MI)	• At any time, chest pain or arrhythmias may occur
Cool skin	
Urine output down	
Narrow pulse pressure	
B/P maintained, lower than baseline	

Treatment of Cardiogenic Shock

- Identify cause
- Manage arrhythmias (brady, tachy) that may be contributing to a decrease in CO
- Reperfusion if STEMI (percutaneous coronary intervention or fibrinolytic therapy)
- Emergent surgery if due to mechanical problem—ruptured papillary muscle, VSD
- See Table 4-7

Table 4-7. Treatment of Cardiogenic Shock

Enhance Effectiveness of Pump	Decrease Demand on Pump
Positive inotropic support	Preload reduction (or optimization)
• Norepinephrine (Levophed)	Afterload reduction
• Dopamine 4–10 mcg/kg/min	Optimize oxygenation
• Dobutamine, milrinone (Primacor)	Mechanical ventilation
AVOID negative inotropic agents!	Treat pain
Vasodilators	IABP for short term support
• May be used in conjunction with Intra-aortic balloon pump therapy (IABP) and positive inotropic agents if in progressive stage with hypotension	Ventricular assist device (VAD), may be used for longer periods of time than IABP

Ventricular Assist Device (VAD)

- You will not be tested on the details of this therapy. However, you need to know it is used in the management of left ventricular heart failure, cardiogenic shock, and cardiac myopathies and it is also used in patients awaiting heart transplant.
- ☆ **Benefits of IABP Therapy**
- You will have at least one question on this.
- Just remember, the balloon does 2 things. It INFLATES and it DEFLATES (Figure 4-9 and Figure 4-10).

Benefits of INFLATION

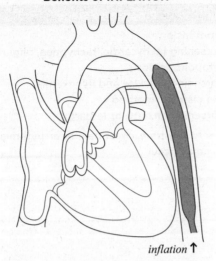

inflation ↑

Figure 4-9. Balloon inflation—increases coronary artery perfusion

→ Inflates at dicrotic notch of the arterial waveform, beginning of diastole

Benefits of DEFLATION

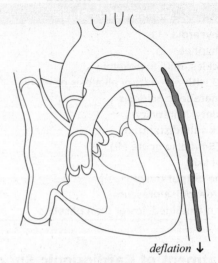

deflation ↓

Figure 4-10. Balloon deflation—decreases afterload

→ Deflates right before systole begins; determined by set TRIGGER for deflation, R-wave of ECG or upstroke of the arterial pressure wave

CARDIAC SURGERY

Who gets coronary artery bypass grafting (CABG)?

- Chronic disabling angina unresponsive to medical therapy, not candidate for PCI
- Left main lesion
- 3-vessel disease

NOTE

The test questions related to heart surgery generally focus on complications and nursing care postoperatively.

Cardiopulmonary Bypass

- Stop the heart during surgery
- Most common cannulation sites:
  - Aorta
  - Right atrium
- The longer the bypass time the more bleeding there is and the more complications postoperatively

Coronary Artery Bypass Procedure

- Priming with isotonic crystalloids (hemodilution), enhances oxygenation by improving blood flow
- Hypothermia (28°–36°C)
- Anticoagulation with large heparin doses
- Circulatory arrest; rapid, during diastole with potassium cardioplegic agent; reinfused at intervals, may be warm or cold cardioplegic agent

Post-Op CABG Assessment for Complications

- Hemodynamic abnormalities
- Arrhythmias
- ☆ Tamponade
- ☆ Pericarditis
- Electrolyte abnormalities
- Hematologic, bleeding
- Pulmonary
- Pain, anxiety
- Renal
- Endocrine (glycemic control)
- Gastrointestinal
- Infection

☆ Post-Op Chest Tube Management
- Maintain patency.
  - Do not allow dependent loops.
  - Milking or stripping chest tubes is not routinely indicated.
    - If clots appear, gently milk chest tubes.
- Mediastinal tubes remove serosanguinous fluid from the operative site; whereas pleural chest tubes remove air, blood, or serous fluid from the pleural space.
- Keep chest tubes lower than patient's chest.
- Do not clamp the system unless changing the drainage system or there is a system disconnect. When the tube is clamped, the connection to the negative chamber is lost.
- Chest tube output >100 mL for 2 consecutive hours.
  - Maintain hemodynamic stability
  - Correct volume status
  - Administer blood products

Valve Surgery (Table 4-8)

Table 4-8. Advantages and Disadvantages of Mechanical and Biological Valves

Mechanical Valve	Biological Valve
Advantages:	Advantages:
• Relatively easy to insert	• Anticoagulation required short term
• Very reliable	• Some cases only ASA
• Lasts longer than biological valve	Disadvantages:
Disadvantages:	• Wears down, especially in high-pressure systems
• High risk of thrombosis	
• Permanent anticoagulation therapy	

Nursing Considerations Post Valve Repair or Replacement

- Avoid a drop in preload. Most patients who have had valvular stenosis or chronic regurgitation have had elevated end-diastolic volumes. Sudden preload normalization may result in hypotension.
- Anticoagulation will be needed for valve replacement; valve repair may require dual antiplatelet therapy (aspirin and clopidogrel).
- Anticipate conduction disturbances since the mitral, tricuspid, and aortic valves are anatomically close to conduction pathways. Temporary or permanent pacing may be needed.

CARDIAC TAMPONADE

- Etiologies: Surgical-related cause (post-op cardiac surgery), medical-related cause (pericarditis), trauma
- Signs and symptoms
  - Restlessness and agitation
  - Hypotension
  - ↑ JVD
  - Equalization of CVP, pulmonary artery diastolic and PAOP
  - Muffled heart tones
  - Enlarging cardiac silhouette and mediastinum on chest radiograph
- ☆ Narrowed pulse pressure, i.e., 82/68
- ☆ Pulsus paradoxus: excessive drop in SBP (>12 mmHg) during inspiration. Cardiac muscle restriction due to tamponade, with inspiration, intrathoracic pressure increases, decreases venous return.
  - Best seen on arterial line waveform as respiratory variation (Figure 4-11).

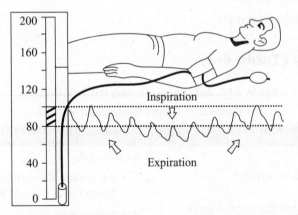

Figure 4-11. Pulsus paradoxus as seen on the arterial waveform

Which valve is at most risk for rupture due to trauma?

- **Aortic valve** because it is most anterior in the chest (Table 4-9)

Table 4-9. Pericarditis vs. Myocardial Contusion

	☆ Medical—Pericarditis	☆ Trauma—Myocardial Contusion
Etiology	Trauma (rare) Viral After an MI Post-op cardiac surgery Radiation Idiopathic Dressler's syndrome—immune response after an MI, surgery, or traumatic injury	Trauma • Worse outcome than pericarditis • Broken vessels bleed into heart, similar to an MI • Cardiac dysrhythmias • Death can occur within the first 48 hours
Signs and symptoms	Chest pain Pain worsens with inspiration Dyspnea Low-grade temp ↑ Sed rate ST elevation in all the leads Cardiac tamponade Post-MI, Dressler's syndrome, may last months	Signs of trauma Chest pain Pain worsens with inspiration Dyspnea Low-grade temp ST elevation in the **area of injury**
Treatment	Symptom relief Analgesics Anti-inflammatory agents NSAIDs Steroid Antibiotics Monitor for worsening symptoms Monitor for constrictive pericarditis Monitor for cardiac tamponade	Monitor for arrhythmias Analgesics as needed

An aneurysm is a localized, blood-filled out-pouching in the wall of an artery. The larger it becomes, the more likely it is to rupture. The cardiovascular blueprint may contain a question about abdominal aortic or thoracic aneurysm.

Etiology of Aneurysms (Figure 4-12)

- Arteriosclerosis
- Hypertension
- Smoking
- Obesity
- Bacterial infections
- Congenital anomalies
- Trauma
- Marfan's syndrome

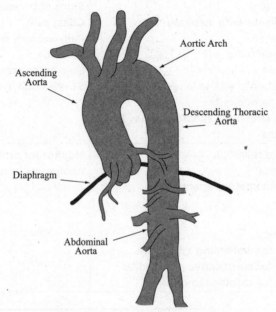

Figure 4-12. Types and locations of cardiovascular-related aneurysms

Abdominal Aortic Aneurysm (75% of all CV-related aneurysms)

- Asymptomatic if small
- Pulsations in abdominal area
- Abdominal or low back pain
- Nausea, vomiting
- Shock

Thoracic Aortic Aneurysms
(25% of all CV-related aneurysms)

- Sudden tearing, ripping pain in chest radiating to shoulders, neck, and back
- Cough
- Hoarseness
- Dysphagia
- Dyspnea
- Dizziness, difficulty walking and speaking
- Widening of mediastinum on chest X-ray

Treatment of Aneurysms

- Aneurysms < 5 cm in diameter and no symptoms
  - Monitor regularly
    - Ultrasound or CT scan
  - Treat hypertension: drug class of choice is beta blockers, which may slow growth
  - People with Marfan's syndrome are often treated sooner
- Thoracic aneurysm causing symptoms or > 6 cm
  - Surgical repair
  - Dissection: SURGERY
  - Aggressive treatment of hypertension and heart rate control
    - Labetalol drip

Aortic Dissection

Blood passes through the inner lining and between the layers of the aorta

- Tear is spiral in nature
- Sudden or gradual
- Ascending aorta or aortic arch
- Life threatening
- Immediate surgical intervention

Now that you have reviewed key cardiovascular concepts, go to the Cardiovascular Practice Questions. Answer the questions, and then check your answers. Continue to review the information until you get at least 80% on the practice questions.

CARDIOVASCULAR PRACTICE QUESTIONS

1. A 59-year-old male is admitted complaining of chest pain and dyspnea. ST elevation and T-wave inversion were seen on the ECG in V2, V3, and V4. IV thrombolytic therapy was started in the ED. Indications of successful reperfusion would include all of the following EXCEPT:

   (A) pain cessation.
   (B) decrease in CK or troponin.
   (C) reversal of ST segment elevation with return to baseline.
   (D) short runs of ventricular tachycardia.

2. Which of the following medication orders should the nurse question for the patient in question 1?

   (A) metoprolol (Lopressor)
   (B) aspirin
   (C) propranolol (Inderal)
   (D) heparin

3. If heart block develops while caring for the patient in question 1, which of the following would it most likely be?

   (A) sinoatrial block
   (B) second degree, Type I
   (C) second degree, Type II
   (D) third degree, complete

4. Appropriate drug therapy for dilated cardiomyopathy is aimed toward:

   (A) decreasing contractility and decreasing preload and afterload.
   (B) decreasing contractility and increasing preload and afterload.
   (C) increasing contractility and increasing both preload and afterload.
   (D) increasing contractility and decreasing both preload and afterload.

5. An 18-year-old is admitted with a history of a syncopal episode at the mall and has a history of an eating disorder. The nurse notes a prolonged QT on the 12-lead ECG and anticipates a reduction in an electrolyte to be the cause. Which of the following is LEAST likely to cause this patient's problem?

   (A) sodium
   (B) magnesium
   (C) potassium
   (D) calcium

6. On the third day after admission for acute MI, a 67-year-old male complains of chest pain and develops a fever. The pain is worse with deep inspiration and is relieved when he leans forward. There are nonspecific ST changes in the precordial leads of the ECG. The nurse anticipates that the patient will most likely need treatment for:

   (A) thoracic aneurysm.
   (B) Dressler's syndrome.
   (C) reinfarction.
   (D) pleuritis.

7. A patient is admitted to the CCU after PCI with stent. Femoral sheath is in place, site is dry with no hematoma. He suddenly complains of severe back pain. Neck veins are flat with head of bed at 30 degrees, heart sounds are normal. Vital signs are B/P 78/48, HR 124 and RR 26. What should the nurse suspect?

   (A) cardiac tamponade
   (B) retroperitoneal bleeding
   (C) coronary artery dissection
   (D) acute closure of the stented coronary artery

8. Your patient admitted with an NSTEMI develops acute shortness of breath, recurrence of chest pain, and a loud systolic murmur at the apex of the heart. Which of the following has most likely occurred?

   (A) The patient has developed acute mitral valve regurgitation.
   (B) The patient has developed acute reinfarction.
   (C) The patient has developed acute mitral wave stenosis.
   (D) The patient has developed acute ventricular septal defect.

9. A patient has just returned from the OR after insertion of a VVI pacemaker. In order to assess function of this pacemaker accurately, the nurse needs to understand that:

   (A) both atrium and ventricle are paced and sensed and may either inhibit or pace in response to sensing.
   (B) the ventricle is paced, ventricular activity is sensed, and pacing is inhibited in response to ventricular sensing.
   (C) both the atrium and ventricle are paced, but only ventricular pacing can be inhibited by a sensed intrinsic ventricular impulse.
   (D) the ventricle is paced in response to a sensed intrinsic atrial impulse or inhibited by a sensed intrinsic ventricular impulse.

10. A patient complains of sudden dyspnea 5 days S/P acute MI (ST elevation in II, III, and aVF, with ST depression in I and aVL). The patient is anxious, diaphoretic, and hypotensive. Examination reveals the development of a loud holosystolic murmur at the apex that radiates to the axilla. The patient has crackles throughout but no S3 at the apex. What is the most likely cause of this patient's deterioration?

(A) right ventricular failure related to right ventricular MI
(B) ventricular septal defect
(C) left ventricular failure due to extension of MI
(D) acute mitral regurgitation due to papillary muscle rupture or dysfunction

11. The patient with diagnosis of cardiogenic shock now requires high dose dopamine (greater than 10 mcg/kg/min) to maintain blood pressure, and the cardiologist is planning to start IABP therapy. This therapy will benefit the patient because it will:

(A) increase afterload with balloon inflation and decrease diastolic augmentation with balloon deflation.
(B) decrease afterload with balloon deflation and increase diastolic augmentation with balloon inflation.
(C) decrease afterload with balloon inflation and decrease diastolic augmentation with balloon deflation.
(D) increase afterload with balloon deflation and decrease diastolic augmentation with balloon inflation.

12. Four days after mitral valve replacement, the patient goes into atrial fibrillation with rapid ventricular response. What should be the nurse's initial action?

(A) Order a 12-lead ECG.
(B) Evaluate the patient for clinical signs of hypoperfusion.
(C) Notify the physician.
(D) Ask the patient to bear down as if having a bowel movement.

13. A patient's 12-lead ECG shows sinus bradycardia at 44 beats/min and ST segment elevation in leads II, III, and aVF. Which of the following treatments for bradycardia for this patient would best resolve the problem?

(A) temporary transvenous pacing
(B) transcutaneous pacing
(C) percutaneous coronary intervention
(D) administration of atropine

14. Which drug would most likely be given to a patient with hypertrophic cardiomyopathy?

(A) metoprolol
(B) digoxin
(C) dopamine
(D) dobutamine

15. A patient is admitted with ST elevation in V2, V3, and V4. Four days after admission, the patient suddenly developed a holosystolic murmur at the lower left sternal border, chest pain, and hypotension. What complication should the nurse expect?

    (A) papillary muscle rupture
    (B) ventricular septal defect
    (C) acute mitral stenosis
    (D) acute reinfarction

16. A postoperative patient on the surgical unit suddenly develops chest pain, extreme weakness, and dyspnea and is found to have ST elevation in II, III, and aVF on the stat ECG. B/P is 92/62, heart rate 58, respiratory rate 28, lungs are clear, and heart sound assessment reveals an S4, no murmurs. In addition to preparing the patient for PCI, which of the following interventions would you anticipate?

    (A) nitroglycerin drip, aspirin
    (B) furosemide (Lasix), atropine
    (C) transcutaneous pacing, morphine
    (D) aggressive fluid administration, right-sided ECG

17. A 52-year-old male presents with complaints of blurred vision and shortness of breath. B/P is 232/136, heart rate 102, respiratory rate 28 with crackles in lower lung fields bilaterally, with S3 and S4 heart sounds on auscultation. Which of the following would be indicated for this patient?

    (A) nitroprusside drip, admit to critical care unit
    (B) digoxin, furosemide
    (C) labetalol drip, admit to a medical unit
    (D) lisinopril, calcium channel blocker

18. An 80-year-old female presents with chief complaint of acute shortness of breath. Clinical exam reveals B/P 180/102, heart rate 105/minute, respiratory rate 32/minute, lungs with crackles bilaterally, pulse oximetry of 88%, S4 on auscultation. ECG revealed sinus tachycardia, left ventricular hypertrophy pattern, chest radiograph showed normal heart size, pulmonary vascular congestion, and echocardiogram showed EF of 55%. Which of the following should be avoided in this patient's treatment plan?

    (A) calcium channel blocker
    (B) digoxin
    (C) low-dose diuretics
    (D) oxygen

19. Mrs. Jones has heart failure. Despite optimal therapy, she gets short of breath when she gets up to walk to the bathroom. Which of the following is the patient experiencing regarding heart failure?

(A) NYHA Class I heart failure, may benefit from an ICD
(B) NYHA Class II heart failure, may benefit from an ICD
(C) NYHA Class III heart failure, may benefit from an ICD
(D) heart failure cannot be classified, further information is needed

20. When the above patient, Mrs. Jones, has an exacerbation of her heart failure, she develops jugular venous distention (JVD), peripheral edema, and abdominal discomfort. These are clinical signs specific to:

(A) acute left ventricular failure.
(B) chronic right ventricular failure.
(C) acute right ventricular failure.
(D) chronic dehydration.

21. The nurse managing a post-op CABG patient assesses a sudden drop in B/P, distended neck veins, muffled heart tones, minimal chest tube output, and a systolic pressure that fluctuates with breathing pattern. The patient most likely needs:

(A) emergent return to the OR.
(B) clamping of the chest tube.
(C) transfusion of PRBCs.
(D) high-dose dopamine.

22. Physical assessment findings indicative of a significant right ventricular (RV) infarction would include:

(A) bibasilar crackles.
(B) flat neck veins with the patient in a Semi-Fowler's position.
(C) jugular venous distention.
(D) tachypnea and frothy sputum.

23. What pulse change might the nurse expect associated with cardiac tamponade?

(A) pulsus alternans
(B) pulsus paradoxus
(C) pulsus magnus
(D) pulsus bisferiens

24. A patient with mitral regurgitation develops atrial fibrillation with a rate of 88, B/P of 118/75. Which of the following may be indicated?

(A) beta blockers and vasopressors.
(B) cardiac glycosides and calcium-channel blockers
(C) beta blockers and calcium-channel blockers
(D) antiarrhythmics and angiotensin-converting enzyme inhibitors

25. Which of the following are predominant signs of left ventricular systolic dysfunction?

   (A) pedal edema, ascites, hepatomegaly, weight gain, ejection fraction less than 40%
   (B) S4, bibasilar crackles, hypertension, ejection fraction greater than 40%
   (C) S3, frequent new cough, bibasilar crackles, ejection fraction less than 40%
   (D) hypertension, murmur, chest pain, weight gain, ejection fraction greater than 40%

26. The nurse was preparing a patient with the diagnosis of STEMI for a percutaneous coronary intervention (PCI). The monitor had previously shown normal sinus rhythm (NSR) and the B/P had been 128/78, chest pain improved from a "9" to a "2" on a 0–10 scale. The monitor alarm sounded, and the rhythm below was observed by the nurse:

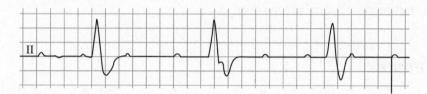

What statement below is TRUE?

   (A) This change is most commonly seen with acute inferior MI. Assess the patient. If serious signs and symptoms develop, begin transcutaneous pacing (TCP).
   (B) This change is most commonly seen with acute anterior MI. Assess the patient. If serious signs and symptoms develop, give atropine.
   (C) This change is most commonly seen with acute inferior MI. Assess the patient. If serious signs and symptoms develop, begin dobutamine.
   (D) This change is most commonly seen with anterior MI. Assess the patient. If serious signs and symptoms develop, begin transcutaneous pacing (TCP).

27. A 58-year-old patient developed chest pain that he scored as an "8." Rapid assessment included profuse diaphoresis, B/P 78/52, heart rate 104/minute, respiratory rate 20/minute, lungs clear, and SpO$_2$ 98%. The patient is currently connected to the bedside monitor with a nasal cannula at 2 L/min in place and intravenous fluids, 0.9 NS at a rate of 10 mL/hour. Which of the following sequences of interventions would be the most appropriate for the nurse at this time?

   (A) Give a chewable aspirin, do an ECG, and start a fluid bolus.
   (B) Give NTG sublingual, increase the FiO$_2$, and give morphine.
   (C) Do an ECG, give NTG sublingual, and give a chewable aspirin.
   (D) Start a fluid bolus, give a chewable aspirin, and do an ECG.

28. The location or type of acute MI is often associated with specific clinical findings. Which of the following statements related to location of MI is TRUE?

   (A) Anterior MI is often associated with heart blocks or bradyarrhythmias.
   (B) Inferior MI is often associated with right ventricular wall infarction.
   (C) Lateral MI is most likely to be associated with posterior MI.
   (D) Posterior MI is most likely to lead to the complication of heart failure.

29. Which of the following statements is accurate regarding heart valves?

(A) The aortic valve is closed during systole.
(B) The mitral valve is closed during systole.
(C) The mitral valve is closed during diastole.
(D) The aortic valve is open during diastole.

30. The following drugs are all considered positive inotropic drugs primarily affecting the beta-1 receptors in the heart, EXCEPT for:

(A) dopamine drip at 12 mcg/kg/min dose.
(B) dopamine drip at 5 mcg/kg/min dose.
(C) dobutamine drip at 7 mcg/kg/min dose.
(D) milrinone at 7 mcg/kg/min dose.

ANSWER KEY

1. **B**	6. **B**	11. **B**	16. **D**	21. **A**	26. **A**
2. **C**	7. **B**	12. **B**	17. **A**	22. **C**	27. **D**
3. **C**	8. **A**	13. **C**	18. **B**	23. **B**	28. **B**
4. **D**	9. **B**	14. **A**	19. **C**	24. **B**	29. **B**
5. **A**	10. **D**	15. **B**	20. **B**	25. **C**	30. **A**

ANSWERS EXPLAINED

1. **(B)** Coronary artery reperfusion due to either PCI or fibrinolysis results in an **elevation** of creatinine kinase (CK) or troponin, NOT a decrease. The theory is that the return of blood flow distal to the occlusion can result in "reperfusion injury" of muscle, elevating cardiac biomarkers. The other 3 choices are indicators of reperfusion.

2. **(C)** The patient in the scenario is having an acute anterior wall MI. A beta blocker is beneficial for an acute MI as these agents decrease the work of the heart and increase the threshold for ventricular fibrillation. Propranolol, although a beta-adrenergic blocker like metoprolol, is NOT a cardioselective beta blocker. It affects beta receptors in heart muscle AND lung tissue. Therefore, it is more likely to cause bronchoconstriction than a cardioselective beta blocker. The other 3 choices (cardioselective beta blocker, anti-platelet, and anticoagulant) are indicated in an acute MI that the patient in the scenario is experiencing.

3. **(C)** The patient is having an acute anterior MI, which is generally due to LAD occlusion. The LAD supplies the HIS bundle, which could result in a second-degree, Type II heart block. The other 3 types of blocks are due to SA node or AV node ischemia, which generally occur with an RCA occlusion (inferior wall MI).

4. **(D)** Dilated cardiomyopathy is likely to result in systolic dysfunction, which decreases contractility, causes compensatory arterial constriction, and results in a higher left ventricular preload. To treat this, therapy is aimed at increasing contractility, decreasing afterload (arterial constriction), and decreasing preload that is too high.

5. **(A)** Abnormal sodium does NOT cause QT prolongation. In contrast, a low magnesium, potassium, or calcium may cause QT prolongation and may result in torsades de pointes ventricular tachycardia and, if self-limiting, transient syncopal episode.

6. **(B)** The pain described in the scenario is typical of the pain caused by pericarditis. Dressler's syndrome is the pericarditis that may result after an acute MI.

7. **(B)** Retroperitoneal bleeding may cause signs of hypovolemia and hypovolemic shock as described in the scenario. It may be a complication of a PCI if the femoral artery is the access site during the procedure. Only this problem results in severe back pain; none of the other 3 choices results in back pain.

8. **(A)** The location of the murmur, at the apex of the heart (midclavicular, 5th ICS), is one clue to this answer. In addition, regurgitation occurs when the valve should be closed and the mitral valve should be closed during systole. Mitral stenosis, choice (C), occurs when the mitral valve is open. Additionally, mitral stenosis cannot be acute, it develops gradually.

9. **(B)** The first letter indicates chamber paced (ventricle). The second letter indicates chamber sensed (ventricle). The third letter indicates the response to sensing (inhibited in response to sensing.)

10. **(D)** The scenario describes a patient having an acute inferior wall MI, which is generally due to occlusion of the RCA. The RCA occlusion may result in papillary muscle dysfunction or rupture of the mitral valve because it supplies the area of the left ventricle where this valve is attached. Although RV infarct could result with RCA occlusion, RV infarct does not result in a systolic murmur at the apex of the heart or lung crackles.

11. **(B)** Cardiogenic shock results in a decrease in cardiac output with a resultant drop in coronary artery perfusion and compensatory vasoconstriction. The deflation of the balloon placed into the descending aorta is beneficial. Deflation decreases afterload and work of the left ventricle. Inflation of the balloon is beneficial because it "boluses" blood into the coronary arteries, increasing perfusion.

12. **(B)** The patient's response to the arrhythmia will determine whether treatment needs to be emergent and what the treatment will be. Vagal maneuvers. e.g., bearing down, are not known to be effective for atrial fibrillation.

13. **(C)** PCI would address the cause of the problem, not only treat signs and symptoms. Selection of the other 3 choices presumes the patient had serious signs and symptoms. Do not read into the questions.

14. **(A)** A decrease in heart rate, provided by a beta blocker such as metoprolol, would increase filling time. In hypertrophic cardiomyopathy, there is a problem with filling. A decrease in heart rate would increase filling time. Diastolic dysfunction does NOT cause a problem with ejection, and the EF is normal. The other 3 choices may be indicated for systolic dysfunction.

15. **(B)** The scenario describes an acute anterior STEMI, generally caused by an occlusion of the LAD. This type of MI is most likely to result in a VSD. Additionally, the location of the murmur is important. Mitral valve disease–related problems do NOT cause murmurs to be loudest at the left sternal border, whereas a VSD would result in a murmur at this location.

16. **(D)** The scenario describes a patient having an acute inferior STEMI, generally due to RCA occlusion. An RCA occlusion may result in an RV infarct, which this patient has signs of (hypotension with clear lungs). The definitive treatment is emergent PCI. Fluid administration will help increase coronary artery perfusion by correcting hypotension and ensure adequate RV preload. The right-sided ECG may help confirm the RV infarct. Nitroglycerin, diuretics, and morphine may decrease preload, which would worsen hypotension.

17. **(A)** The patient has signs of organ dysfunction (heart failure) secondary to extreme hypertension. Therefore, he has hypertensive crisis or emergency. The B/P needs to be emergently decreased. Most often this treatment is best done in an ICU setting.

18. **(B)** The patient presents with signs of heart failure due to diastolic dysfunction (hypertension, left ventricular hypertrophy, EF > 40%). These patients have a problem with FILLING, not ejecting. Digoxin, a positive inotrope, may increase wall stress and worsen filling of the left ventricle.

19. **(C)** The patient has symptoms with minimal activity, which describes NYHA Class III. This would qualify her for an ICD.

20. **(B)** The signs described are those of chronic right-sided heart failure. Acute right ventricular failure may result in JVD but not peripheral edema or abdominal discomfort (which is due to liver engorgement).

21. **(A)** The signs described in the scenario are those of cardiac tamponade. The treatment for cardiac tamponade for the post-op open heart surgery patient is return to the OR to drain the pericardial fluid that has accumulated. Development of the problem in other patient populations would necessitate an emergent pericardiocentesis to drain the fluid.

22. **(C)** A right ventricular infarction large enough to cause RV failure causes a problem with RV emptying, leading to an elevated right atrial pressure causing distended jugular vein distention. Choices (A) and (D) are signs of left ventricular failure. Choice (B) is a sign of dehydration.

23. **(B)** Pulsus paradoxus is fluctuation of the systolic blood pressure with inspiration and expiration by more than 12 mmHg, best seen when an arterial line is in place. Inspiration increases thoracic pressure. When combined with fluid surrounding the heart in cardiac tamponade, inspiration further decreases venous return to the heart, leading to drop systolic pressure by > 12 mmHg during the inspiratory phase of breathing. Choice (A), pulsus alternans is characterized by a change in amplitude of the systolic waveform from beat to beat, usually indicative of severe left ventricular failure. Choice (C), pulsus magnus, is a bounding pulse. Choice (D), pulsus bisferiens, is a double pulse and is not covered by the CCRN test.

24. **(B)** The scenario describes development of atrial fibrillation with a controlled ventricular response and stable B/P. Even with a normal B/P, the development of atrial fibrillation drops the cardiac output by 20% to 25% due to a loss in "atrial kick" provided by normal sinus rhythm. A cardiac glycoside (such as digoxin) may be beneficial as it is a weak positive inotrope that may compensate for the loss of atrial kick and calcium-channel blockers will keep the rate controlled. Pressors are not needed in this case. Use

of both beta blockers and calcium-channel blockers would decrease the rate too much. ACE inhibitors would offer no benefit in this case.

25. **(C)** S3 heart sound in an adult is indicative of high left ventricular pressure, cough, and lung crackles are signs of pulmonary edema secondary to elevated left ventricular end-diastolic pressure (PAOP). The EF is less than 40% in systolic heart failure.

26. **(A)** The patient clinical status describes a stable B/P but development of a bradyar-rhythmia, specifically a complete heart block with a ventricular rate of 30/minute. This is usually seen with RCA disease, generally associated with inferior MI. Patient assessment will determine patient treatment. Transcutaneous pacing would be an appropriate treatment for an unstable patient with this arrhythmia.

27. **(D)** The clinical description may be that of acute coronary syndrome complicated by hypotension. Addressing the hypotension is a priority as this is further decreasing coronary artery perfusion. A fluid bolus would address hypotension, and no contraindications seem to be present for a fluid bolus as lungs are clear. Aspirin is indicated for acute chest pain and could be given while preparing to do the ECG, which is needed to help make the diagnosis.

28. **(B)** Because most inferior MIs are due to RCA occlusion and the RCA also supplies blood to the right ventricular muscle wall, inferior MI is associated with RV infarct.

29. **(B)** During systole (left ventricular ejection) the aortic valve is open, allowing for ejection, and the mitral valve is closed at this time. The mitral valve is open during filling (diastole).

30. **(A)** At high doses (> 10 mcg/kg/min), dopamine stimulates alpha receptors in arteries and causes vasoconstriction. The other 3 drugs/doses affect mainly beta-1 receptors in the heart, producing a positive inotropic effect.

Pulmonary Concepts

5

*The difference between a successful person and others is not a
lack of strength, not a lack of knowledge, but rather a lack of will.*

—Vince Lombardi

PULMONARY TEST BLUEPRINT

Pulmonary 18% of total test   **27 Questions**

➜ Acute lung injury (e.g., ARDs, RDs)
➜ Acute pulmonary embolism
➜ Acute respiratory failure
➜ Acute respiratory infections (e.g., acute pneumonia, bronchiolitis)
➜ Air leak syndromes (e.g., pneumothorax, pneumopericardium)
➜ Aspirations (e.g., aspiration pneumonia, foreign body)
➜ COPD, asthma, chronic bronchitis, emphysema
➜ Pulmonary hypertension
➜ Status asthmaticus
➜ Thoracic surgery
➜ Thoracic trauma (e.g., fractured ribs, lung contusions, tracheal perforation)

PULMONARY TESTABLE NURSING ACTIONS

☐ Identify and monitor normal and abnormal physical assessment findings
☐ Interpret ABGs
☐ Monitor patient for response to pulmonary medications (e.g., bronchodilators,
mucolytics)
☐ Recognize indications for and manage patients requiring:

○ Artificial airway
○ Bronchoscopy
○ Chest tubes
○ Conventional modes of mechanical ventilation
○ High-frequency mechanical ventilation
○ Noninvasive positive pressure ventilation (e.g., BIPAP, CPAP, high-flow nasal
cannula)
○ Oxygen therapy delivery devices
○ Prevention of complications related to mechanical ventilation (e.g., barotrauma,
VAP)

- ○ Pulmonary therapeutic interventions (e.g., airway clearance, intubation, weaning, extubation)
  - ○ Respiratory monitoring devices (e.g., sPO_2, SvO_2, $EtCO_2$) and report values
  - ○ Therapeutic gases (e.g., nitric oxide, heliox, CO_2)
  - ○ Thoracentesis
- ☐ Recognize signs and symptoms of respiratory emergencies, initiate interventions, and seek assistance as needed
- ☐ Monitor patient and follow protocols for thoracic and ENT surgery

> Plan on spending approximately 27 hours studying the pulmonary section since there will be 27 questions related to pulmonary. The first half of this section reviews pulmonary physiological concepts that may appear on the exam. These concepts are the basis of the specific pulmonary disorders and treatments that are covered in the second half of this section, which reviews pulmonary disorders.

PULMONARY ASSESSMENT AND PHYSIOLOGY

Ventilation

- Ventilation is the movement of air in from the atmosphere and out from the body to maintain appropriate concentrations of O_2 and CO_2.
- Central control (brain stem): primary control
  - ○ Senses blood pH, decrease in pH → ventilation is stimulated
  - ○ Decrease pH = acidosis results in increase rate and/or depth of breathing
- Peripheral control (PaO_2 "sensors" in aortic arch): secondary control
  - ○ Senses PaO_2 of blood, decrease in PaO_2 → ventilation stimulated
  - ○ Decrease in PaO_2 = hypoxemia, results in increase rate and/or depth of breathing
  - ○ Chronic $PaCO_2$ retainers rely on mild hypoxemia for ventilator drive. If PaO_2 is corrected to normal, may result in decreased drive to breathe (ventilate)
- What is the clinical indicator of ventilation? How do you know your patient is ventilating normally?
  - ○ Need to know the **$PaCO_2$** (NOT the PaO_2)
- What is minute ventilation?
  - ○ Tidal volume Vt × respiratory rate (RR)—easily seen on the ventilator of the patient requiring mechanical ventilation.
  - ○ Normal ventilation is ~ 4L/minute
  - ○ An increase in minute ventilation = an increase in **work of breathing**
- What is the primary muscle of ventilation?
  - ○ Diaphragm!
  - ○ Anything that affects "health" of the diaphragm (deconditioning, hypoxemia, acidosis, hypophosphatemia) will adversely affect ventilation

- What is the position for optimal ventilation?
  - Upright sitting position
  - Supine position is NOT good for ventilation; if a patient is in respiratory distress, the worst position for the patient is flat on his back!

Dead Space Ventilation (concept covered on the exam)

- Volume of air that does not participate in gas exchange
  - Anatomic dead space: ~ 2 mL/kg of Vt
    - We all have this; it is normal
    - No gas exchange at level of nose down to alveoli
  - Alveolar dead space: pathologic, non-perfused alveoli, PE
  - Physiologic dead space = Anatomic dead space + alveolar dead space
- ☆ A **pulmonary embolus** results in increased alveolar dead space! A clot in the pulmonary circulation (a pulmonary embolus): no blood flow past alveoli in that area of the pulmonary circulation (Figure 5-1).

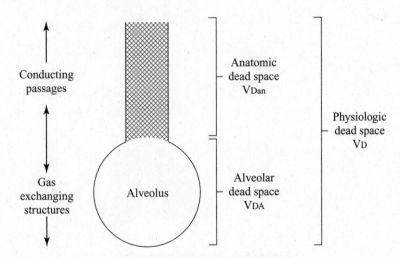

Figure 5-1. Dead space ventilation

Pulmonary Perfusion

The main function of the pulmonary system is gas exchange. For gas exchange to occur normally, there needs to be ventilation. However, movement of air alone is not enough for normal gas exchange. There needs to be perfusion, movement of blood past alveoli.

- Pulmonary perfusion is movement of blood through pulmonary capillaries.
- Any decrease in blood flow past alveoli (e.g., pulmonary embolus, low cardiac output states) will affect the ventilation/perfusion ratio and gas exchange.
- Normal ventilation/perfusion ratio:

$$\frac{4 \text{ L ventilation/min (V)}}{5 \text{ L perfusion/min (Q)}}$$

Ideal lung unit = 0.8 ratio, normal V/Q ratio

Any problem that alters ventilation (V) or perfusion (Q) can result in abnormal gas exchange if compensatory mechanisms are not successful. For example, a low cardiac output, even though not a pulmonary problem, can result in poor gas exchange.

■ You will not be expected to calculate V/Q ratios for the exam. However, you will need to know that the pulmonary problems (discussed in this section) will result in abnormal V/Q ratios, from mild to extreme, depending on the extent of the problem.

EFFECT OF GRAVITY ON PULMONARY PERFUSION

■ In the upright position, most pulmonary blood is in the lower lung lobes (see A in Figure 5-2). when lying supine, most pulmonary blood is posterior (see B in Figure 5-2). Rarely are ALL lung units perfused, but an example would be vigorous exercise (as in C in Figure 5-2).

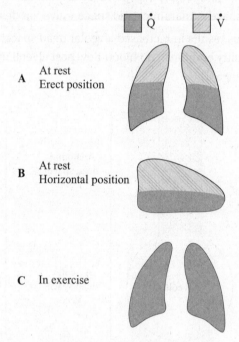

◻ Q̇   ◻ V̇

A   At rest
    Erect position

B   At rest
    Horizontal position

C   In exercise

Figure 5-2. Perfused lung units

■ What are the clinical implications?
☆ Want the "good" lung down
  ○ Large right lung pneumonia: if patient is turned to the right (bad lung), more blood goes to the right, patient may become hypoxemic
  ○ This patient should not be turned to the right side

V/Q Ratio

☆ Normal V/Q ratio
  ○ When there are no problems with either ventilation or perfusion, the patient will have normal gas exchange on room air (Figure 5-3).

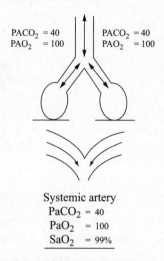

PACO$_2$ = 40 PACO$_2$ = 40
PAO$_2$ = 100 PAO$_2$ = 100

Systemic artery
PaCO$_2$ = 40
PaO$_2$ = 100
SaO$_2$ = 99%

Figure 5-3. Normal V/Q ratio, FiO$_2$ 0.21

- Abnormal V/Q ratio
  - When there is a problem with ventilation or perfusion, there is a V/Q mismatch.
  - The patient will develop hypoxemia on room air. However, provision of oxygen will generally correct the hypoxemia until the etiology can be determined and addressed (Figure 5-4).
  - Treatment of V/Q mismatch
    - Give O$_2$
    - Identify and treat underlying problem

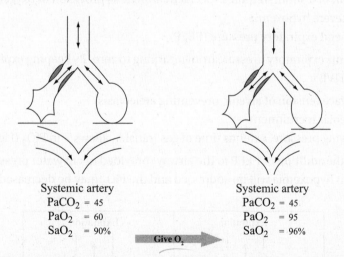

Systemic artery
PaCO$_2$ = 45
PaO$_2$ = 60
SaO$_2$ = 90%

Give O$_2$ →

Systemic artery
PaCO$_2$ = 45
PaO$_2$ = 95
SaO$_2$ = 96%

Figure 5-4. V/Q mismatch, i.e., pneumonia, pulmonary embolism

- ☆ Shunt
  - An extreme V/Q mismatch; even provision of 100% FiO$_2$ will NOT correct the hypoxemia (Figure 5-5).
  - ARDS is an example of a shunt.
  - Treatment of a shunt
    - Give O$_2$ (usually 100%)
    - PEEP: increases alveolar recruitment, prevents alveolar collapse

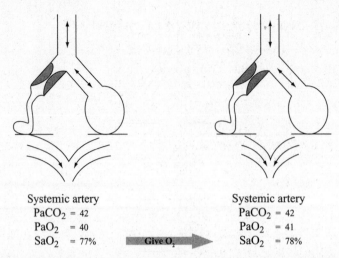

Systemic artery
PaCO$_2$ = 42
PaO$_2$ = 40
SaO$_2$ = 77%

Give O$_2$ →

Systemic artery
PaCO$_2$ = 42
PaO$_2$ = 41
SaO$_2$ = 78%

Figure 5-5. Shunt, i.e., acute respiratory distress syndrome (ARDS)

- A shunt is movement of blood from the right side of the heart to the left side of the heart without getting oxygenated; venous blood to the arterial side
- Normal physiologic shunt: thebesian veins of the heart empty into the left atrium. This is why the normal oxygen saturation on room air is 95% to 99%; cannot be 100% on room air due to this shunt. (With supplemental oxygen, 100% saturation can be achieved.)
- Anatomic shunt: example, ventricular or atrial septal defect.
- ☆ Pathologic shunt: ARDS. Blood goes through lungs but does NOT get oxygenated resulting in **refractory hypoxemia**.

    ○ Treatment of a shunt: requires special treatment as provision of oxygen alone will not correct severe hypoxemia

    ○ Positive-end expiratory pressure (PEEP)

    – Prevents expiratory pressure from returning to zero. By keeping expiratory pressure POSITIVE it . . .

    – ↓ Surface tension of alveoli, preventing atelectasis

    – ↑ Alveolar recruitment

    – ↑ Driving pressure, extends time of gas transfer, allows ↓ in FiO$_2$ (Figure 5-6)

    – With the addition of PEEP to the airway (provided in cm water pressure, i.e., 10 cm, 15 cm) hypoxemia will be addressed and the FiO$_2$ may be decreased from 100%

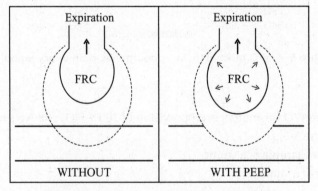

Figure 5-6. Visual representation of PEEP

Assessment of Oxygenation in the Critically Ill

Adequate oxygenation is the delivery of O_2 to meet tissue demands at the **cellular** level. In order to achieve this, each of the following needs to occur:

- Adequate ventilation
- Transfer of O_2 across alveolar-capillary membrane
- Presence of hemoglobin to carry O_2
- Adequate cardiac output to deliver O_2 to the tissue bed
- Release of O_2 from the hemoglobin molecule
- Ability of cells to utilize O_2

At the cellular level, sufficient oxygen is needed for production of adenosine triphosphate (ATP), which is needed for cell energy and life. See Figure 5-7 to see how oxygen is needed for aerobic metabolism with production of sufficient ATP for cell life. Without sufficient oxygen at the cellular level, lactic acid is produced (LACTIC ACIDOSIS), which is the evidence of anaerobic metabolism, organ failure, and eventual cell death.

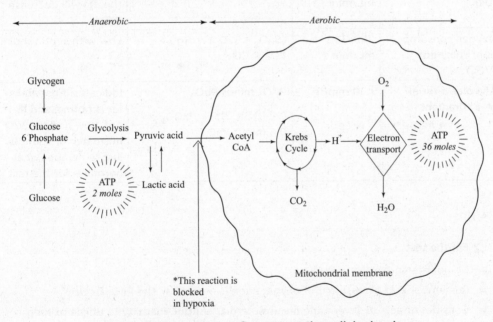

Figure 5-7. Importance of oxygen at the cellular level

It is NOT sufficient to examine only PaO_2 and SaO_2!! For example, the patient with severe sepsis/septic shock may have a normal PaO_2, SaO_2, hemoglobin, clear lungs, adequate ventilation, and oxygen delivery, yet a lactate level of 10. This is lactic acidosis. Why? Oxygen utilization is affected by severe sepsis/septic shock and results in anaerobic metabolism at the cellular level. Table 5-1 lists clinical indicators of oxygenation in the critically ill.

Table 5-1. Indicators of Oxygenation

Parameter	Normal	How Calculated/Measured	Clinical Relevance
Arterial oxygen (PaO_2)	80–100 mmHg on room air	Directly measured	Less than 80, hypoxemia (mild, moderate, severe)
Saturation of arterial oxygen (SaO_2)	95–99% on room air	Directly measured	Direct relationship to PaO_2, amount of hemoglobin combined with O_2
Mixed venous oxygen saturation (SvO_2)	60–75%	Direct measurement (Pulmonary artery)	Most sensitive indicator of oxygenation at the cellular level
Oxygen content (CaO_2)	15–20 mL/100 mL blood	$CaO_2 = (Hgb \times 1.39 \times SaO_2) + (PaO_2 \times 0.003)$	Severe anemia may result in hypoxia
Oxygen delivery (DO_2)	900–1100 mL/min	$CaO_2 \times CO \times 10$	Pump problems (heart) will decrease DO_2
Oxygen consumption, utilization (VO_2)	250–350 mL/min	$(SaO_2 - SvO_2) \times Hgb \times 13.9 \times CO$	Low with septic shock
Alveolar-arterial (A-a) gradient	< 10 mmHg	PAO_2 minus PaO_2 $(\%FiO_2 \times 715) - PaCO_2 \div 0.8$ minus PaO_2	Indicates if gas transfer is normal and if not, how bad the V/Q mismatch or shunt is; just remember what normal is for the test

☆ For the test:

➤ Do not memorize the formulas

➤ Remember that assessment of oxygenation is more than the PaO_2 or SaO_2

➤ Consider effects of severe anemia, low cardiac output, inability to utilize oxygen even when delivery is adequate (e.g., severe sepsis)

Most critically ill patients have continuous monitoring of oxygen saturation (SaO_2) noninvasively measured with the use of bedside pulse oximetry (SpO_2). Although the normal SaO_2 on room air is 95% to 99%, the goal for most critically ill patients is to maintain the SpO_2 at 90% or greater, usually with supplemental oxygen. Note from the curve depicted in Figure 5-8 that when the SaO_2 is less than 90%, the PaO_2 is less than 60 mmHg. When the PaO_2 is less than 60 mmHg, cells begin to have difficulty maintaining aerobic metabolism (without compensation, i.e., increase in heart rate or oxygen delivery).

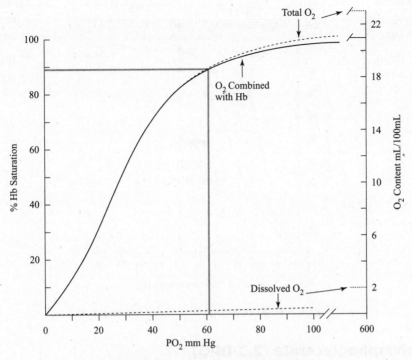

Figure 5-8. PaO$_2$/SaO$_2$ relationship

For the CCRN test, you will need to understand a high-level concept, the **oxyhemoglobin-dissociation curve**. Certain clinical conditions make hemoglobin "hold on" to oxygen molecules (curve shifts to the LEFT). Other conditions allow hemoglobin to "release" the oxygen more easily to the tissue (curve shifts to the RIGHT). See Table 5-2 for conditions that shift the curve to the left and right and Figure 5-9 for an illustration of the oxyhemoglobin-dissociation curve.

Table 5-2. Clinical Conditions Causing a Shift of the Oxyhemoglobin Dissociation Curve

Shift to the Left	Shift to the Right
Alkalosis (low H$^+$) Low PaCO$_2$ Hypothermia Low 2,3-DPG	Acidosis (high H$^+$) High PaCO$_2$ Fever High 2,3-DPG
Remember left is aLkaLosis, coLd, Low Bad for patient; SaO$_2$ high but O$_2$ stuck to Hgb	Good for tissues; SaO$_2$ low but O$_2$ easily released to tissues

- Conditions that cause a shift to the left result in a higher SaO$_2$, but the tissues do not get needed O$_2$ as readily.
- Conditions that cause a shift to the right result in a somewhat lower SaO$_2$, but the tissues receive O$_2$ more readily.

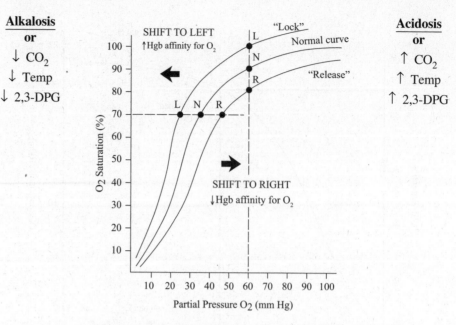

Figure 5-9. Oxyhemoglobin-dissociation curve

2,3-Diphosphoglycerate (2,3-DPG)

- What is 2,3-DPG? It is an organic phosphate found in RBCs that has the ability to alter the affinity of Hgb for oxygen.
  - Decreased 2,3-DPG results in hemoglobin holding on to O_2 (Table 5-3)
  - Increased 2,3-DPG results in hemoglobin more readily releasing O_2 (Table 5-3)

Table 5-3. Effect of 2,3-DPG on Hgb Affinity for Oxygen

Decreased 2,3-DPG	Increased 2,3-DPG
Multiple blood transfusions of banked blood	Chronic hypoxemia (high altitudes, chronic HF)
Hypophosphatemia	Anemia
Hypothyroidism	Hyperthyroidism
Result: Less O_2 available to tissues	Result: More O_2 available to tissues

Carbon Monoxide Poisoning

- Carbon monoxide (CO) has a greater affinity to hemoglobin than does oxygen, approximately 230 times greater (Figure 5-10)!
- In the presence of CO, oxygen cannot be carried → tissue hypoxia.
- Do NOT use pulse oximetry to monitor oxygenation status for the patient with CO poisoning. The pulse oximeter cannot differentiate between CO and O_2. Therefore, an SpO_2 of 95%, in the presence of CO poisoning, means only that the hemoglobin is saturated with a total of 95% molecules.
  - If the CO level of the blood is 40%, the maximum amount of O_2 that can be carried by hemoglobin is 60%.

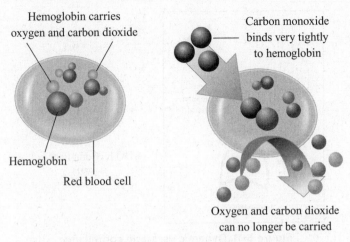

Figure 5-10. Carbon monoxide effects on hemoglobin

Carboxyhemoglobin levels and associated clinical presentation:

- 0–5% Normal
- < 15% Often in smokers, truck drivers
- 15–40% Headache, some confusion
- 40–60% Loss of consciousness, Cheyne-Stokes respirations
- 50–70% Mortality > 50%

☆ Treatment
- 100% FiO_2 until symptoms resolve and carboxyhemoglobin level is < 10%
- Hyperbaric oxygen chamber if available, generally within 30 minutes

Lung Compliance

Think of compliance as the degree of elasticity of tissue. Therefore, a decrease in compliance increases resistance, or stiffness.

- **Static compliance:** measurement of the elastic properties of the **lung**

  Tidal volume ÷ **plateau pressure** (minus PEEP)

  ○ Note that an increase in plateau pressure will decrease compliance

- **Dynamic compliance:** measurement of the elastic properties of the **airways**

  Tidal volume ÷ **peak inspiratory pressure** (minus PEEP)

  ○ Note that an increase in peak inspiratory pressure will decrease compliance

- Normal for both is ~ 45–50 mL/cm H_2O
- Patients with pulmonary problems that involve mainly the airways, i.e., asthma, have a decrease in dynamic compliance, but static compliance remains normal (Figure 5-11).
- Patients with pulmonary problems that involve mainly the lungs, i.e., pneumonia, ARDS, have a decrease in static compliance, but their dynamic compliance may also decrease as the lung pressures may transmit up to the airways (Figure 5-11).

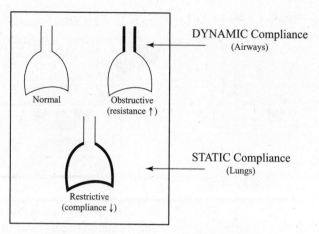

Figure 5-11. Dynamic vs. static compliance

TIP

⭐ For the test, remember that decreased compliance increases the work of breathing.

- Status asthmaticus
  - ○ Static compliance (lungs) would be normal
  - ○ Dynamic compliance would be low
- ARDS
  - ○ Static compliance would be low
  - ○ Dynamic compliance would also be low

ACID-BASE INTERPRETATION

ABGs WILL be tested on the CCRN test. You need to understand the 4 major acid-base abnormalities as well as states of compensation—uncompensated, partial compensation, and full compensation. Not only will you need to know how to interpret the ABG, you will need to know what the clinical implications are for the patient and the treatment if any. All RNs are taught ABGs in nursing school, then usually again when they enter critical or acute care, but from my greater than 30 years of experience teaching critical care nurses, an average of 25% who attend the CCRN Review Course get the ABG question wrong on the pretest that I give. How did you do on the ABG question in the Pretest of this book? A succinct review of acid-base interpretation is given below (Table 5-4). ABGs are provided with answers so that you can practice, as needed.

Table 5-4. Normal ABG Parameters

Parameter	Normal Range	Absolute Normal
pH	7.35–7.45	(7.40)
PCO_2	35–45 mmHg	(40 mmHg)
HCO_3	22–26 mmol/kg	(24 mmol/kg)
BE	–2 to +2	(0)
PO_2	80–100 mmHg	
SaO_2	95–99% (on room air)	

The information that follows will focus on acid-base interpretation, not oxygenation, which is covered in other areas of this book.

General Points Related to Acid-Base Balance

- Remember that the pH represents the hydrogen ion (H^+) concentration of the blood.
- Due to the Henderson-Hasselbalch equation, when the H^+ concentration is increased, the pH decreases, and when the H^+ concentration is decreased, the pH increases. There is an inverse relationship between the H^+ and the pH, so don't get confused!
- Think of $PaCO_2$ as an acid. When it increases, there is acidosis. When it decreases, there is alkalosis.
  - The $PaCO_2$ is controlled by the lungs. It is the **respiratory** parameter.
  - The lungs can change the $PaCO_2$ within minutes (rapid change).
- Think of HCO_3 as a base. When it is greater than normal, alkalosis may be present. When it is less than normal, acidosis may be present.
  - The HCO_3 is controlled by the kidneys. It is the **metabolic** parameter.
  - The kidneys alter the HCO_3 over hours to days (slow change).

Table 5-5. Four Primary Acid-Base Disorders and Expected Compensatory Change

Imbalance	pH*	Primary Change	Compensatory Change
Respiratory acidosis	< 7.35	↑ $PaCO_2$	↑ HCO_3
Metabolic acidosis**	< 7.35	↓ HCO_3	↓ $PaCO_2$
Respiratory alkalosis	> 7.45	↓ $PaCO_2$	↓ HCO_3
Metabolic alkalosis	> 7.45	↑ HCO_3	↑ $PaCO_2$

*In the presence of FULL compensation, the pH will enter the normal range.
**Metabolic acidosis may also be evaluated by the anion gap (see below) and the venous CO_2 (which will be lower than normal in the presence of metabolic acidosis).

ANION GAP

The anion gap is the difference between positive and negative anions. In most instances of metabolic acidosis, there is an increase in the anion gap. In several types of metabolic acidosis, though, the anion gap remains normal.

Calculation of anion gap (you will NOT need to do this for the test), but know what is normal:

$$(Na^+ + K^+) - (Cl^- + HCO_3^-)$$

- Normal is 5–15 mEq/L
- The anion gap is helpful in determining cause and/or response to treatment of metabolic acidosis (Table 5-6). For instance, if the patient with DKA presents with an anion gap of 25, one would expect the anion gap to decrease gradually as the patient responds positively to treatment. Since electrolytes are assessed frequently, the acidosis can be monitored by monitoring the anion gap without getting frequent ABGs.

NOTE

You will not need to know how to calculate the anion gap for the test.

Table 5-6. Problems Associated with an Anion Gap

Problems Associated with an Increase in Anion Gap	Problems Associated with a Normal Anion Gap
Ketoacidosis	Saline infusion (hyperchloremic acidosis)
Uremia	TPN
Salicylate intoxication	Diarrhea
Methanol	Ammonium chloride
Alcoholic ketosis	Acute renal failure, sometimes chronic
Unmeasured osmoles: ethylene glycol, paraldehyde	Note that problems that cause a normal anion gap metabolic acidosis are less
Lactic acidosis: shock, hypoxemia	common problems.

ACID-BASE COMPENSATION

- Compensation is the body's way of attempting to return the pH to normal (7.35–7.45).
  - Uncompensated
  - Partial compensation
  - Full compensation: **rare** in critically ill, suspect mixed disorder if present
  - Tables 5-7, 5-8, 5-9, and 5-10

Table 5-7. Examples of Compensation for Respiratory Acidosis

Uncompensated	Partial Compensation	Full Compensation
pH 7.30	pH 7.32	pH 7.35
$PaCO_2$ 50	$PaCO_2$ 50	$PaCO_2$ 50
HCO_3 24	HCO_3 29	HCO_3 31

Table 5-8. Examples of Compensation for Respiratory Alkalosis

Uncompensated	Partial Compensation	Full Compensation
pH 7.55	pH 7.50	pH 7.45
$PaCO_2$ 25	$PaCO_2$ 25	$PaCO_2$ 25
HCO_3 22	HCO_3 18	HCO_3 16

Table 5-9. Examples of Compensation for Metabolic Acidosis

Uncompensated	Partial Compensation	Full Compensation
pH 7.30	pH 7.32	pH 7.35
$PaCO_2$ 35	$PaCO_2$ 33	$PaCO_2$ 30
HCO_3 16	HCO_3 16	HCO_3 16

Table 5-10. Examples of Compensation for Metabolic Alkalosis

Uncompensated	Partial Compensation	Full Compensation
pH 7.50	pH 7.47	pH 7.45
$PaCO_2$ 45	$PaCO_2$ 48	$PaCO_2$ 50
HCO_3 32	HCO_3 32	HCO_3 32

COMBINED ACID-BASE DISORDERS ... SELDOM SEEN ON THE TEST

Occurs when 2 single disorders are present simultaneously to produce the **same** abnormality

- Combined respiratory and metabolic acidosis:

  pH   7.21
  $PaCO_2$ 50
  HCO_3 12

- Combined respiratory and metabolic alkalosis:

  pH   7.59
  $PaCO_2$ 30
  HCO_3 33

MIXED ACID-BASE DISORDERS ... SELDOM SEEN ON THE TEST

- Simple acid-base disorders result from a single process such as metabolic acidosis.
- In many critically ill patients, multiple acid-base disturbances exist concurrently and result in complex, mixed acid-base disorders.
- For example, a septic shock patient may present with respiratory alkalosis **and** metabolic acidosis.
- Complex formulas can be applied to determine whether the compensating parameter ($PaCO_2$ or HCO_3) has compensated more than predicted for the primary problem, indicating a mixed disorder is present. You will not need to know these formulas for the test.

SYSTEMATIC ASSESSMENT OF ACID-BASE

1. Evaluate the pH → determine whether normal, acidemic, or alkalemic
2. Evaluate respiratory then renal parameters → determine which, if either, is abnormal
3. Determine state of compensation
4. Evaluate for mixed disorder
5. Assess oxygenation (PaO_2, SaO_2)

PRACTICE ABGs

> **Directions:** Interpret each of the following ABGs, the primary problem, and the compensation. The answers can be found on page 104.

ABG	Interpretation
1. pH 7.48 $PaCO_2$ 32 HCO_3 24	1. _____
2. pH 7.32 $PaCO_2$ 48 HCO_3 25	2. _____
3. pH 7.30 $PaCO_2$ 38 HCO_3 18	3. _____
4. pH 7.28 $PaCO_2$ 60 HCO_3 29	4. _____
5. pH 7.49 $PaCO_2$ 40 HCO_3 30	5. _____

6. pH 7.28 PaCO$_2$ 70 HCO$_3$ 33   6. _____

7. pH 7.50 PaCO$_2$ 49 HCO$_3$ 38   7. _____

8. pH 7.31 PaCO$_2$ 32 HCO$_3$ 15   8. _____

9. pH 7.30 PaCO$_2$ 50 HCO$_3$ 25   9. _____

10. pH 7.48 PaCO$_2$ 40 HCO$_3$ 30   10. _____

11. pH 7.38 PaCO$_2$ 80 HCO$_3$ 47   11. _____

PULMONARY DISORDERS

About 11 pulmonary topics are included in the CCRN exam blueprint. However, some topics are more likely to be included on the test than others. It is highly recommended that you study ARDS, status asthmaticus, pneumonia, and pulmonary embolism in order to do well on the pulmonary questions. The physiological concepts reviewed above are the foundation for all of the pulmonary disorders. Specific pulmonary disorders likely to be seen on the test are reviewed below.

ACUTE RESPIRATORY FAILURE

- Acute respiratory failure is defined as a **rapidly** occurring inability of the lungs to maintain adequate oxygenation of the blood with or without impairment of carbon dioxide (CO$_2$) elimination. Specifically, the ABG demonstrates:
  - PaO$_2$ of 60 mmHg or less, with or without an elevation of PaCO$_2$ to 50 mmHg or more with pH < 7.30

- As seen from the definition, the primary problem may be one of hypoxemia (Type 1) or hypercarbia (Type 2), or both (Type 3). See Table 5-11 for the specific problems that result in each type of acute respiratory failure.

Table 5-11. Types of Acute Respiratory Failure

Type 1 Hypoxemic	Type 2 Hypercapneic	Type 3 Combined
Pneumonia	CNS depression due to drugs (opiates, sedatives)	ARDS
ARDS	↑ ICP	Asthma
Atelectasis	COPD (including asthma)	COPD
Pulmonary edema	Flail chest	
Pulmonary embolism (massive)	ALS	
Interstitial fibrosis	Guillain-Barré syndrome	
Asthma	Multiple sclerosis	
	Myasthenia gravis	
	Spinal cord injury	

- Clinical signs/symptoms of acute **hypoxemic** respiratory failure
  - Pulmonary: tachypnea, adventitious breath sounds, accessory muscle use
  - Cardiac: tachyarrhythmias (initial), bradyarrhythmias (late), hypertension or hypotension, cyanosis (central, e.g., lips, earlobes)
  - Neurological: anxiety, agitation
- Clinical signs/symptoms of acute **hypercapneic** respiratory failure
  - Pulmonary: shallow breathing, bradypnea, lungs may be clear or with adventitious breath sounds
  - Neurological: progressive decreased level of consciousness (lethargic, obtunded, stuporous, unresponsive)

Prompt identification and treatment may prevent a catastrophic outcome! Etiology of the signs/symptoms may not be the primary focus initially.

Treatment of Acute Respiratory Failure

- Maintain airway and improve ventilation
  - Positioning (upright)
  - Suctioning
  - Bronchodilator therapy for wheezing
  - Noninvasive ventilation
  - Intubation, mechanical ventilation if needed
  - Repeat ABGs as needed
- Optimize oxygenation
  - Adjust FiO_2 to keep SaO2 ~ > 0.90
  - Decrease FiO_2 to 0.50 or less ASAP
  - Do not allow hypoxemia to occur to "prevent O_2 toxicity"
  - Use PEEP/CPAP as needed
  - Pulse oximetry to monitor response to therapy
- Circulation, cardiac output
  - Manage hypotension
  - Address cardiac arrhythmias
- Identify etiology, target treatment accordingly
- Emotional support

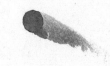

Use of Noninvasive Ventilation for the Management of Acute Respiratory Failure

Noninvasive ventilation (NIV), when used for the appropriate patient, has been shown to decrease morbidity and mortality. There are 2 main types of NIV. Generally, though, the exam does not cover the details related to type of NIV. More importantly, understand those who would NOT benefit from the therapy. Occasionally, a patient may initially be a good candidate for NIV but then due to change in condition, the patient should be intubated with an endotracheal tube.

- CPAP—Continuous positive airway pressure
  - Indicated for patients with hypoxemic respiratory failure who have increased work of breathing, e.g., cardiogenic pulmonary edema
  - Settings include FiO_2 and 1 pressure setting in cm H_2O pressure
- BiPAP—Bilevel positive airway pressure
  - Indicated for patients with hypoxemic and/or hypercapneic respiratory failure
  - Settings include FiO_2 and 2 pressure settings, the inspiratory pressure (IPAP) and the expiratory pressure (EPAP)
  - IPAP assists ventilation and EPAP assists oxygenation

ADVANTAGES OF NIV

- Buys time for medical treatment to take effect
- Reduces work of breathing (WOB)
- Decreases preload and afterload
- Improves oxygenation
- Improves ventilation (BiPAP)
- Reduces atelectasis
- Prevents intubation and resultant risks

- ☆ Contraindications for NIV
  - Hemodynamic instability or life-threatening arrhythmias
  - Copious secretions
  - High risk of aspiration
  - Impaired mental status (unable to protect airway)
  - Suspected pneumothorax
  - Inability to cooperate
  - Life-threatening refractory hypoxemia (PaO_2 <60 with FiO_2 1.00)

CHRONIC OBSTRUCTIVE PULMONARY DISEASE (COPD): ACUTE EXACERBATION

- COPD includes emphysema, asthma, bronchitis (more detail on status asthmaticus is in the next section)
- In general with each type of COPD, it is easier for air to enter the pulmonary system than exit, inspiration is easier than exhalation.
- Physiologic consequences include:
  - Dynamic hyperinflation occurs due to too much air in lungs.
  - Air trapping and auto-PEEP are common.
  - Expiratory flow rates are LOW
  - An acute exacerbation results in a V/Q mismatch due to a problem with ventilation, an increase in the $PaCO_2$
  - May have chronic CO_2 retention; if so, will have partial or complete compensation and high HCO_3 on the ABG

- Signs of an acute exacerbation of COPD include:
  - Worsening dyspnea
  - Increase in sputum purulence
  - Increase in sputum volume
  - Hypercapnea, hypoxemia
- Management of an acute exacerbation of COPD includes:
  - Titrate FiO_2 to $PaO_2 > 60$ mmHg or $SaO_2 > 90\%$ with care not to overcorrect hypoxemia and decrease respiratory drive
    - Must address **severe** hypoxemia; do not withhold oxygen only because hypoventilation may occur . . . cells still need oxygen
  - Bronchodilator therapy
    - Inhaled short-acting beta agonist (SABA), e.g., albuterol
    - Inhaled anticholinergic
  - Corticosteroid therapy
  - Antibiotic therapy (when pneumonia is thought to be the trigger)
  - Proceed with mechanical ventilatory support if needed (noninvasive or invasive)
    - Multiple studies have shown that non-invasive ventilation (NIV) is beneficial in patients with acute exacerbation of COPD

STATUS ASTHMATICUS

- Status asthmaticus is airway hyper-reactivity that produces severe airway narrowing that is refractory to aggressive bronchodilator therapy, which may result in respiratory failure. Status asthmaticus can be fatal as evidenced by the pathophysiology diagram in Figure 5-12 below.

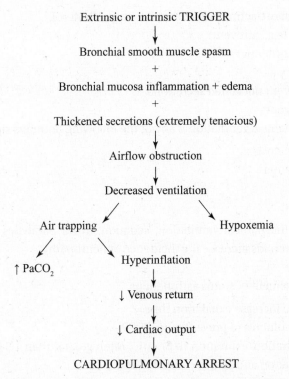

Figure 5-12. Pathophysiology of status asthmaticus

Clinical Presentation of Status Asthmaticus

- Dyspnea, tachypnea
- Cough, chest tightness
- Accessory muscle use
- Wheezing → decreased breath sounds → absent breath sounds . . . ominous sign!
- V/Q mismatch
- Chest X-ray may have flattened diaphragm (sign of air trapping)
- Tachycardia
- Pulsus paradoxus ≥ 15 mmHg (severe is > 18 mmHg)
- Anxiety → ↓ LOC
- May have elevated WBC, eosinophils
- Peak flow rate < 80% of predicted, < 50% is severe
- History of previous intubations (higher mortality)
- Table 5-12 describes ABG changes

Table 5-12. ABG Progression in Status Asthmaticus (on Room Air)

Stage 1	Normal PaO_2, respiratory alkalosis (↓ $PaCO_2$)
Stage 2	Mild hypoxemia, respiratory alkalosis (↓ $PaCO_2$)
Stage 3	Worsening hypoxemia, normalization of pH and $PaCO_2$
Stage 4	Severe hypoxemia, respiratory acidosis

Management of Status Asthmaticus

- Measure presenting peak flow rate (PFR)
  - Admit to hospital if PFR is 50–70%
  - Admit to ICU if PFR < 50%
- Bronchodilator: short-acting beta-2 agonists (e.g., albuterol)
- Anticholinergics (e.g., atrovent)
- Corticosteroids (systemic)
- O_2, pulse oximetry
- Hydration to prevent thickened secretions
- Avoid sedation agents
- Intubation, mechanical ventilation if any of the following ominous signs occurs:
  - Respiratory acidosis
  - Severe hypoxemia
  - Silent chest
  - Change in LOC
- If intubated on mechanical ventilation, sedation, avoid paralytics because paralytics combined with steroids increase the incidence of neuropathy

- ☆ Ventilator management of status asthmaticus
  - Use low rate to increase exhalation time
  - Use low tidal volumes to prevent auto-PEEP
  - Increase inspiration/expiration (I/E) ratio, often greater than 1:3–4, to allow time for optimal exhalation and prevent auto-PEEP

- Pulmonary embolism is a partial or complete obstruction of the pulmonary capillary bed by a blood clot or other substance such as fat, air, amniotic fluid, or foreign material with disruption of blood flow to an area of the lung (Table 5-13 and Figure 5-13).

  ○ Massive: > 50% occlusion

  ○ Submassive: < 50% occlusion

  ○ 80–90% result from DVT

Table 5-13. Risk Factors for Venous Thromboembolism (VTE)

Strong	Moderate	Weak
Fracture (hip or leg)	Arthroscopic knee surgery	Bedrest > 3 days
Hip or knee replacement	Central venous lines	Prolonged sitting
Major trauma	Chemotherapy	Increasing age
Spinal cord injury	HF or respiratory failure	Laparoscopic surgery
	Hormone replacement therapy	Obesity
	Malignancy	Pregnancy, antepartum
	Oral contraceptives	Varicose veins
	Stroke	
	Pregnancy, postpartum	
	Previous VTE	

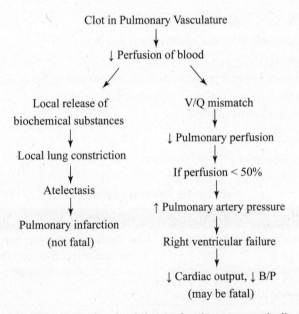

Figure 5-13. Pathophysiology of pulmonary embolism

Although pulmonary embolism (PE) may be due to a variety of causes, the two types most likely to be covered on the test are venous embolism and fat embolism. See Table 5-14 for the signs and symptoms of PE.

Types of PE

- **Venous—DVT**
- **Fat emboli—Long bone, pelvis**
- Air emboli—Surgery, IV lines
- Catheter embolization
- RA/LA or RV embolus—Afib/flutter (left atrial leading to stroke is more common)
- Amniotic fluid (rare)—Amniocentesis, abruptio placenta, or abortion
- Tumor EMBOLI—Malignancy causes increase in thrombin
- Septic Emboli—Bacteria/Viral

Table 5-14. Signs and Symptoms of PE

	If massive . . .
Dyspnea, tachypnea Tachycardia, chest pain Right-sided S_3 or S_4 Anxiety, apprehension Cough, hemoptysis, crackles Syncope **Petechiae (fat emboli)** Low-grade fever Respiratory alkalosis	Hypoxemia Hypotension EKG changes-RBBB, right axis deviation on ECG, tall peaked P-waves in lead II, RV strain pattern, ST elevation in V_1 and V_2 Cardiopulmonary arrest—PEA

Diagnosis of PE

- Pulmonary angiography—gold standard!
- V/Q scan: "high" probability, "low" probability, not definitive
- High-speed CT scan
- D-dimer: good rule-out test; if positive, means clot present in the body, therefore if symptoms ARE due to PE, expect D-dimer to be positive.
- Venous Doppler (helps with source)

TIP

☆ **A PE will increase alveolar dead space!**

Note: ~ 2/3 PE never get diagnosed!

Table 5-15 lists mechanical and pharmacological ways to prevent PE.

Table 5-15. Prevention of PE

Mechanical	Pharmacological
Graduated compression stockings (GCS) and/or Intermittent pneumatic compression (IPC) Use continuously except while ambulating!	Low–molecular weight heparin (LMWH): enoxaparin (Lovenox) **DAILY** Low-dose unfractionated heparin: **t.i.d.**

Treatment of PE

- Maintain adequate airway, ventilation, oxygenation
- Fluids!
- Anticoagulation
  - Heparin (80 units/kg IVP and then 18 units/kg/hr drip) or
  - Low–molecular weight heparin (1 mg/kg q 12 hrs)
  - Coumadin **on the first treatment day** if able

- Fibrinolytic therapy: **for all patients with hemodynamic compromise with low risk for bleeding**
- Maintain cardiac output (inotropes, fluids)
- Analgesics
- IVC filter for selected patients
- May require long-term anticoagulation

NOTE

You will not need to know drug doses for the test.

PULMONARY HYPERTENSION

Pulmonary hypertension (PH) is included on the test blueprint. However, you are less likely to see questions covering this topic than status asthmaticus, PE, pneumonia, and ARDS. Keep this in mind when studying.

- Defined as a MEAN pulmonary artery pressure greater than 25 mmHg at rest and PAOP less than 16 at rest with secondary right heart failure
  - The normal pulmonary artery mean pressure is ~ 20 mmHg. Because the RV normally pumps into a low-pressure system, the wall of the RV is thin compared to that of the left ventricle (LV). Pulmonary hypertension results in right ventricular failure, cor pulmonale.
- 5 Groups defined by the World Health Organization (WHO)
  - Group 1—Pulmonary artery hypertension (PAH); sporadic and hereditary due to localized small pulmonary muscular arterioles, i.e., collagen vascular diseases, drug/toxin induced
  - Group 2—Pulmonary hypertension (PH) due to left heart disease; LVF, valvular heart disease
  - Group 3—PH due to lung diseases or hypoxemia
  - Group 4—PH due to chronic thromboembolic problems
  - Group 5—PH due to unclear or multifactorial, e.g., sarcoidosis

Signs and Symptoms

- Exertional dyspnea, lethargy, and fatigue due to an inability to increase cardiac output with activity
- Progression to RV failure, chest pain, syncope with exertion, and peripheral edema
- Passive hepatic congestion may cause anorexia and ABD pain
- Ortner's syndrome—cough, hemoptysis, and hoarseness
- Systolic ejection murmur, increased intensity of pulmonic component of S2, diastolic pulmonic regurgitation murmur, right-sided murmurs, and gallops are augmented with inspiration
- RV hypertrophy, elevated JVD, hepatomegaly, peripheral edema, ascites, and pleural effusion

Treatment of Pulmonary Hypertension

- Treat the underlying cause as able
- Each "group" has specific treatments based on cause

- All regimens should consider diuretics, oxygen, anticoagulants, digoxin, and exercise training
- Dilators used (calcium-channel blockers, phosphodiestrase-5 inhibitors, e.g., sildenafil (Viagra) or tadalafil (Cialis)
- Patients refractory to all medical interventions—lung transplantation (bilateral or heart-lung transplant) or possible atrial septostomy (right to left shunt)

PNEUMONIA

Pneumonia is an acute inflammation of the lung parenchyma caused by an infectious agent that can lead to alveolar consolidation.

Causative agents:

1. Bacterial
2. Viral
3. Fungal
4. Parasitic

Pneumonia may also be classified according to where it developed:

- Community acquired (CAP)
    - Outside the hospital
    - Risk factors will help decide treatment
    - Pathogens: *Streptococcus pneumoniae*, *Legionella pneumophila*, *Klebsiella pneumoniae*, *Haemophilus influenzae*, *Staphylococcus aureus*, *Mycoplasma pneumoniae*, *Pseudomonas aeruginosa*
- Hospital acquired (HAP)
    - Acute care
    - Long-term care
    - Nursing home
    - Ventilator-associated (VAP) . . . now referred to as ventilator-associated condition/event
    - By definition, develops 48 hours or more after admission
    - Common pathogens: *P. aeruginosa*, *Escherichia coli*, *K. pneumoniae*, Acinetobacter baumannii, *Staphylococcus aureus* (especially diabetes and head trauma), MRSA
    - Hospital acquired pneumonia has higher mortality than CAP

Risk Factors for Pneumonia

Multiple factors will increase risk:

- Age
- Preexisting pulmonary disease
- Smoking
- ↓ LOC
- Artificial airways
- Chronic illness
- Malnutrition

- Immunocompromise
- Increased secretions
- Atelectasis
- Immobility
- Depressed cough or gag reflexes
- Concurrent antibiotic therapy
- Aspiration
- Spread from another site (gut, wound)
- Multisystem organ dysfunction

Signs and Symptoms of Pneumonia

- Chills, diaphoresis, fever, malaise
- Tachycardia, chest pain
- Confusion (esp. elderly)
- Productive cough
- Use of accessory muscles
- Dehydration
- Over area of consolidation on the chest:
  - ↑ Tactile fremitus
  - Dull to percussion
  - Bronchial breath sounds or diminished breath sounds
  - Bronchophony (louder/clearer)
  - Egophony ("e" to "a")
  - Whispered pectoriloquy (whisper heard better with stethoscope)

Diagnosis of Pneumonia

- CXR: Consolidation or diffuse patchy infiltrates
- Sputum culture with gram stain
- Blood cultures
- WBC: high but may be normal or low in immunocompromised or elderly
- WBC differential: increased bands > 10%
- ABGs: hypoxemia
- Thoracentesis for effusions

Treatment of Pneumonia

- Optimize Oxygenation and Ventilation
  - Titrate FiO_2
- ☆ Positioning—GOOD lung
  - – O
  - – W
  - – N
  - Bronchial hygiene, chest physiotherapy
  - Noninvasive ventilation or Intubation/mechanical ventilation as needed
  - Bronchoscopy (with lavage, if needed)
  - Mobilize, clear secretions

- Identify organism
  - Sputum culture and sensitivity
  - Blood cultures
- Antibiotic therapy
  - Empiric therapy → choice based on likely organism based on pt. assessment, type of pneumonia, if resistant or not
  - Timing: 1st dose within 4 hours, if admitted, should be given in the ED
  - Organism-specific therapy as soon as results of C&S available
- System support
  - Hydration
  - Fever management
  - Glucose control
  - Nutrition
- General preventative measures
  - Smoking cessation
  - Pneumonia vaccine < 65
  - Flu vaccine

Prevention of Hospital-Acquired Pneumonia

- Hand hygiene
- Keep HOB elevated 30°
- Prevent bacterial translocation from GI tract: use the gut, feed patient
- Oral hygiene!
- Educate: common institution pathogens, rates of nosocomial pneumonia
- Use evidence-based confirmation of feeding tube placement

  - Confirm with X-ray prior to using for feeding.
  - Mark exit site with indelible marker for future reference.
  - Assess patency every 4 hours.
  - Observe for a change in length of the external portion of the feeding tube (as determined by movement of the marked portion of the tube).
  - Review routine chest and abdominal X-ray reports to look for notations about tube location.
  - Observe changes in volume of aspirate from feeding tube.
  - If pH strips are available, measure pH of feeding tube aspirates if feedings are interrupted for more than a few hours.
  - Observe the appearance of feeding tube aspirates if feedings are interrupted for more than a few hours.
  - Obtain an X-ray to confirm tube position if there is doubt about the tube's location.

Prevention of Ventilator Associated Pneumonia (VAP)

All of the interventions to prevent hospital-acquired pneumonia plus:

- Drain accumulated condensate from tubing.
- Prevent backflow of tubing condensate into endotracheal tube (ETT).
- Change ventilator tubing only when contaminated.

- Utilize aseptic technique for ETT, tracheostomy suctioning.
- Adherence with mouth care protocol.
- Brush teeth to remove plaque.
- Keep ETT cuff inflated.
- Perform subglottal suctioning prior to cuff deflation.
- Utilize ETT with port for continuous subglottal suctioning.

ASPIRATION

Aspiration of toxic substances into the lung with injury to the lung resulting from the chemical, mechanical, and/or bacterial characteristics of the aspirate

- Oropharyngeal is most common!
- May or may not involve an infection
- May be acute or chronic: micro or massive
- Table 5-16 shows management techniques

Due to the anatomy of the right mainstem bronchus (shorter, wider, and with less of an angle), most aspirations occur in the RIGHT lung. Although aspirations may occur in both lungs, they seldom are isolated solely to the left lung.

Etiology of Aspiration

- Altered level of consciousness
- Drug, alcohol abuse
- Depressed gag, cough, or swallowing reflexes
- Presence of feeding tubes (all types)
- Improper patient positioning
- Presence of artificial airways
- Ileus or gastric distention
- History of dysphagia, GERD, esophageal strictures, $\downarrow$GI motility
- Increased secretions

Signs and Symptoms of Aspiration

- Acute respiratory distress
- Presence of gastric contents in oropharynx
- Tachycardia
- Hypoxemia
- Crackles
- Copious secretions due to alveolar edema
- Hypotension (massive fluid shifts may occur)

Table 5-16. Emergent Management of Aspiration

Witnessed Aspiration	All Aspirations
Place patient in slight Trendelenburg, on right side to aid drainage Suction mouth and pharyngeal areas Bronchoscopy for large particles	O_2, titrate up as needed Intubation/mechanical ventilation as needed Monitor for onset of noncardiogenic pulmonary edema (ARDS) Monitor for ↓ B/P

ACUTE RESPIRATORY DISTRESS SYNDROME (ARDS) AND ACUTE LUNG INJURY (ALI)

TIP

☆ The test always includes several questions on this topic! Study accordingly.

ARDS or ALI is a syndrome caused by a variety of acute conditions that trigger an inflammatory response resulting in an increase in permeability of the pulmonary capillary membrane that allows a transudation of proteinaceous fluid into the interstitial and alveolar spaces. It may also be referred to as "noncardiogenic pulmonary edema." Damage to Type II alveolar cells is one of the pathological consequences. Since these are the cells responsible for the production of surfactant, massive atelectasis occurs.

Acute lung injury (ALI) is similar to ARDS with less severe of a shunt resulting in hypoxemia.

- All of the criteria in Table 5-17 must be present for the diagnosis of ARDS/ALI. The pulmonary edema is not due to heart failure. Hypoxemia is REFRACTORY, meaning the FiO_2 is increased to the maximum of 100% and hypoxemia is still present.

NOTE

PEEP treats a shunt by preventing alveolar collapse; it does not necessarily decrease pulmonary shunting.

- Because a shunt is present, PEEP needs to be provided in order to increase alveolar recruitment and treat the refractory hypoxemia.

Table 5-17. Differentiation of ARDS and ALI

ARDS	ALI
Acute onset with precipitating event Bilateral infiltrates consistent with pulmonary edema $PaO_2/FiO_2 \leq 200$ mmHg, regardless of the level of PEEP PAOP* ≤ 18 mmHg	Acute onset, with precipitating event Bilateral infiltrates consistent with pulmonary edema PaO_2/FiO_2 between 201 and 300 mmHg, regardless of the level of PEEP PAOP* ≤ 18 mmHg

*PAOP = pulmonary artery occlusive pressure

PaO_2/FiO_2 Examples

- Patient is receiving 50% FiO_2 and PaO_2 is 90:

$$90 \div 0.50 = 180$$

- Patient is receiving 30% FiO_2 and PaO_2 is 110:

$$110 \div 0.30 = 367$$

- Patient is receiving room air and PaO_2 is 62:

$$62 \div 0.21 = 295$$

- Patient is on 100% FiO_2 and PaO_2 is 95:

$$95 \div 1.00 = 95$$

Remember: Not only PaO_2/FiO_2 is considered to diagnose ALI or ARDS; the other 3 factors also need to be present.

Surfactant

- Phospholipid/lipoprotein produced by Type II alveolar cells
- Stabilizes alveoli, "keeps them open"
- Increases lung compliance
- Eases work of breathing
- Therefore, with ARDS (destruction of Type II alveolar cells):
  - Massive atelectasis, alveolar collapse
  - Decreased compliance
  - Increased work of breathing
  - Decreased functional residual capacity (FRC)

Figure 5-14 and Tables 5-18 and 5-19 show the pathophysiology, etiology, and signs and symptoms of ARDS and ALI.

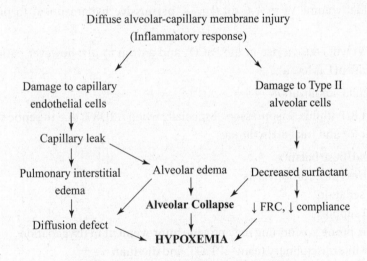

Figure 5-14. Pathophysiology of ARDS/ALI

Table 5-18. Etiology of ARDS/ALI

"Direct" Injury	"Indirect" Injury
Aspiration	Sepsis
Pneumonia	Shock
Pulmonary contusion	Head injury
Fat/air embolism	Non-thoracic trauma
O_2 toxicity	Blood transfusion
Inhalation injury	Pancreatitis
Drowning	Burns
Transthoracic radiation	Heart bypass
	DIC

Table 5-19. Signs and Symptoms of ARDS/ALI

Early	Late
Tachycardia	Tachycardia, episodes of bradycardia
Apprehension, restlessness	Agitated
Mild dyspnea	Extreme dyspnea
Respiratory alkalosis	Respiratory and metabolic acidosis
Few crackles	Crackles, wheezes
Chest X-ray → isolated infiltrate or "ground glass" appearance	Chest X-ray → white out/bilateral infiltrates
PaO_2 on room air ~ 60	PaO_2 on room air ~ 30

Treatment of ARDS/ALI

☆ Pulmonary stabilization strategies

- ○ Intubation with mechanical ventilation
- ○ PEEP, usually 15 cm H_2O or greater; monitor for barotrauma, ↓cardiac output, treat hypotension, but cannot stop PEEP
    - – Note: Disconnection of the ventilator circuit (and PEEP) will result in alveolar derecruitment and hypoxemia that may not be readily corrected
- ○ Limit plateau pressure to 30 cm H_2O or less
- ○ Limit tidal volume Vt to 4–6 mL/kg → "permissive hypercapnea" to prevent volutrauma
    - – Low Vt will cause a rise in the $PaCO_2$ and a drop in pH; however patients tend to tolerate pH as low as 7.2

- Cardiovascular stabilization
    - ○ Support B/P (fluids, vasopressors, especially when ARDS is due to septic shock)
    - ○ Monitor for and treat arrhythmias

- Monitor acid/base balance
- DVT and stress ulcer prophylaxis
- Analgesia, sedation
- Nutritional support
- Nitric oxide, prone positioning may provide improvement in oxygenation
- Coordinate interdisciplinary team—PT, OT, and dietitian
- Prevent, identify organ failure
- Emotional support (patient, family)
- Monitor for complications
- Steroids? **NO!**

Complications of ARDS/ALI

The mortality from ARDS is still around 30%, although patients do not die from hypoxemia. Instead, they die from multisystem organ dysfunction.

- Multisystem organ failure (renal, GI, CNS)
- Secondary infections
- Pulmonary embolus
- Ileus
- Skin breakdown
- Malnutrition
- Barotrauma: pneumothorax, subcutaneous emphysema

PNEUMOTHORAX

Air leak syndromes—pneumothorax (Figures 5-15 and 5-16 and Table 5-20) and pneumopericardium—are included in the Adult CCRN test blueprint. A simple, unilateral pneumothorax is generally not life threatening unless it occurs in a patient with end-stage chronic lung disease. A tension pneumothorax, however, may be life threatening. Therefore, you must know the difference between the two. Chest tube care is also included in the test blueprint.

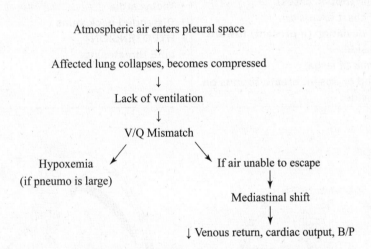

Atmospheric air enters pleural space
↓
Affected lung collapses, becomes compressed
↓
Lack of ventilation
↓
V/Q Mismatch
↓ ↘
Hypoxemia (if pneumo is large)   If air unable to escape
↓
Mediastinal shift
↓
↓ Venous return, cardiac output, B/P

Figure 5-15. Pathophysiology of pneumothorax

Types of Pneumothorax

- Spontaneous
- Traumatic
    - Open (penetrating chest trauma)
    - Closed (blunt chest trauma)
    - Iatrogenic (due to therapeutic or diagnostic procedures) (Figure 5-16)
- ☆ **Tension**
    - Air unable to exit → mediastinal shift
    - Life-threatening

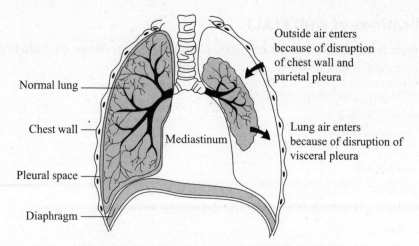

Normal lung

Chest wall

Mediastinum

Pleural space

Diaphragm

Outside air enters because of disruption of chest wall and parietal pleura

Lung air enters because of disruption of visceral pleura

Figure 5-16. Pneumothorax (no mediastinal shift)

Table 5-20. Signs and Symptoms of Pneumothorax

Spontaneous or Traumatic	Tension
Depends on size of pneumothorax and depends on underlying lung disease if any • Dyspnea, tachypnea • Chest pain (not all cases) • Unequal chest excursion • Tracheal deviation (if present) **toward** affected side • Hypoxemia (if large) • Decreased or absent breath sounds on affected side	Similar to traumatic EXCEPT • Tracheal deviation **away from affected side** (Figure 5-18) • Tachycardia • **Distended neck veins** • **HYPOTENSION** • LIFE threatening!

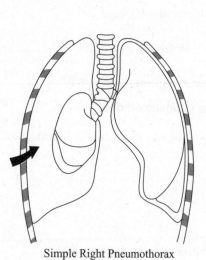

Simple Right Pneumothorax

Figure 5-17. Right pneumothorax (no tension)

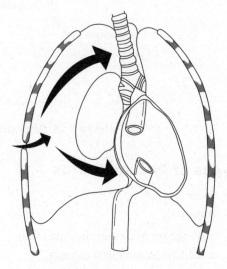

Right Tension Pneumothorax

Figure 5-18. Right tension pneumothorax, mediastinal shift

HEMOTHORAX

- Usually due to trauma, lung collapse, and blood in pleural or mediastinal space

  - Dullness to percussion
  - Absent breath sounds on affected side
  - Tracheal deviation towards unaffected side

Treatment of Pneumothorax

- Pneumothorax > 20%

  - Chest tube: reestablish negative pleural pressure
  - Supplemental O_2
  - Treat pain, if needed

- Pneumothorax < 20%

  - O_2
  - Monitor for lung re-expansion
  - If with underlying lung disease, may need chest tube

☆ Chest Tube Assessment and Management

- Close assessment of respiratory status, should improve after chest tube insertion
- Pain assessment, treatment
- Entry site—dressing assessment
- Tubing—no dependent loops!
- Drainage collection chamber

  - Keep lower than chest

- Water seal chamber

  - Tidaling with deep inspiration, normal
  - Air leak

    - Bubbling in water seal chamber, not normal
    - May be present postoperatively; if there has been no leak and now there is bubbling, notify physician
    - Avoid high airway pressures with chest tubes in place to avoid air leak

- Suction control chamber: gauge or water level determines amount of suction, NOT the wall suction source
- Clamp only when changing system, with inadvertent disconnection, or with physician order.

  - Clamping cuts off the negative pressure water seal chamber; expanded lung may re-collapse

Endotracheal Tube Placement

- Confirmation of correct placement is done immediately after intubation
  - Waveform capnography is most accurate
  - End-tidal CO_2 detector
  - Auscultation
- Cuff inflation to 20 cm H_2O pressure
- Obtain a chest radiograph for placement confirmation, should be **3–5 cm above the carina**
- Assess and document tube placement at the level of the lip for ongoing assessment of correct placement
- If tube migrates down, it most often migrates to the right lung due to anatomy of the mainstem bronchi (right is shorter, wider, with less angle than the left)
- Get ABGs within 20 to 30 minutes of intubation to assess acid-base status
- The endotracheal tube:
  - Is narrow, increases airway resistance, similar to breathing through a straw
  - ETT has a greater degree of dead space ventilation than a tracheostomy tube

Volume and Pressure Ventilation

- Ventilator breaths may be delivered at a set volume (most common for adults) or at a set pressure
- The main focus of the test is how the ventilator settings may differ depending on the primary problem of the patient, e.g., in ARDS or asthma

VENTILATOR MODES

- Assist-control (AC) mode
  - Patient receives the set tidal volume at the set breath rate and all breaths triggered by the patient's spontaneous effort above the set rate
    - For example, if the AC is set at a rate of 12 breaths/min, at a tidal volume of 700 mL and the patient's total rate per minute is 20, the tidal volume of the 8 extra breaths initiated by the patient is 700 mL because the extra breaths are sensed by the machine and the set tidal volume (700 mL) is given
  - All breaths are machine breaths
  - Provides full ventilatory support
  - Not used as a weaning mode unless being alternated with periods of spontaneous breathing (reducing the A/C rate does nothing if the patient is spontaneously breathing)
  - Can result in overventilation and/or hyperinflation of the lungs at higher spontaneous breathing rates

- Synchronized intermittent mandatory ventilation (SIMV) mode
  - Patient receives the set tidal volume at the set breath rate and all breaths above the set rate are spontaneous breaths at the patient's own tidal volume
    - For example, if the SIMV is set at a rate of 12 breaths/min, at a tidal volume of 700 mL and the patient's total rate per minute is 20, the tidal volume of the 8 extra breaths will vary from breath to breath because the breaths spontaneously initiated by the patient are at the patient's own tidal volume
  - All machine breaths are synchronized with the patient's breathing effort
  - Provides full or partial ventilatory support
  - Reducing the SIMV rate will allow the patient to assume more of the work of breathing
  - Spontaneous breaths may be pressure supported

VENTILATOR SETTINGS

Positive End Expiratory Pressure (PEEP)

- Positive pressure applied to the airways at end exhalation
- Increases lung volume at end exhalation (FRC), creating more surface area for gas exchange; increases alveolar recruitment
- Can be applied to patients via artificial airways, full face mask, nasal mask, and nasal prongs (neonates)
- Think oxygenation!

Continuous Positive Airway Pressure

- PEEP applied to a spontaneously breathing patient
- Patient receives no machine breaths
- Patient assumes all of the work of breathing
- Usually the last step in the weaning process
- All breaths may be pressure supported
- Patient may fatigue if left on for an extended period of time

PRESSURE SUPPORT VENTILATION

- Patient receives an increase in airway pressure during inspiration to augment (boost) spontaneous tidal volume
- Patient triggered mode (if patient is paralyzed and/or sedated, PSV will not be triggered on)
- Rate, tidal volume, inspiratory flow rate, and inspiratory time are determined by the patient's effort
- Cannot use PSV with assist/control mode
- Frequently used during weaning to **reduce the work of breathing** and overcome imposed work of ETT and ventilator circuit

Breath Rate: determined by $PaCO_2$, generally 12 to 16/minute on full support

Tidal Volume (Vt): determined by patient ideal body weight and problem

- Generally 8–10 mL/kg
- For ARDS, in order to prevent "volutrauma," 4–6 mL/kg

Fraction of inspired oxygen (FiO_2) generally set at 100% on intubation and then adjusted down according to PaO_2; goal is to decrease to 50% or less as soon as able

Ventilator Alarms

- Alarms are set for patient safety

High-Pressure Limit Alarms Are Caused By:

- Agitation
- Coughing
- Secretions
- Aspiration
- Kinked/occluded ETT or ventilator circuit
- Bronchospasm or mucosal edema
- Decreasing lung compliance (ARDS)
- Pneumothorax

Low Pressure Limit Alarms Are Caused By:

- Ventilator circuit disconnection or leak
- Inadequate tidal volume
- Cuff leak
- Chest tube leak

If unable to troubleshoot an alarm, what should you do?

- Disconnect the ventilator from the airway, and ventilate with a bag/valve device.
- A bag/valve device should be at the bedside of every patient receiving mechanical ventilation and with the mask available as well in the case of loss of the artificial airway.

See Table 5-21.

Table 5-21. Principles of Ventilator Management for Select Patient Problems

ARDS	Asthma
Plateau (static) pressure (< 30 cm) Low tidal volume (4–6 mL/kg) High PEEP (15–20 cm)	Provide short inspiratory time and long expiratory time • Low rate • Low Vt • High peak flow rate Monitor for auto-PEEP

WEANING FROM MECHANICAL VENTILATION

Criteria for weaning, spontaneous breathing trial:

- Original reason for intubation resolving
- Resting minute ventilation (ideally < 10 L/min)
- Spontaneous tidal volume (ideally > 5 mL/kg)
- Negative inspiratory force (NIF) (ideally > –25 cm H_2O)
- Rapid shallow breathing index (respiratory rate/Vt) (ideally < 100 breaths/min/L)
- Vital capacity (ideally 3 to 5 liters)
- ABGs/oxygenation acceptable with FiO_2 50% or less

Criteria for stopping the spontaneous breathing trial:

- Respiratory rate > 35/min
- Respiratory rate < 8/min
- SpO_2 < 88%
- Respiratory distress
- Mental status change
- Acute cardiac arrhythmia

Now that you have reviewed key pulmonary concepts, go to the Pulmonary Practice Questions. Answer the questions, and then check your answers. Continue to review the information until you get at least 80% on the practice questions.

PULMONARY PRACTICE QUESTIONS

1. Which of the following developments would indicate that the patient receiving noninvasive ventilation may require intubation with an endotracheal tube?

    (A) need for increase in FiO_2 from 0.30 to 0.40
    (B) dry cough and fever
    (C) change in mental status with difficulty to arouse
    (D) positive blood cultures

2. The patient was discharged from the medical unit 7 days ago following an acute ischemic stroke and is now anxious and complaining of severe shortness of breath. Patient demonstrates tachycardia, tachypnea, hypotension, SpO_2 88% on 3 L/nasal cannula, and temp = 37.9°C. Breath sounds are present, clear, and equal bilaterally. Chest X-ray is clear. ABGs reveal a respiratory alkalosis. Based on this history and assessment, which of the following problems exists and which interventions do you anticipate?

    (A) increased dead space ventilation, fibrinolytic therapy
    (B) decreased dynamic compliance, bronchodilators
    (C) infection, antibiotics
    (D) shunt, PEEP therapy

3. The patient receiving mechanical ventilation has a peak inspiratory pressure of 70 cm H_2O and a plateau pressure of 35 cm H_2O. What intervention would be most beneficial?

    (A) Increase FiO_2.
    (B) Administer morphine.
    (C) Obtain stat ABGs.
    (D) Administer a bronchodilator.

4. Which of the following is an appropriate intervention for a patient with status asthmaticus on a ventilator?

    (A) Decrease peak flow rate.
    (B) Increase tidal volume.
    (C) Check for auto-PEEP.
    (D) Increase breath rate.

5. Which of the following interventions has been demonstrated to decrease ventilator-acquired pneumonia?

    (A) Provide sedation.
    (B) Maintain head of the bed 20° or greater.
    (C) Adhere to a mouth care protocol.
    (D) Deflate endotracheal tube cuff prior to suctioning.

6. A 49-year-old male, 70 kg, is admitted to ICU with smoke inhalation and ARDS. He is receiving mechanical ventilation with the following ventilator settings: $FiO_2 = 0.80$, assist control mode, 10 breaths/min, Vt 400 mL, PEEP 15 cm pressure. Arterial blood gases are as follows: pH 7.39, $PaCO_2$ 42, PaO_2 96, HCO_3 22, and O_2 sat 98%. Which of the following interventions is appropriate?

   (A) Decrease the FiO_2.
   (B) Increase the tidal volume.
   (C) Decrease the PEEP.
   (D) Make no changes.

7. The following is TRUE related to lung compliance:

   (A) an increase in peak inspiratory pressure will decrease static compliance.
   (B) a decrease in compliance increases the work of breathing.
   (C) static compliance is decreased with an asthma exacerbation.
   (D) the plateau pressure is used to calculate dynamic compliance.

8. Clinical features of ARDS includes each of the following EXCEPT:

   (A) bilateral chest infiltrates on X-ray.
   (B) PAOP > 18 cm H_2O.
   (C) refractory hypoxemia.
   (D) tachypnea.

9. Your patient has mild tachypnea, productive cough, bronchial breath sounds in the right mid and lower lobes, dull to percussion over the right lower chest, SpO_2 92% on 0.40 FiO_2. Which of the following interventions would be appropriate for this patient?

   (A) Contact the physician for an order for a bronchodilator.
   (B) Noninvasive ventilation.
   (C) Avoid turning to the right side.
   (D) Maintain in a supine position.

10. Drug therapy most likely to be prescribed for a patient with status asthmaticus includes which of the following drug categories?

    (A) bronchodilators and anticoagulants
    (B) corticosteroids and diuretics
    (C) antibiotics and expectorants
    (D) bronchodilators and corticosteroids

11. The following interventions may improve oxygenation EXCEPT for:

    (A) increase the FiO_2.
    (B) give PRBCs.
    (C) give fluids or pressors to increase low B/P.
    (D) increase ventilator rate.

12. While monitoring a patient post-thoracotomy, the nurse suspects hypoventilation. Which characteristic best defines hypoventilation?

(A) $PaCO_2$ > 45 mmHg
(B) respiratory rate < 12
(C) pH < 7.35
(D) PaO_2 < 60 mmHg

13. The patient admitted with a carboxyhemoglobin level of 45% is lethargic, complains of a headache, is receiving 100% O_2 per face mask, and is noted to have an SpO_2 of 100%. Which of the following is indicated?

(A) Administer hydrocodone with acetaminophen.
(B) Continue the FiO_2 of 1.00.
(C) Decrease the FiO_2.
(D) Intubate and initiate mechanical ventilation.

For questions 14 and 15

A 38-year-old female is admitted with respiratory failure secondary to viral pneumonitis. She is receiving mechanical ventilation and suddenly becomes restless, tachypneic, tachycardic, and hypotensive. The high-pressure ventilator alarm is continuous, and pulse oximetry (SpO_2) decreases to 0.83. Breath sounds are diminished on the right with tracheal deviation to the left.

14. Based on the information above, what condition is likely developing?

(A) ARDS (acute respiratory distress syndrome)
(B) hemothorax
(C) tension pneumothorax
(D) pulmonary embolism

15. Treatment for the patient described above would likely include which of the following?

(A) morphine and furosemide
(B) addition of PEEP
(C) vasopressors
(D) chest tube

For questions 16 and 17

A 63-year-old male is admitted with acute respiratory distress. Symptoms include marked shortness of breath and circumoral cyanosis. He is awake and complains of shortness of breath. He has a history of COPD (chronic obstructive pulmonary disease). Blood gases reveal the following information:

pH	7.22
$PaCO_2$	62
PaO_2	54
SaO_2	81%
HCO_3	25
FiO_2	30%

16. Based on the information above, what condition is likely developing?

   (A) congestive heart failure
   (B) ARDS
   (C) acute respiratory failure
   (D) pulmonary emboli

17. What would be the priority treatment indicated at this time?

   (A) Increase the FiO_2.
   (B) Intubate and initiate mechanical ventilation.
   (C) Postural drainage treatment.
   (D) Administer a bronchodilator.

_____

18. Which of the following may be an effect of mechanical ventilation and PEEP (positive end-expiratory pressure)?

   (A) atelectasis
   (B) oxygen toxicity
   (C) ARDS
   (D) reduced cardiac output

19. The following is NOT a clinical finding seen in pneumonia:

   (A) a chest X-ray with an area of consolidation.
   (B) hypoxemia refractory to O_2 administration with a need for PEEP.
   (C) normal WBCs with increased immature neutrophils (bands).
   (D) bronchial breath sounds, diminished breath sounds, or crackles on auscultation.

20. Which of the following would be the earliest sign of hypoventilation?

   (A) respiratory rate of 20/minute
   (B) anxiety
   (C) decreased level of consciousness
   (D) SpO_2 of 85%

21. A 70 kg patient with ARDS is intubated and mechanically ventilated. The patient is on a continuous vecuronium infusion to maintain a twitch of "1." Peak inspiratory pressure is 55 cm H_2O, and the plateau pressure is 50 cm H_2O. The PaO_2 is 60. The physician orders the following ventilator settings: assist control mode, rate 12/minute, tidal volume 700 mL, FiO_2 1.00, PEEP 15. The nurse knows that:

(A) continuous positive airway pressure (CPAP) is an appropriate mode for the patient receiving vecuronium.
(B) a tidal volume of 700 mL is inappropriate for this patient.
(C) the PEEP should be decreased to 5 cm H_2O pressure to improve oxygenation.
(D) the plateau pressure is appropriate for this patient.

22. In caring for the postoperative patient with a chest tube, care of the patient needs to include:

(A) loop tubing right above the collection chamber.
(B) place the collection chamber on the IV pole when turning the patient.
(C) clamp the chest tube during patient transport.
(D) report sudden bubbling in the negative pressure chamber.

23. A patient with acute exacerbation of COPD is minimally responsive, tachypneic, and tachycardic. ABG results include pH 7.20, $PaCO_2$ 68, PaO_2 65. The nurse anticipates the next intervention will be:

(A) initiate noninvasive ventilation.
(B) endotracheal intubation.
(C) begin low-flow oxygen per nasal cannula.
(D) administer sodium bicarbonate to correct acidosis.

24. A patient with a known history of asthma is admitted with asthma exacerbation. The critical care nurse needs to be aware of the potential clinical signs that may indicate a need for intubation and initiation of mechanical ventilation. Which of the following would indicate a possible need for intubation?

(A) difficult to arouse
(B) respiratory alkalosis
(C) bilateral wheezing
(D) SaO_2 92%

25. Which one of the following factors would DECREASE the release of oxygen from hemoglobin at the tissue level?

(A) temp 39°C
(B) increased levels of 2.3-DPG
(C) arterial pH of 7.30
(D) massive transfusion of stored, banked blood

26. The trauma patient with multiple long-bone fractures suddenly develops agitation, tachypnea, tachycardia, and mild hypoxemia. Lungs are clear, and petechial rash is noted on the upper body. Which of the following is suspected?

   (A) acute respiratory distress syndrome
   (B) fat embolism
   (C) deep-vein thrombosis
   (D) delirium

27. The arterial blood gas (ABG) is pH 7.32, $PaCO_2$ 33, HCO_3 16. Based on this ABG, what might be the patient's problem?

   (A) anxiety
   (B) shock
   (C) drug overdose
   (D) electrolyte imbalance

ANSWER KEY

1. **C**	6. **A**	11. **D**	16. **C**	21. **B**	26. **B**
2. **A**	7. **B**	12. **A**	17. **A**	22. **D**	27. **B**
3. **D**	8. **B**	13. **B**	18. **D**	23. **B**	
4. **C**	9. **C**	14. **C**	19. **B**	24. **A**	
5. **C**	10. **D**	15. **D**	20. **C**	25. **D**	

ANSWERS EXPLAINED

1. **(C)** Noninvasive ventilation is not safe for the patient unable to protect the airway. A depressed level of consciousness increases the risk of airway obstruction or aspiration. Choice (A) can be provided with NIV. The other choices do not put the patient receiving NIV at greater risk for a poor outcome.

2. **(A)** The scenario describes a patient who is experiencing a pulmonary embolism (PE). Signs of hypotension and hypoxemia indicate that it is a massive PE. The PE increases dead space ventilation due to the drop in pulmonary perfusion. Fibrinolytic therapy (tissue plasminogen activator) is indicated for massive PE. For any of the other choices to be correct, the patient would have abnormal breath sounds.

3. **(D)** The clinical picture is one of asthma. Asthma is an airway problem resulting in bronchospasm, which increases airway pressure as evidenced by elevated inspiratory pressure while the lung pressure itself (plateau pressure) remains normal. Symptoms would be relieved with a bronchodilator; the other selections would not relieve these symptoms.

4. **(C)** The patient with asthma has difficulty with expiration. Therefore, with each breath, air may get trapped with resulting elevation in end-expiratory pressure even without PEEP being set on the ventilator. This may decrease cardiac output because it decreases venous return. The other interventions would all increase the air trapping.

5. **(C)** Mouth care decreases bacterial colonization in the mouth, which decreases the possibility of microaspiration of bacteria into lower airways. Each of the other 3 choices have NOT been found to decrease the incidence of ventilator-acquired pneumonia. Sedation should be minimized, head of bed should be greater than 30 degrees, and the ETT cuff should not be deflated prior to suctioning but, instead, prior to ETT removal. (At that time, the mouth and subglottal space should be well suctioned.)

6. **(A)** The goal is to get the FiO_2 down to 50% or less ASAP for the patient who requires high FiO_2. This patient's oxygenation status would allow a decrease in FiO_2. During acute ARDS, the tidal volume needs to be low to prevent "volutrauma" and PEEP needs to be maintained to limit atelectasis.

7. **(B)** Decreased compliance increases "stiffness" and therefore requires more work to ventilate. Choice (A) is not correct because an increase in peak inspiratory pressure will decrease dynamic compliance. Choice (C) is not correct because asthma decreases dynamic (airway) compliance, not static (lung) compliance. Choice (D) is not correct because dynamic compliance is calculated using the peak inspiratory pressure. The plateaus pressure is calculated using the static pressure.

8. **(B)** If the PAOP is high, the pulmonary edema is most likely cardiac in origin. Whereas in ARDS, the pulmonary edema is noncardiogenic in origin. The other 3 choices are all present in ARDS (bilateral infiltrates, refractory hypoxemia, and tachypnea).

9. **(C)** The clinical scenario is one of right-sided pneumonia. Therefore, the right side is the "bad" side. Due to effects of gravity on perfusion, the patient generally does better with the "good" lung DOWN. With the "bad" lung down, there is increased risk of worsening hypoxemia. Choice (A) is not correct because the patient is not wheezing. Therefore, there is no indication for a bronchodilator. Choice (B) is not correct because condition does not warrant NIV. Choice (D) is not correct because the best position for the patient with a pulmonary problem is sitting upright, not flat.

10. **(D)** The patient with asthma needs a bronchodilator to treat the bronchospasm caused by smooth muscle contraction around the airways and steroids to treat the airway inflammation. There is no indication for anticoagulants, diuretics, or antibiotics to treat asthma.

11. **(D)** An increase in breath rate will influence the $PaCO_2$ (ventilation), not oxygenation. The other 3 choices will improve oxygenation at the tissue level. An increase in the FiO_2 provides more oxygen at the alveolar-capillary membrane. Blood transfusion will increase oxygen content by increasing hemoglobin, which is the carrier of oxygen. An increase from low blood pressure will increase oxygen delivery.

12. **(A)** The best clinical indicator of effective ventilation is the $PaCO_2$. Although a breath rate less than 12 may indicate hypoventilation, it is not as sensitive an indicator as $PaCO_2$. In addition, breath rate does not include the other determinant of effective ventilation (depth of ventilation or tidal volume). Although a low pH may indicate hypoventilation, it may also indicate metabolic acidosis, and hypoxemia (PaO_2 less than 80 mmHg on room air) may be present during hyperventilation.

13. **(B)** If the patient has a CO level of 45%, the best SaO_2 achievable is 55% since saturation of hemoglobin cannot be greater than 100% total. The patient needs 100% FiO_2 until CO levels have returned to normal and symptoms (alteration in level of consciousness, headache) are relieved. Opiates may depress the level of consciousness and mask

the patient's response to FiO_2. A decrease in FiO_2 would decrease the driving forces of oxygen and prolong abnormal CO levels. Intubation would not help oxygenation since the same FiO_2 can be provided with a face mask. Intubation would be indicated for a ventilation problem, and the patient does not have signs of hypoventilation.

14. **(C)** The clinical scenario describes a pneumothorax. Because of hypotension and tracheal deviation to the opposite side of the pneumothorax, the pneumothorax is a life-threatening tension pneumo with symptoms due to mediastinal shift. If ARDS was the problem, the patient would have bilateral crackles. If a hemothorax was the problem, there would generally be a history of trauma, not infection. Mediastinal shift (tracheal deviation to the opposite side and hypotension) is not usually present with a hemothorax. If the problem was a PE, the breath sounds would be equal bilaterally.

15. **(D)** The treatment for a tension pneumothorax is a chest tube (generally after emergent needle decompression). None of the other choices is of any benefit for a tension pneumothorax.

16. **(C)** Not enough information is provided to make a choice other than (C). Acute respiratory failure is an ABG diagnosis, and this ABG meets requirements of acute respiratory failure. Do NOT read into questions.

17. **(A)** The patient has severe hypoxemia that needs to be addressed first in order to prevent all of the associated effects of severe hypoxemia. Although the patient is not ventilating normally, the elevated $PaCO_2$ is less of a problem as indicated by the patient's mental status. The level of consciousness is not depressed. There is no indication in the scenario for choices (C) or (D).

18. **(D)** Initiation of mechanical ventilation (even without PEEP) that delivers positive pressure breaths results in a mild increase in intrathoracic pressure with a resultant decrease in venous return. PEEP increases intrathoracic pressure even more and causes a decrease in venous return. Mechanical ventilation and/or PEEP do not cause any of the other 3 choices.

19. **(B)** Pneumonia results in a V/Q mismatch, not a shunt. Therefore, administration of oxygen will correct the hypoxemia. PEEP is not required as it is for a shunt (ARDS). The worse the pneumonia, the greater the FiO_2 requirement will be. The other 3 choices are possible clinical indicators of pneumonia.

20. **(C)** As ventilation decreases, the $PaCO_2$ rises and affects the brain by decreasing the level of consciousness from lethargy, to obtunded, to stupor, to comatose state. Although the patient MAY have hypoventilation with a respiratory rate of 20/minute, it would not be considered a typical sign. Anxiety and SpO_2 are more signs of hypoxemia than early hypoventilation.

21. **(B)** Because the patient has ARDS, low tidal volumes (4–6 mL/kg) are indicated (permissive hypercapnea) in order to prevent volutrauma. Because the patient is 70 kg, a Vt of 700 mL is too high. CPAP requires that the patient has a spontaneous breathing effort. Therefore, CPAP is not appropriate for this patient. The patient with ARDS requires high PEEP to prevent atelectasis and hypoxemia. Therefore, a decrease in PEEP would worsen hypoxemia. The plateau pressure should be kept at 30 cm H_2O or less. Therefore, this patient's plateau pressure is too high and a decrease in the Vt may help decrease plateau pressure.

22. **(D)** Sudden bubbling in the negative pressure chamber is an indication of a possible air leak and should be reported to the physician. All of the other 3 choices should be avoided when caring for the patient with a chest tube. Loops will increase pressure in the system. The collection chamber needs to be kept below the level of the chest at all times. Clamping the tube cuts off the negative pressure provided by the negative pressure chamber and could result in lung re-collapse.

23. **(B)** Due to the patient's decreased level of consciousness, the need for improved ventilation is a priority. NIV would address the hypoventilation but would not be considered safe for the patient with minimal responsiveness. Providing oxygen alone would not address the main problem (hypoventilation), which in this case is worse than the problem of hypoxemia. The patient has respiratory acidosis and should not be treated with sodium bicarbonate.

24. **(A)** A depressed level of consciousness may be an indication of hypoventilation (respiratory acidosis) and a precursor to respiratory arrest for the patient with asthma exacerbation. Respiratory alkalosis and bilateral wheezing are common early manifestations during an asthma exacerbation. Mild hypoxemia should be treated with an increase in FiO_2 but is not considered ominous unless severe.

25. **(D)** Banked blood does not have normal 2,3-DPG. Low levels of 2,3-DPG shift the oxyhemoglobin dissociation curve up to the left, which will decrease hemoglobin release of oxygen at the tissue level. The remaining 3 choices—fever, increased levels of 2,3-DPG, and acidosis—all shift the curve to the right, which increases release of oxygen from hemoglobin.

26. **(B)** The clinical scenario is one of pulmonary embolism. With the history of long-bone fracture and development of petechiae, fat embolism is most likely. ARDS does not present with clear lungs. DVT does not always result in a PE. If it did, though, the PE would be due to a blood clot and petechiae would not be present. Delirium may result in agitation but not the other symptoms.

27. **(B)** The low pH indicates acidosis. The low bicarbonate indicates the acidosis is metabolic, and the low $PaCO_2$ indicates hyperventilation has started in order to compensate. The only option that causes metabolic acidosis is shock. Anxiety generally causes respiratory alkalosis. Opiate drug overdose results in respiratory acidosis, and electrolyte imbalance (low chloride) causes metabolic alkalosis.

ANSWERS TO PRACTICE ABGs

1. Respiratory alkalosis, no compensation
2. Respiratory acidosis, no compensation
3. Metabolic acidosis, no compensation
4. Respiratory acidosis, partial compensation
5. Metabolic alkalosis, no compensation
6. Respiratory acidosis, partial compensation
7. Metabolic alkalosis, partial compensation
8. Metabolic acidosis, partial compensation
9. Respiratory acidosis, no compensation
10. Metabolic alkalosis, no compensation
11. Mixed disorder, respiratory acidosis, metabolic alkalosis

Neurology Concepts

6

You have brains in your head. You have feet in your shoes.
You can steer yourself any direction you choose.

—Dr. Seuss

NEUROLOGY TEST BLUEPRINT

Neurology 12% of total test   **18 Questions**

→ Aneurysm
→ Brain death (irreversible cessation of whole brain function)
→ Congenital neurological abnormalities (e.g., AV malformation)
→ Encephalopathy (e.g., anoxic, hypoxic, ischemic, metabolic, infectious)
→ Head trauma (e.g., blunt, penetrating skull fractures)
→ Hydrocephalus
→ Intracranial hemorrhage/intraventricular hemorrhage (e.g., subarachnoid, epidural, subdural)
→ Neurologic infectious disease (e.g., viral, bacterial)
→ Neuromuscular disorders (e.g., muscular dystrophy, Guillain-Barré, myasthenia gravis)
→ Neurosurgery
→ Seizure disorders
→ Space-occupying lesions (e.g., brain tumors)
→ Stroke (e.g., ischemic, hemorrhagic)

MULTISYSTEM TESTABLE NURSING ACTIONS

☐ Identify and monitor normal and abnormal physical assessment findings.
☐ Recognize and monitor normal and abnormal neurological diagnostic test results (e.g., ICP, head CT scan, lumbar puncture).
☐ Recognize indications for and monitor/manage patients requiring neurological monitoring devices and drains.
☐ Manage patients receiving medications (e.g., mannitol, hypertonic saline, sedation, neuromuscular blockade, anticonvulsants), and monitor response.
☐ Recognize signs and symptoms of neurological emergencies (e.g., increased intracranial pressure, herniation, decreased LOC, seizure), initiate interventions and seek appropriate consultation.
☐ Monitor patient and follow protocols pre-, intra- and post-procedure (e.g., ICP catheter insertion, lumbar puncture).
☐ Monitor patients, and follow protocols for neurosurgery.

Neurology comprises 12% of the Adult CCRN Test with 18 questions. Therefore, you will need to study for approximately 18 hours.

NEUROLOGY ANATOMY

The brain is enclosed within the skull with the "higher" centers above the transtentorial shelf and the brain stem below the transtentorial shelf (Figure 6-1). Although the skull protects the brain, the inner surface and shelf have jagged edges that can tear brain tissue in the event traumatic injury causes movement of the brain within the skull. If brain swelling occurs, the brain has nowhere to expand except down toward the foramen magnum.

- There are 2 "holes" in the skull, the transtentorial notch (small) and the foramen magnum (large) through which the brain stem is attached to the spinal cord.

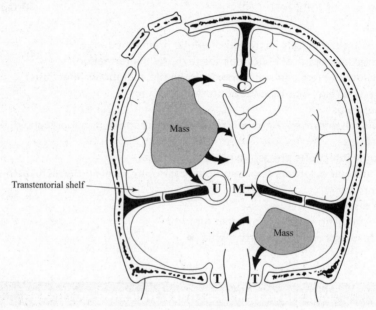

Figure 6-1. Brain anatomy

Cranial Nerves

- You do not need to memorize all of the cranial nerves for the test. However, several cranial nerves may be incorporated in the questions. (Figure 6-2)
  - I (olfactory): smell, often affected with a basilar skull fracture
  - II (optic): sight, NOT pupil reaction
  - III (oculomotor): pupillary function, flows out of midbrain (in brain stem) and traverses the transtentorial notch; therefore with an increase in intracranial pressure, parasympathetic stimulation is blocked, sympathetic stimulation predominates = dilated pupil on the side of the injury
  - V (trigeminal): corneal reflex, chewing
  - VIII (vestibulocochlear): intactness of this cranial nerve is tested by Doll's eyes and cold caloric exams

- IX (glossopharyngeal): swallow, gag
- X (vagus): pharyngeal/laryngeal movement
- All cranial nerves arise from the brain stem except cranial nerves I and II which arise from above the brain stem.

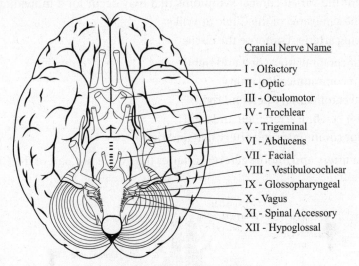

Figure 6-2. Cranial nerves

Blood Supply to the Brain

- Basal vertebral: supplies lower areas, brain stem
- Carotids: supply upper areas (Figure 6-3)
  - Left internal carotid is dominant for most people

Brain Function Based on Anatomic Location

- Frontal lobe: Personality, abstract thought, long-term memory
- Temporal lobe: Hearing, sense of taste and smell, interpretations
- Occipital lobe: Vision, visual recognition, reading comprehension
- Parietal lobe: Object recognition by size, weight, shape; body part awareness
- Cerebellum: coordination, balance, gait

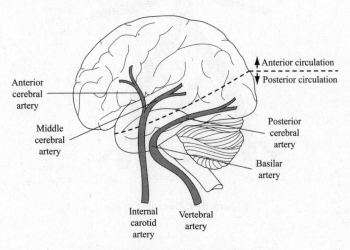

Figure 6-3. Blood supply to the brain

- The Circle of Willis is a circulatory anastomosis comprised of various arteries that supply blood to the brain. A well-developed Circle of Willis allows collateral blood flow to one area from another area in the event of an occlusion. (Figure 6-4)
- Less than 50% of the population has a well-developed, intact Circle of Willis, which accounts for the varied clinical symptoms that may occur for 2 individuals who have a stroke in the same area of the Circle of Willis.
- The following arteries compose the circle:
  - Anterior cerebral artery (left and right)
  - Anterior communicating artery
  - Internal carotid artery (left and right)
  - Posterior cerebral artery (left and right)
  - Posterior communicating artery (left and right)
- The basilar artery and middle cerebral arteries (MCA) are **not** part of the Circle of Willis.

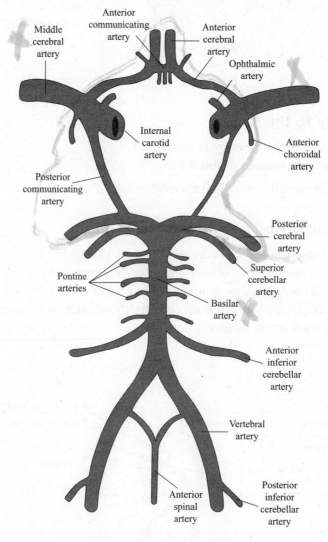

Figure 6-4. Circle of Willis

Components of a Neuro Assessment

MENTAL STATUS

- Level of consciousness (LOC): **change in LOC is always the first sign of a neuro problem** (except for an epidural hematoma that may cause pupil changes before an LOC change). The following are included in LOC assessment:

  - Arouseability—voice, shake, pain
    - Each of these should be applied one at a time in order to identify any subtle change, i.e., don't shout and shake at the same time
    - When assessing for pain, apply a central stimulus, e.g., sternal rub, trapezius squeeze, orbital pressure for a full 30 seconds before you state there is no response

  - Orientation—time, place, person
    - Generally the first to become abnormal is time, then place, and lastly person

  - The RAS is a network of neurons connecting the brain stem (lower RAS) to the cortex (higher RAS)
  - The upper RAS is responsible for awareness; the lower part of the RAS is responsible for the sleep-wake cycle
  - If the lower RAS is damaged, coma occurs; if only the upper portion of the RAS is damaged, the patient loses awareness but still wakes up and goes to sleep

- Speech/language: Broca's area in the left hemisphere

  - Expressive aphasia
  - Receptive aphasia

- Memory: short term usually becomes abnormal before long term
- Attention span/thought content/judgment
- Personality: occasionally the first sign of a problem, before LOC changes, the patient's personality may change, e.g., in brain tumors

MOTOR FUNCTION

- **Decussation** (crossing) of motor fibers occurs in the medulla; motor problems are contralateral to the problem.
- Strength, movement are indicators of motor function.
- Pronator drift may be evident before strength changes are detected
  - Ask the patient to close eyes, hold out both arms with palms up, and hold for 15 seconds
  - If one arm drifts down, that arm has weakness
- Abnormal flexion or distention (Figure 6-5)
- Flaccid: **medulla** dysfunction

TIP

☆ **Consciousness depends on an intact cerebral cortex and reticular activating system (RAS).**

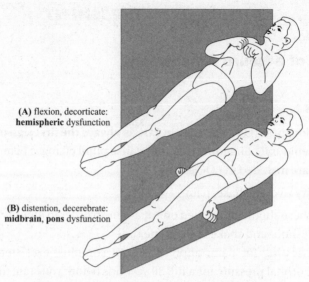

(A) flexion, decorticate: **hemispheric** dysfunction

(B) distention, decerebrate: **midbrain, pons** dysfunction

Figure 6-5. Abnormal flexion or distention

SENSORY FUNCTION

- Deficits generally the same side(s) as motor deficits

PUPILLARY ASSESSMENT

- Pupillary response assesses cranial nerve III (oculomotor) function, pupil constriction and accommodation
- Sympathetic effect on pupils: dilate
- Parasympathetic effect on pupils: constrict
- 17% of population has unequal pupils
- Changes occur on the side of the injury, ipsilateral

REFLEXES

- Babinski: positive is abnormal in adults (toes flair up toward the head when bottom of the foot is stroked); due to pressure on pyramidal/motor tracts in cerebrum, found on opposite side of damage
- Brain-stem reflexes are assessed if all other reflexes are absent and brain death is suspected
  - ○ Cough, gag, corneal
  - ○ Oculocephalic reflex assessment, "doll's eyes"
    - – Doll's eyes, assesses cranial nerves 3, 6, and 8
    - – The C-spine is first cleared; the patient's eyes are held open and eye movement is watched as the head is rapidly turned from side to side
    - – Positive: eyes move in the opposite direction of head turn
    - – Positive reflex is good: "it's good to be a doll" (Figure 6-6)

A is normal: eyes reflexively turn opposite of the side the head is turned

TIP

"It's good to be a doll," to have positive doll's eyes. This is normal.

A

B is abnormal: eyes turn to the same side the head is turned

B

C is abnormal: eyes stay midpoint, do not move to either side when head is turned

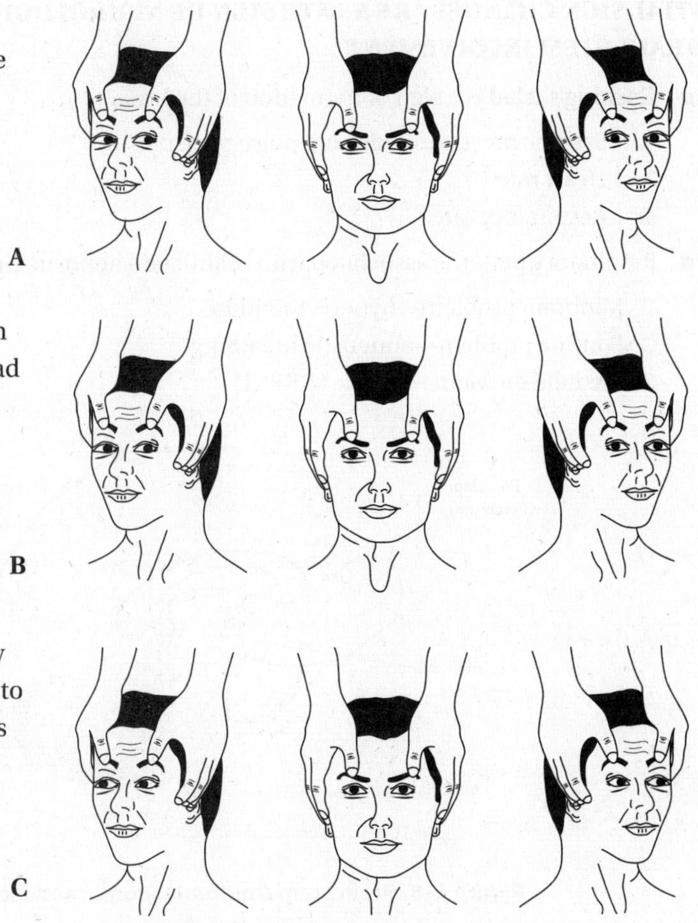

C

Figure 6-6. Assessment of oculocephalic reflex (doll's eyes)

○ Oculovestibular reflex assessment (Figure 6-7)

   – The patient's eyes are held open while ice water is injected slowly into the ear canal and the eye response is observed (cold calorics)

   – Positive: eyes move toward the side of the ice water injection

   – Positive reflex is good

A is normal

B is abnormal

C is abnormal, absent response

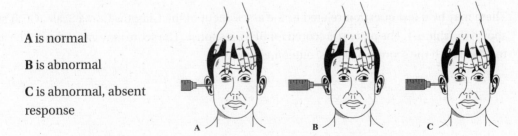

Figure 6-7. Assessment of oculovestibular reflex (cold calorics)

VITAL SIGN CHANGES ARE A LATE SIGN OF NEUROLOGICAL INJURY, BRAIN-STEM INVOLVEMENT

■ **Cushing's triad** is a sign of herniation of the brain:

1. ↑ Systolic pressure, **widening** pulse pressure
2. ↓ Heart rate
3. ↓ Respiratory rate

■ Respiratory patterns associated with brain-stem abnormalities (Figure 6-8)

○ Midbrain problem—hyperventilation
○ Pontine problem—apneustic breathing
○ Medulla problem—ataxic, ARREST!

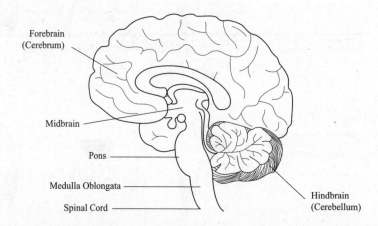

Figure 6-8. Brain stem (midbrain, pons, medulla oblongata)

MISCELLANEOUS ASSESSMENTS

■ Trauma, drainage
■ Meningeal irritation
■ Abnormal ICP waveforms
■ Radiology studies
■ Chemistries, ABGs, urine osmolality
■ Cerebrospinal fluid (CSF) assessment

There **may be a test question** related to the assessment of the Glasgow Coma Scale (GCS) as shown in Table 6-1. The patient is scored for BEST response. The score may vary from 15 (best) to 3 (worst). If the score is 8 or less, outcome is poor.

Table 6-1. Glasgow Coma Scale

Best Eye Opening	Score
Spontaneously	4
To speech	3
To pain	2
No response	1
Best Verbal Response	**Score**
Oriented	5
Confused conversation	4
Inappropriate words	3
Garbled sounds	2
No response	1
Best Motor Response	**Score**
Obeys commands	6
Localizes stimuli	5
Withdrawal from stimulus (normal flexion)	4
Abnormal flexion (decorticate)	3
Abnormal extension (decerebrate)	2
No response	1

Which is worse, obtunded or stuporous? Stuporous—patient cannot speak. Remember, "O" comes before "S", "O" is better!

➤ Obtunded, can speak, mumble words
➤ Stuporous, does not speak, moan, grimace

Homonymous Hemianopsia

■ Homonymous hemianopsia is loss of vision in half the field of each eye (*hemi-* = half, *anopia* = of each field); See Figure 6-9

■ Indicates damage to the **optic nerve** cranial nerve II

■ Occurs opposite the side (contralateral) of the problem, e.g., stroke, tumor

■ Results in neglect of affected side

■ Instruct patient to turn head to the unaffected side

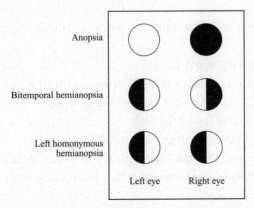

Figure 6-9. Examples of visual field defects

Summary of Neuro Assessment

- Whether the pathology is a tumor, a hematoma, an infarct, or swelling, several general assessment principles apply:
  - Eyes deviate toward the pathology
  - Pupil changes are ipsilateral, same side as pathology
  - Visual changes (homonymous hemianopsia) are contralateral, opposite side of pathology
  - Motor changes are contralateral side of pathology
  - Babinski is contralateral, opposite side of pathology
  - If pathology on both sides, bilateral Babinski

BRAIN HERNIATION

- Brain herniation occurs when swelling within the brain becomes so severe that structures of the brain are squeezed to the point where blood cannot get up into the brain and death may occur.
- Although there are several types of brain herniation, the CCRN test generally focuses on either **uncal or transtentorial (central)** herniation. (Figure 6-10)

1. **Uncal***
2. **Central***
3. Cingulate
4. Transcalvarial
5. Upward
6. Tonsillar

*Most likely to be covered on the CCRN Exam

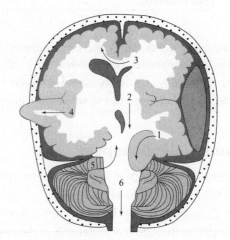

Figure 6-10. Types of brain herniation

Uncal Herniation

- Displacement of temporal lobe (uncus) against the brain stem and 3rd cranial nerve (oculomotor, pupil)
- Lateral shift, **no** initial change in LOC
- Compresses (knocks off) parasympathetic innervation to affected side, blown (dilated) pupil on same side (ipsilateral) seen **before** change in LOC
- Babinski: on opposite side (contralateral)
- Slight weakness, pronator drift to opposite side
- Stupor, coma, posturing, bilateral fixed and dilated pupils, death
- Most often caused by **epidural hematoma** that occurs in temporal area, some strokes

Central Herniation

- Swelling on both sides, downward displacement of hemispheres
- Usually due to diffuse edema, slower development
- Slight change in LOC and then coma
- First both pupils are small (1–3 mm) then parasympathetic innervation on both sides is suppressed and both pupils dilate.
- Babinski bilaterally
- Death
- May be caused by cerebral edema secondary to encephalopathy or stroke

ENCEPHALOPATHY

- Encephalopathy is a nonspecific term for any diffuse disease of the brain that alters brain function or structure.

Etiology

- Hypoxic
- Metabolic
- Hepatic
- Drugs
- Infection

Signs

- Minor to major, can result in swelling, ↑ intracranial pressure (ICP)

  - Loss of memory and cognitive ability
  - Personality changes, agitation
  - Inability to concentrate, lethargy, and progressive loss of consciousness
  - Seizures
  - Coma
  - Brain death

Treatment

- Identify etiology and treat
- Keep patient safe
- Avoid conditions that may increase ICP

Questions on the test related to stroke generally focus on clinical presentation typical of a right-sided or left-sided stroke (Table 6-2).

Table 6-2. Types of Stroke

Embolic, Ischemic	Hemorrhagic
TIA (transient ischemic attack), 24 hrs	Intracerebral
Cerebral infarct	Subarachnoid
	AV malformation

Stroke Assessment

RIGHT BRAIN BLEED, INFARCT

- Eyes deviate toward the pathology—RIGHT
- LEFT sided-muscle weakness, paralysis
- LEFT homonymous hemianopsia
- LEFT Babinski
- Emotional lability

LEFT BRAIN BLEED, INFARCT

- Eyes deviate to the LEFT
- RIGHT-sided weakness, paralysis
- RIGHT homonymous hemianopsia
- RIGHT Babinski
- Aphasia (expressive, receptive, or global) if left hemisphere dominant
- In most people, the dominant internal carotid artery is on the left

Treatment of Acute Ischemic Stroke

NEUROLOGICAL EMERGENCY! "TIME IS BRAIN."

- Rule out hypoglycemia (which may mimic stroke symptoms)
- Assess ABCs
- Assess B/P: Do not treat acutely unless systolic B/P > 220 or diastolic > 120.
    - Sudden decrease in blood pressure will decrease perfusion to an area of the brain that already has lost perfusion, may increase size of ischemic area
- IV, O_2, cardiac monitoring
- Baseline labs
- CT Scan within 25 minutes of arrival (or symptom onset)

DECISION POINT!

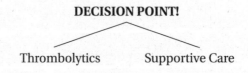

Thrombolytics   Supportive Care

Eligibility Criteria for Use of Tissue Plasminogen Activator (tPA) for Acute Ischemic Stroke

INCLUSION CRITERIA FOR USE OF tPA

- Onset < 4.5 hours
- CT negative
- No contraindications

EXCLUSION CRITERIA FOR USE OF tPA

- Evidence of hemorrhage
- Stroke or head trauma in past 3 months
- Any history of intracranial hemorrhage
- Major surgery in past 14 days
- Active bleeding in past 21 days
- MI in past 3 months
- Seizure at onset of stroke (history of seizure disorder is OK)
- Platelets <100,000/mm^3
- Serum glucose <50 mg/dL
- INR > 1.7 if on warfarin, noncompressible arterial puncture
- Spontaneous clearing of symptoms or only minor (NIH Stroke Score 1) symptoms
- Persistent blood pressure elevation (systolic ≥ 185 mmHg, diastolic ≥ 110 mmHg)

tPA Administration

- Administer tPA 0.9 mg/kg total (maximum 90 mg), with 10% of total dose as bolus

  ○ 75 kg: 0.9 mg × 75 = 67.5 total (or 68)
  ○ Bolus =10% of 68 = 6.8 mg
  ○ Infuse remainder (61.2 mg) over 60 min

> **NOTE**
>
> **Dosing is not usually included on the test.**

- Goal B/P for 1st 24 hours after tPA: systolic < 180 mmHg and diastolic < 105 mmHg (IV labetalol is usually the drug of choice for B/P control for this patient population)

Post-tPA Infusion Care

- Close neuro assessment: what is the worst complication?

  ○ Intracerebral hemorrhage: watch for change in level of consciousness (LOC)

- Close B/P assessment: goal, systolic < 180 mmHg and diastolic < 105 mmHg
- Bleeding precautions
- Supportive care (will probably be left with some neuro deficits although not as severe as if tPA not used)

Pontine Infarct Stroke Characteristics . . . Think "P"!

- **Ap**neustic breathing pattern
- **P**inpoint **p**upils
- **P**arasympathetic innervation (pontene, lose sympathetic innervation)

- Due to trauma, rupture of aneurysm, tumor—5% of all strokes
  - Aneurysm most common, often of the middle cerebral artery (Figure 6-11)
- May develop hydrocephalus due to inability of arachnoid villi to reabsorb CSF
- Usually seen in those 50 to 70 years of age when due to aneurysm, incidence increases with age

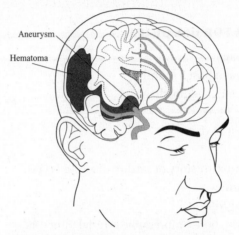

Figure 6-11. Subarachnoid hemorrhage

- The patient's Hunt and Hess grading score (Table 6-3) on presentation with SAH helps predict outcome and immediate treatment.
- The test may provide a clinical scenario and expect you to know the score, or the score may be given and the test will expect you to know the patient's presenting neurological status.
- Note that LOC does not change until the score is III or greater.

Table 6-3. Hunt and Hess grading scale

Grade/Score	Neurologic Status
I	Asymptomatic or mild headache, slight nuchal rigidity
II	Awake, alert, severe headache, stiff neck, cranial nerve palsy*
III	Drowsy or confused, stiff neck, mild focal neuro deficit
IV	Stuporous, moderate or severe hemiparesis, perhaps mild posturing
V	Coma, posturing

*Diplopia, ptosis, dilation

Classic Triad of Symptoms for Aneurysm Rupture

1. Sudden explosive headache
2. Decreased LOC
3. Nuchal rigidity, + Kernig's sign (explained in the meningitis section)
- May have prominent U wave on ECG
- Surgery?

  - Within 48 hours if Grade I, II, III
  - Perhaps delayed if IV or V

Complications of Subarachnoid Hemorrhage (SAH)

- **Hydrocephalus** may develop since the chorionic villi in the subarachnoid space reabsorbs CSF. If chorionic villi are blocked, CSF may not be able to be reabsorbed.
- Rebleed and vasospasm are manifested by change in level of consciousness (Table 6-4).

Table 6-4. Comparison of Rebleed and Vasospasms

Rebleed	Vasospasm
Possible 7 to 10 days after the initial bleed, peak incidence on days 4–8 Greatest cause of death Amicar, an antifibrinolytic agent, prevents rebleed	Incidence 40–60%, symptoms in 20–30% Usually occurs 5–7 days **post-bleed** (not post-op) Diagnosed by transcranial Doppler and/or arteriogram Associated with hyponatremia "Triple H therapy" may be used to prevent vasospasm

- Vasospasm results in brain ischemia, may be a devastating complication (Figure 6-12)

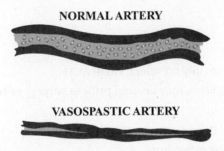

NORMAL ARTERY

VASOSPASTIC ARTERY

Figure 6-12. Comparison of normal and vasospastic artery

TREATMENT OF VASOSPASM

- Transluminal ballooning
- "Triple H therapy": Note that this therapy has recently become controversial. Therefore, it will not likely appear on the test. However, you should review the concept anyway.
  - **Hypervolemia**: crystalloids, colloids to keep CVP 10, PAOP 16–18
  - **Hemodilution**: Fluids to reduce hematocrit to ~ 30%
  - **Hypertension**: Pressors to keep SBP 160–200
    - Effectiveness of "triple H therapy" is now in question. However, **hypotension should definitely be avoided.**
- Prevent vasospasm by providing:
  - Calcium-channel blocker nimodipine (Nimotop), 60 mg every 4 hours, for aneurysmal SAH

ARTERIOVENOUS MALFORMATION (A-V MALFORMATION)

- An A-V malformation is a developmental (congenital) vascular anomaly composed of a tightly tangled mass of dilated vessels that shunt arterial blood into the venous side without the usual connecting capillaries
- Genetic, symptoms usually appear in young adults

Signs and Symptoms

- Hemorrhage—most common (50–70%), usually small AVMs
- Seizures—2nd most common, usually large AVMs
- Other symptoms
  - Headache
  - Progressive neurological deficits
  - Possible hydrocephalus
  - **Neuropsychiatric manifestations**—(less common) due to vascular steal syndrome, diversion of blood causes ischemia to adjacent normal tissues

Treatment

- Surgery is curative.
- Radiation is curative but only for select, small AVMs.
- Embolization is not curative, may be used prior to surgery or radiation to decrease risk of bleeding.
  - Minimally invasive, done via femoral artery
  - Heparin given during procedure

BRAIN TUMORS

- Principles of pathology (right hemisphere, left hemisphere) already discussed apply in terms of symptoms.
- Seizures are an early manifestation.
- Mortality remains high.
- Benign tumors may cause death.
- The one neuro problem that **steroid therapy**, such as decadron, can prevent is elevated ICP.

INCREASED INTRACRANIAL PRESSURE (ICP)

The concept of increased ICP is very likely to be included in the test you take. It is important to remember that there are many causes of increased ICP: medical, surgical, and trauma. Therefore, any patient with a neurological problem may develop signs of increased ICP.

- The first sign of an increase in ICP is **change in level of consciousness (LOC)** since the "higher" centers of the brain show symptoms first and then progress down toward the brain stem.

Intracranial Pressure Overview

- Normal is ~ 0–10 mmHg
- 10–20 mmHg is moderately high
- Increased is > 20 mmHg
- Cerebral perfusion pressure, especially in the presence of elevated ICP, is more important than ICP alone and demonstrates the important relationship between the MAP and ICP
- Cerebral perfusion pressure (CPP) is mean arterial pressure (MAP) minus ICP:

$$CPP = MAP - ICP$$

  - Average CPP is 80–100 mmHg
  - Minimum for perfusion is 50 mmHg
  - Brain death is < 30 mmHg
  - With elevated ICP, maintain CPP ~ 70 mmHg
  - Hypotension in the presence of elevated ICP can be devastating

> **Examples:** Note that with the same ICP, the patient with hypotension has poor brain perfusion, whereas the patient with the higher MAP, even with the ICP of 30 mmHg, has better cerebral perfusion.
>
> | A | B |
> |---|---|
> | MAP = 110 | MAP = 55 |
> | ICP = 30 | ICP = 30 |
> | CPP = 80 | CPP = 25 |

Signs and Symptoms of Increased ICP

- Altered LOC
- Restlessness/agitation
- Headache
- Nausea and vomiting
- Seizures
- Cranial nerve palsies (most commonly III, VI–X)
- Visual dysfunction
- Papilledema
- Pupillary changes
- Motor dysfunction (weakness, flexor and/or extensor posturing, flaccidity)
- Cushing's triad

ICP MONITORING

- ICP monitoring may be done with a fiber-optic catheter or a fluid-filled system.
- Indications include head trauma with GCS 8 or less on presentation and post-op neurosurgery.
- When using the fluid-filled system, the level of the transducer should be at the external auditory meatus, which is at the level of the foramen of Monro.

- In addition to the pressure value, there are 3 types of ICP waves (Figure 6-13):
  ○ C waves
  ○ B waves
  ○ A waves

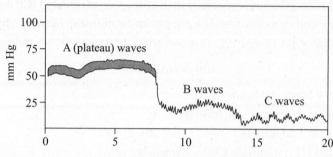

Figure 6-13. ICP waves

Wave Interpretation

- A waves are "awful"
- B waves are "bad"
- C waves are "common"
- In order to be significant, pressure and wave changes need to be sustained over several minutes
- Cerebral vasospasm results in A waves and high ICP

Strategies to Lower ICP

- Decrease volume: mannitol/furosemide/3% saline, patient position (upright to facilitate venous drainage from the brain)
- Prevent dilation of cerebral vessels: prevent acidosis (low pH causes dilation of arteries)
- Reduce cerebrospinal fluid (CSF): ventriculostomy
- Prevent secondary brain injury

  ○ Airway: control pH
  ○ Breathing: prevent hypoxemia
  ○ Circulation: prevent hypotension

- Prevent agitation, pain

  ○ Propofol has been demonstrated to reduce ICP by as much as 15 mmHg

- Why would 0.45 NS or D5W be contraindicated for a patient with ↑ ICP?

  ○ These are hypotonic fluids. Therefore, they would rapidly leave the vascular compartment and go intracellular. In the brain, which already has an increase in ICP, cell "swelling" would exacerbate the problem.
  ○ Use isotonic fluids.

- Should hyperventilation be used to decrease ICP?

  ○ No! Hyperventilation will cause an alkalosis (pH will rise). This will result in cerebral vasoconstriction, which WILL lower ICP. The bad news, however, is that the vasoconstriction also reduces cerebral blood flow.
  ○ Keep pH low normal, ~ 7.35

Summary . . . In the Presence of Elevated ICP

- Avoid:

  o Acidosis—causes vasodilation, ↑ ICP

  o Alkalosis—causes vasoconstriction, ↓ flow to head

  o Hypotonic solution—fluid moves from vasculature into cells

  o Hyperextension, flexion of neck—prevents optimal jugular venous outflow

  o PEEP—↑ thoracic pressure, prevents optimal jugular venous outflow

  o Low protein—↓ serum oncotic pressure, fluid displaced from vasculature into intracellular space; Feed!!

  o Restraints—↑ agitation

  o Agitation, noxious stimuli—↑ ICP

  o Fever—cerebral hypermetabolism, ↑ ICP

These may all contribute to elevated ICP.

TRAUMATIC BRAIN INJURY (TBI)

Overview

- **Traumatic brain injury (TBI)** is a blunt (closed) or penetrating insult to the brain from an external mechanical force.

  o Causes primary brain injury and potential secondary brain injury

  o Results in temporary or permanent impairments of cognitive, physical, and psychosocial function.

- Etiologies of TBI: **falls** (40%); **blunt trauma** (16%); **motor vehicle accidents** (14%); **assaults** (11%); **unknown/other** (19%)

- Severity according to GCS within 1st 48 hours

  o Severe TBI   3–8

  o Moderate TBI   9–12

  o Mild TBI   13–15

- Types of TBI

  o Diffuse: concussion, diffuse axonal injury (DAI)

  o Focal: contusions, intracranial hematomas, skull fractures, open head injuries

- CT of head is diagnostic test of choice

Intracranial Hematomas, Hemorrhage

Hematomas may develop above the dura (epidural, Figure 6-14), below the dura (subdural, Figure 6-15), and within the brain tissue itself (intracerebral). Usually at least one question on the CCRN test is about intracranial hematomas.

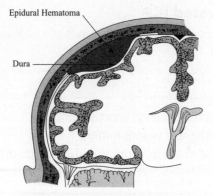

Figure 6-14. Epidural hematoma

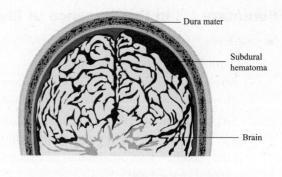

Figure 6-15. Subdural hematoma

☆ Epidural Hematoma

- Usually due to meningeal artery bleed secondary to temporal bone trauma with bleeding between skull and dura (Figure 6-16)
- **Rapidly** developing symptoms
- More common in younger population, not common in elderly
- 20–30% of all intracerebral hematomas

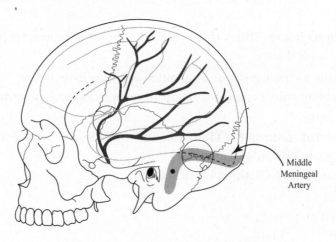

Figure 6-16. Middle meningeal artery

NOTE

What type of herniation results from an epidural hematoma? Uncal!

CLINICAL PRESENTATION

- Headache
- Irritability—confusion
- Vomiting
- Ipsilateral pupil dilation, often BEFORE decreased LOC
- Contralateral hemiparesis/hemiplegia
- Decreasing LOC

TREATMENT

- Emergent surgery to evacuate hematoma (burr hole)
- Monitor and treat increasing ICP

Subdural Hematoma

- May occur due to trauma or spontaneously with bleeding between dura and arachnoid membrane
- More prevalent in elderly or alcoholics (falls)
- 50–70% of all intracerebral hematomas
- Unlike an epidural hematoma, which is always acute, subdural hematoma may be:
  - Acute (within 24 hours)
  - Subacute (within 2 weeks)
  - Chronic (> 2 weeks)

CLINICAL PRESENTATION

- Similar to epidural hematoma, although less vomiting and pupil change does not usually preceed change in LOC
- May develop more slowly

TREATMENT

- Close neuro assessment for signs of increased ICP
- Surgery to evacuate hematoma

Intracerebral Hematoma

- May be due to a gunshot wound, severe acceleration-deceleration injury, or laceration of brain from depressed skull fracture
- May be non-traumatic (stroke)
- 2–20% of all hematomas

CLINICAL PRESENTATION

- Varies greatly due to area of brain involved
- May or may not have increased ICP

TREATMENT

- Surgery if large and neuro status is deteriorating

SKULL FRACTURE

Types of Skull Fracture (Figure 6-17)

- Linear does not require surgery
- Open, depressed:
  - Most surgeons prefer to elevate depressed skull fractures if the depressed segment is **greater than 5 mm** below the inner table of adjacent bone
  - Indications for immediate elevation are gross contamination, dural tear with pneumocephalus, and an underlying hematoma
  - Comminuted is fracture with bone fragmentation, usually depressed

☆ Basilar is linear fracture that occurs in the floor of the cranial vault (skull base), results in **meningeal tear**

- ○ Most likely to be covered on the test
- ○ Requires more force to cause than other areas of the neurocranium
- ○ Rare, occurs in approximately 4% of severe head injury patients

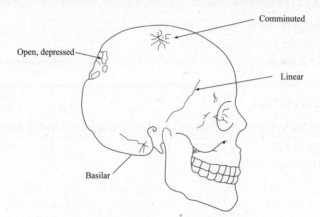

Figure 6-17. Types of skull fractures

Signs, Symptoms of Basilar Skull Fracture

- Raccoon eyes (Figure 6-18)
- Battle's sign, discoloration at back of ear (Figure 6-19)
- Otorrhea, fluid from ear, due to meningeal tear (Figure 6-19)
- Rhinorrhea, due to meningeal tear (Figure 6-18)

  - ○ No nose blowing!

- Lose cranial nerve 1, no sense of smell (may be temporary or permanent)

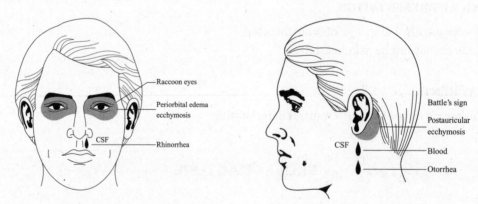

Figure 6-18. Raccoon eyes, rhinorrhea   **Figure 6-19.** Battle's sign, otorrhea

Nursing Implications

- Determine whether ear or nose drainage is spinal fluid:

  - ○ Check for sugar; if positive, it is spinal fluid
  - ○ Put drainage on a 4 × 4

    - – If spinal fluid, will see a clot surrounded by a **yellow** halo, **"halo sign"**

- Cover ear or nose with dry sterile gauze, do not pack in

Treatment

- Don't block CSF drainage
- Surgical repair ONLY if CSF leakage is persistent
- Risk of meningitis, monitor for infection; antibiotics ONLY if sign of infection
- Do not insert a nasogastric tube, may displace up to brain, reason not quite clear, use orogastric tube

SEIZURES

Overview

- Most general tonic-clonic seizures are self-limiting, last less than 3 minutes
- Normal ventilation does not occur during tonic-clonic seizure, therefore the $PaCO_2$ may be elevated immediately post-seizure
- Protect airway, turn to side
- Maintain patient safety
- Stop seizure
  - Lorazepam (Ativan): 0.05–0.15 mg/kg at 1 mg/min, max ~ 8 mg or
  - Diazepam (Valium): 0.25 mg/kg at 2–5 mg/min, max ~ 30 mg
- Prevent seizure
  - Phenytoin (Dilantin): 15–20 mg/kg at 50 mg/min, max 1 gram
  - Phenobarbital: 5 mg/kg at 50 mg/min
- Seizure may be followed by a postictal period with transient signs of decreased LOC
- What if Dilantin level is therapeutic and patient seizes?
  - Give Lorazepam!
- How are benzodiazepines reversed?
  - Romazicon! Romazicon has a shorter half-life than some benzodiazepines, therefore sedation effects may recur.
- After a generalized tonic-clonic seizure, the patient may experience a postictal state of decreased level of consciousness.

NOTE

Dosages are not usually covered on the test.

Status Epilepticus (Table 6-5)

- Seizure activity of 5 minutes (time revised from 30 minutes) or more caused by a single seizure or a series of seizures with no return of consciousness between seizures
- Not responsive to usual therapy
- Causes
  - Withdrawal from anticonvulsant meds
  - Acute alcohol withdrawal
  - Toxic levels of drugs
  - CNS infections
  - Brain tumors/CNS trauma
  - Metabolic disorders—hypoglycemia, hepatic failure, hyponatremia, hypocalcemia, hypomagnesemia
  - Stroke

☆ Table 6-5. Pathophysiology of Status Epilepticus

Early	Late (30 minutes)
↑ Cerebral blood flow	Cerebral blood flow unable to meet
Tachycardia, hypertension	demands
$PaCO_2$ ↑, PaO_2 ↓	Arrhythmias (hyperkalemia)
↑ Glucose (stress response)	Hypoglycemia
↑ K^+ (destruction of skeletal muscle cells)	↑ ↑ K^+ and CKs
	Rhabdomyolysis (extremely high CKs)
	Ventricular fibrillation

☆ Death is due to **cerebral hypermetabolism.**

MENINGITIS

Cerebrospinal Fluid (CSF) Overview

- CSF produced in choroid plexus (4th ventricle), absorbed by arachnoid villi
- Normal glucose is 60% of serum glucose
- Normal protein is 20–45 mg/dL protein
- Normal LP pressure is 80–180 cm H_2O

For the test, you will need to know signs of meningeal irritation and the difference between bacterial and viral meningitis (Table 6-6).

Table 6-6. The Difference Between Bacterial and Viral Meningitis

Bacterial Meningitis	Viral Meningitis
↑↑ Protein	↑ Protein
↓ Glucose	Normal glucose (60% of serum glucose)
↑↑ WBCs	↑ WBCs
Purulent CSF	Clear CSF
Opening pressure >180 cm H_2O (measurement done with lumbar puncture)	Opening pressure (lumbar puncture) often normal

Both bacterial and viral have one or more signs of meningeal irritation:

Headache + nuchal rigidity + Brudzinsky sign + Kernig's sign

Nuchal rigidity

- Flex head to chest, pain and stiffness

Brudzinski's sign (Figure 6-20A)

- Chin to chest, legs come up

Kernig's Sign (Figure 6-20B)

- Legs up and out, pain in neck and leg

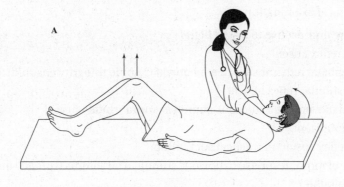

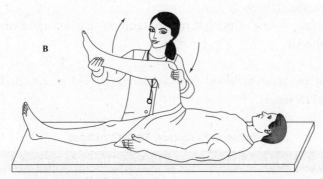

Figure 6-20. Brudzinski's (A) and Kernig's (B) signs

Treatment: Antibiotics for bacterial meningitis

The following topics (brain death, Guillain-Barré syndrome, myasthenia gravis, and muscular dystrophy) are included in the neuro test blueprint but are less likely than the previous information to be included on the test.

BRAIN DEATH

Brain death is the complete, irreversible cessation of function of the cerebrum, cerebellum, and brain stem.

Determination of Brain Death

- First, confirm the following
  - ○ Coma is irreversible and cause known
  - ○ Neuro-imaging explains coma
  - ○ CNS depressant drug effect absent (if indicated toxicology screen)
  - ○ No evidence of residual paralytics (electrical stimulation if paralytics used)
  - ○ Absence of severe acid-base, electrolyte, endocrine abnormality
  - ○ Normothermia or mild hypothermia (core temperature 36°C)
  - ○ Systolic blood pressure 100 mm Hg or greater
  - ○ No spontaneous respirations

- Perform clinical examination
  - Pupils are nonreactive to bright light
  - Corneal reflex absent
  - Oculocephalic reflex absent (tested only if C-spine integrity ensured)
  - Oculovestibular reflex absent
  - No facial movement to noxious stimuli at supraorbital nerve
  - Gag reflex absent
  - Cough reflex absent to tracheal suctioning
  - Absence of motor response to noxious stimuli in all 4 limbs (spinally mediated reflexes are permissible)
- Perform apnea test (Table 6-7)
- Perform confirmatory tests (optional, may be required at institutions where "whole brain" criteria are applied)
  - EEG
  - Absence of intracranial blood flow as demonstrated by cerebral angiography or transcranial Doppler

Table 6-7. Apnea Test Protocol

Apnea Test Prerequisites	When to Terminate Test Early
Core temp > 36.5°C	Spontaneous respiratory movements noted
SBP > 90 mmHg	SBP < 90
$PaCO_2$ > 35	SpO_2 falls below 85%
Absence of drugs to cause respiratory depression	Unstable cardiac arrhythmias occur
Preoxygenation prior to ventilator; disconnection for 20 minutes at 100%	
PaO_2 may be normal or supranormal after preoxygenation period	

☆ After 8–12 minutes, do an ABG, reconnect the ventilator, and interpret the test results.

Interpretation of Apnea Test Results

Apnea Test **Positive**—Supports Brain Death

- Absent respiratory movements
- $PaCO_2 \geq 60$ mmHg or $PaCO_2 \geq 20$ mmHg over baseline

Apnea Test **Negative**—Does Not Support Brain Death

- Respiratory movements observed

Apnea Test **Indeterminate**

- Test terminated prior to achieving a $PaCO_2 \geq 60$ mmHg or 20 mmHg above baseline
- $PaCO_2$ is < 60 mmHg or < 20 mmHg over baseline

GUILLAIN-BARRÉ SYNDROME (GBS)

Etiology

- Viral agent (parainfluenza 2, measles, mumps, herpes zoster) 50% of the cases
- Recent vaccination (flu shot) 15% of cases
- Recent surgical procedure 5% of cases
    - Demyelination of lower motor neurons affects spinal and cranial nerves
    - **Ascending** paralysis, usually symmetrical, return occurs proximally; diaphragmatic involvement may result in ventilatory failure
    - Protein in CSF
    - No alteration in consciousness

Treatment

- Monitor:
    - Vital capacity for impending respiratory failure
    - Urine OP for urinary retention
- Intubation, mechanical ventilation for respiratory failure
- Corticosteroids
- Intravenous immunoglobulin instead of plasma exchange
- Plasmapheresis exchange—complete exchange of plasma with the removal of abnormal circulating antibodies that affect the myelin sheaths; removal of these antibodies will lessen the severity and duration of GBS

MYASTHENIA GRAVIS: "GRAVE MUSCULAR WEAKNESS"

- Myasthenia gravis is an autoimmune attack of neuromuscular junction
- Clinical presentation
    - Progressive skeletal muscle weakness
    - Early: easily fatigued
    - Later: paralysis
    - 70% have ocular dysfunction
        - Ptosis, diplopia, difficulty keeping eye closed
    - Dysarthria, dysphagia
- Myasthenia Gravis Crisis
    - Treatment of myasthenia crisis depends on which of the 2 types of crises the patient is experiencing (Table 6-8).

Table 6-8. Myasthenic vs. Cholinergic Crisis in Myasthenia Gravis

Myasthenic Crisis	Cholinergic Crisis
Due to undiagnosed/under-treatment or acute exacerbation Deficiency of acetylcholine (an excitatory neurotransmitter)	Due to overtreatment Excess of acetylcholine

How are the 2 crises differentiated? The patient is given the "tensilon test" (Table 6-9).

Table 6-9. Tensilon Test

Myasthenic Crisis	Cholinergic Crisis
Tensilon 2 mg IV ↓ Clinical improvement	Tensilon 2 mg IV ↓ Increased muscle weakness ↓ SLUDGE • Salivation • Lacrimation • Urination • Defecation • Gastrointestinal distress • Emesis

During the administration of the tensilon, the patient is asked to hold arms out (Figure 6-21) in order to detect weakness.

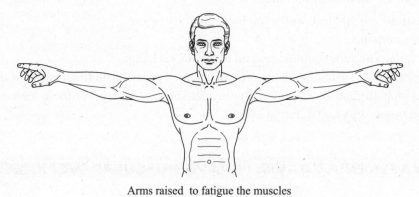

Arms raised to fatigue the muscles

Figure 6-21. Tensilon administration

Treatment

- Pyridostigmine (Mestinon, cholinesterase inhibitor); it prevents cholinesterase from breaking down acetylcholine
- Corticosteroids, immunosuppressants
- Removal of the thymus gland
- Plasmapheresis
- IV immune globulin

MUSCULAR DYSTROPHY

- The muscular dystrophies are an inherited group of progressive myopathic disorders resulting from defects in a number of genes required for normal muscle function (Table 6-10)
- Causes progressive muscle weakness (myopathy) and atrophy (loss of muscle mass) due to defects in one or more genes required for normal muscle function
- Most often, weakness starts near the trunk and spreads to the extremities, affecting the legs before the arms
  - Duchenne
  - Becker
  - Other

Table 6-10. Comparison of Duchenne and Becker Muscular Dystrophy

Duchenne Muscular Dystrophy (DMD)	Becker Muscular Dystrophy
Onset very young, wheelchair-bound by 12 years of age Most patients with DMD die in their late teens or twenties as a result of respiratory infections or cardiomyopathy	Onset is usually later and symptoms are usually milder than DMD Children can usually walk until they are approximately 15 years old, with some people continuing to walk as adults Usually survive into their mid-40s. The most common cause of death is heart failure from cardiomyopathy

Treatment

- Steroids
- Pneumococcal, influenza vaccines
- Monitor heart function
  - ACEI/beta blockers
- Baseline pulmonary function tests
- Nocturnal ventilatory support
- Caution with anesthesia/sedation
  - More prone to malignant hyperthermia

Now that you have reviewed key neurology concepts, go to the Neurology Practice Questions. Answer the questions, and then check your answers. Continue to review the information until you get at least 80% on the practice questions.

NEUROLOGY PRACTICE QUESTIONS

1. Which of the following about pupillary response is TRUE?

    (A) Pupil change is the first sign of an increase in intracranial pressure.
    (B) Sympathetic stimulation produces dilation of the pupil.
    (C) The optic nerve is responsible for pupil size.
    (D) Bilateral dilatation of the pupil is an early sign of increased intracranial pressure.

2. Consciousness is dependent upon an intact

    (A) reticular activating system (RAS) and cerebral cortex.
    (B) occipital lobe and midbrain.
    (C) medulla and meningeal artery.
    (D) cerebellum and pons.

3. A patient presented with a **left** cerebral hemispheric ischemic stroke. The patient would most likely have which of the following?

    (A) left Babinski reflex
    (B) eye deviation to the right
    (C) left homonymous hemianopsia
    (D) right pronator drift

4. Which of the following interventions would the nurse consider to be inappropriate for the patient with increased ICP?

    (A) maintaining the $PaCO_2$ level at ~ 35 mmHg
    (B) feeding the patient via a feeding tube
    (C) log roll when turning the patient
    (D) administering 5% dextrose/water at 83 mL an hour

5. A patient has a history of a fall while skiing, hitting the right side of his head. He presented with a nose fracture, developed a sudden episode of emesis, and dilated right pupil, followed by a decrease in level of consciousness. Which of the following should the nurse anticipate?

    (A) emergent lumbar puncture to assess pressure
    (B) emergent surgery for septal deviation
    (C) emergent treatment for uncal herniation
    (D) emergent treatment for subdural hematoma

6. Examination of the CSF in bacterial meningitis will reveal all EXCEPT which of the following?

    (A) cloudiness
    (B) decreased glucose
    (C) decreased protein
    (D) increased pressure

7. Five days after a subarachnoid hemorrhage, the patient experienced a decrease in level of consciousness. The CT scan is negative for rebleed. The patient will most likely benefit from:

(A) return to the operating room.
(B) aggressive fluid administration.
(C) aminocaproic acid (Amicar).
(D) osmotic diuretic, e.g., mannitol.

8. A 71-year-old female presented with a possible stroke, responsive to verbal stimuli, blood pressure 180/110, pupils equal and reactive. Her level of consciousness suddenly decreases. Upon examination of her eyes, you note the left pupil is large and nonreactive to light. Blood pressure is 192/114, blood glucose level is 90 mg/dL. Based on the information above, what has likely occurred?

(A) Second cranial nerve (optic) compression.
(B) The patient is having a hypoglycemic reaction.
(C) Increasing MAP (mean arterial pressure) has decreased cerebral perfusion pressure.
(D) Increasing ICP has compressed the third (oculomotor) cranial nerve.

9. A 32 year old is admitted with raccoon eyes. You notice clear fluid draining from his nose. The most appropriate intervention would be to:

(A) tape rolled sterile gauze under the nose.
(B) insert a nasogastric tube to prevent vomiting.
(C) suction the nasopharynx as needed.
(D) insert nasal packing until the physician arrives.

10. A patient presented with a scalp laceration and a 6 mm depressed skull fracture, no neuro changes. Which of the following is true regarding the care of this patient?

(A) The patient should be held for observation for 24 hours before being discharged.
(B) The patient may be discharged with instructions to return in 48 hours.
(C) The patient needs a prescription for antibiotic therapy.
(D) The patient needs immediate surgery.

11. A 53-year-old woman presents with complaints of "the worse headache I have ever had." She is said to have a Grade I aneurysm. Which of the following describes a Grade I aneurysm?

(A) minimal headache, no neurological deficits
(B) mild to severe headache, minimal neurological deficits
(C) stuporous, mild to severe hemiparesis
(D) comatose, decerebrate posturing

12. Which of the following is TRUE of brain tumors?

    (A) Benign tumors do not cause death.
    (B) Steroids are contraindicated.
    (C) Seizures are often an early symptom.
    (D) Mortality has been dramatically reduced.

13. The nurse suspects brain death for the patient 3 days after admission with hepatic encephalopathy. Which of the following is most definitive of brain death?

    (A) coma
    (B) absent corneal, cough, gag reflexes
    (C) positive Babinski
    (D) posturing

14. Increased intracranial pressure may be caused by many disorders—ischemic or hemorrhagic stroke, traumatic brain injury, hypoxic encephalopathy, intracranial hematoma, tumor, infection, among others. Which of the following would most likely prevent a further increase in intracranial pressure or decreased cerebral perfusion?

    (A) maintain $PaCO_2$ 25 mmHg to 35 mmHg
    (B) maintain neck flexion
    (C) prevent/treat agitation/pain
    (D) keep head of bed flat

15. Priority interventions for a patient with a generalized tonic-clonic seizure with a normal serum phenytoin level include:

    (A) turn patient to side, administer phenytoin (Dilantin).
    (B) monitor seizure duration, assess level of consciousness.
    (C) monitor seizure duration, insert a bite block.
    (D) turn patient to side, administer lorazepam (Ativan).

16. Your patient has had a right hemispheric stroke. Which of the following clinical presentations is most typical for this patient?

    (A) eyes deviate right, left homonymous hemianopsia, left-sided weakness, right pupil dilation
    (B) eyes deviate right, right homonymous hemianopsia, left-sided weakness, right pupil dilation
    (C) eyes deviate left, left homonymous hemianopsia, right-sided weakness, left pupil dilation
    (D) eyes deviate left, right homonymous hemianopsia, right-sided weakness, left pupil dilation

17. The patient has been diagnosed with Guillain-Barré and is anxiously asking numerous questions. Which of the following would be CORRECT regarding this diagnosis?

   (A) Coma will be prevented with plasmapheresis.
   (B) Weakness will occur on one side of the body.
   (C) It was most likely caused by a recent bacterial infection.
   (D) Lung vital capacity will be closely monitored.

18. Which of the following patients would most likely require neurosurgery?

   (A) patient with metabolic encephalopathy
   (B) patient with subdural hematoma
   (C) patient with meningitis
   (D) patient with basilar skull fracture

ANSWER KEY

1. **B**	4. **D**	7. **B**	10. **D**	13. **B**	16. **A**
2. **A**	5. **C**	8. **D**	11. **A**	14. **C**	17. **D**
3. **D**	6. **C**	9. **A**	12. **C**	15. **D**	18. **B**

ANSWERS EXPLAINED

1. **(B)** The reason an increase in ICP will eventually cause pupil dilation is that compression of the oculomotor nerve (on the side of the injury or pathology) decreases parasympathetic stimulation, which allows sympathetic stimulation to predominate, resulting in pupil dilation. Pupil changes occur AFTER a change in level of consciousness (except for uncal herniation). The optic nerve is responsible for vision. Bilateral pupil dilation is a late (not early) sign of an increase in ICP.

2. **(A)** The lower end of the reticular activating system is in the brain stem and is responsible for sleep-wake cycles. If damaged, coma will occur. The cerebral cortex is also responsible for consciousness. Choices (B), (C), and (D) are responsible for functions other than consciousness.

3. **(D)** Reflex, motor, and vision changes are contralateral to the injury or pathology. Eyes deviate toward the side of injury. A pronator drift is a subtle, early sign of motor weakness.

4. **(D)** 5% dextrose/water is a hypotonic solution that will easily leave the vascular space. By osmosis, the solution will displace to the intracellular space, resulting in cell swelling (including brain cell swelling) and an increase in ICP. The other choices are all appropriate for the patient with increased ICP and will not make the ICP worse.

5. **(C)** The patient has signs of an epidural hematoma, most likely to the right temporal area and possible uncal herniation. This is one neurological problem that causes pupil dilation BEFORE sustained change in level of consciousness.

6. **(C)** Protein is increased in bacterial meningitis, not decreased. Cloudiness, decreased glucose, and increased pressure—choices (A), (B), and (D), respectively—are all typical of bacterial meningitis.

7. **(B)** The 2 major complications of subarachnoid hemorrhage are rebleed and vasospasm. In this case, rebleed was ruled out. This patient most likely has vasospasm and aggressive fluid administration is indicated. Choice (A) does not help vasospasm. Choice (C) may be indicated for a rebleed. A diuretic—choice (D)—will decrease vascular volume and may worsen vasospasm.

8. **(D)** Left pupil dilation is a sign of cranial nerve III, oculomotor compression on the side of the pathology due to an increase in ICP. Choice (A), optic nerve compression, affects vision. Choice (B), hypoglycemic reaction, would not result in pupil dilation. Choice (C), an increase in MAP, would increase the cerebral perfusion pressure (CPP), not decrease CPP.

9. **(A)** The patient most likely has a basilar skull fracture that causes a meningeal tear with potential for CSF drainage from the nose (or ear). The CSF should be allowed to drain. Choices (B), (C), and (D) may be harmful.

10. **(D)** With a skull depression of 6 mm, the patient will require surgery to elevate the skull from brain tissue. The other 3 choices will not prevent the potential complications that might occur.

11. **(A)** The patient has signs of a subarachnoid hemorrhage secondary to an aneurysm. Hunt and Hess grading of a Grade I is choice (A). Choice (B) is a Grade II. Choice (C) is a Grade IV. Choice (D) is a Grade V. This patient's prognosis, according to the Hunt and Hess score, is good.

12. **(C)** Seizures are often an early symptom. The other 3 choices are NOT truly related to brain tumors.

13. **(B)** Cough, gag (cranial nerve IX) and corneal (cranial nerve V) are brain-stem reflexes and absence reflects loss of brain-stem activity, all present in brain death. While coma is present in brain death, it represents loss of function of the reticular activating system, which is higher than the brain stem. Babinsky reflex and posturing are not present in brain death.

14. **(C)** When an increase in ICP is suspected, it is important to prevent anything that may worsen the ICP. Agitation and/or pain will further increase ICP. The other 3 choices are not indicated when an increase in ICP is suspected or known. Choice (A), hyperventilation, may decrease ICP by causing an alkalosis and cerebral constriction. However, it will decrease cerebral perfusion. Choice (B) will prevent venous drainage from the head. Choice (D) will not optimize venous drainage from the head.

15. **(D)** Turning the patient helps to protect the airway and prevent pulmonary aspiration. Lorazepam will help stop the current seizure. Choice (A), which includes administration of phenytoin, is not an immediate priority. However, it will be given to prevent future seizure activity after the current seizure is controlled. Choice (B), monitor seizure duration, is correct. However, assessment of level of consciousness is not possible during a generalized tonic-clonic seizure. Choice (C) is not correct because an attempt

to insert a bite block may cause more problems by displacing the tongue back and occluding the airway.

16. **(A)** Eyes deviate to the side of the pathology. Visual and motor problems occur opposite the side of pathology. Pupil change occurs on the side of pathology. The other 3 choices are not completely accurate.

17. **(D)** The patient with Guillain-Barré develops ascending, bilateral weakness/paralysis that may affect the main muscle of ventilation, the diaphragm. Therefore, vital capacity is monitored regularly in order to identify impending respiratory failure. Choice (A) is not correct since coma is not typical of Guillain-Barré. Choice (B) is not correct because weakness is bilateral, not unilateral. Choice (C) is not correct because bacterial infection does not usually lead to Guillain-Barré. Instead, viral infections have been associated with the problem.

18. **(B)** A subdural hematoma requires evacuation unless it is very small without clinical signs. Metabolic encephalopathy, meningitis, and basilar skull fracture are all managed medically, not surgically.

Multisystem Concepts

7

By failing to prepare, you are preparing to fail.

—Benjamin Franklin

NOTE

Hypovolemic shock is included in the cardiovascular blueprint but is covered in this section with multisystem problems.

MULTISYSTEM TEST BLUEPRINT

Multisystem 8% of total test   **12 Questions**

→ Asphyxia
→ Distributive shock (e.g., anaphylaxis)
→ Multi-organ dysfunction syndrome (MODs)
→ Multisystem trauma
→ Sepsis/septic shock
→ Systemic inflammatory response syndrome (SIRS)
→ Toxic ingestions/inhalations (e.g., drug/alcohol overdose)
→ Toxin/drug exposure

MULTISYSTEM TESTABLE NURSING ACTIONS

☐ Recognize and monitor normal and abnormal diagnostic test results (e.g., lab, radiology)

☐ Recognize indications for and manage patients undergoing:

  ○ Continuous sedation
  ○ Procedural sedation
  ○ Therapeutic hypothermia

☐ Assess patient's pain

☐ Manage patients receiving:

  ○ Medications (e.g., pain medications, reversal agents) and monitor response
  ○ Nonpharmacological methods for pain relief and monitor response

☐ Recognize signs and symptoms of multisystem emergencies (e.g., shock states, trauma), initiate interventions, and seek assistance as needed

As you can see from the CCRN test blueprint, multisystem includes 12 questions. Therefore plan on studying this content for approximately 12 hours before taking the final practice test.

Overview

- Although blood pressure (hypotension) is generally thought of when discussing shock (Figure 7-1), shock is actually a **cellular disease** due to either inadequate perfusion (oxygen demand is greater than oxygen delivered) or the inability of cells to utilize the delivered oxygen (oxygen utilization, consumption).

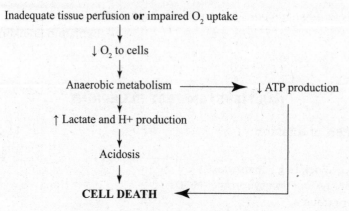

Figure 7-1. Pathophysiology of shock

- There are 3 phases of all types of shock

  1. Compensatory
  2. Progressive
  3. Refractory

- The rapidity with which the patient progresses through these stages varies depending on many factors.

- During the **compensatory phase** of shock (Figures 7-2 and 7-3), the blood pressure (B/P) is maintained due to 2 mechanisms, stimulation of the sympathetic nervous system and activation of the renin-angiotensin-aldosterone system (RAAS).

Sympathetic Nervous System Activation

Decrease in cardiac output/circulating volume or increased oxygen utilization

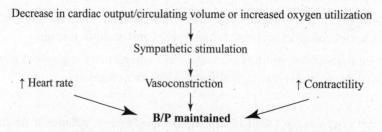

Figure 7-2. Physiology of compensatory phase of shock

Renin-Angiotensin-Aldosterone System (RAAS)

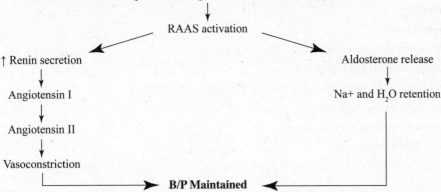

Figure 7-3. Physiology of compensatory phase of shock

Clinical Signs/Symptoms of Shock Phases

COMPENSATORY PHASE OF SHOCK (BLOOD PRESSURE MAINTAINED)

- Tachycardia
- Tachypnea, respiratory alkalosis
- Normal PaO_2
- Oliguria
- Skin pale, cool (except in early sepsis)
- Restlessness, anxiety
- Complaints of thirst
- **B/P maintained!**

PROGRESSIVE PHASE OF SHOCK (COMPENSATORY MECHANISMS FAILING)

- **Hypotension**
- Worsening tachycardia, tachypnea, oliguria
- Metabolic acidosis
- Decreased PaO_2
- Clammy, mottled skin
- Further change in LOC
- May complain of nausea

REFRACTORY PHASE OF SHOCK

- Not responsive to interventions
- Severe systemic hypoperfusion, **multisystem organ dysfunction**
- May survive shock, die from failure of one or more organs
  - Pulmonary (ARDS)
  - Kidney (acute tubular necrosis)
  - Heart (failure, ischemia)
  - Hematologic (disseminated intravascular coagulation)
  - Neurological (encephalopathy, stroke)
  - Liver (failure)

Types of Shock

- Hypovolemic
- Septic
- Anaphylactic
- Cardiogenic (covered in cardiac section)
- Neurogenic (not covered on test)
- Obstructive (covered in cardiac and pulmonary sections)
  - Tension pneumothorax
  - Massive pulmonary embolism
  - Cardiac tamponade

HYPOVOLEMIC SHOCK

- Critical reduction in the circulating intravascular volume leading to inadequate tissue perfusion
- Most common type of shock
  - Internal causes—third spacing, pooling in intravascular compartments
  - External causes—hemorrhage, GI or renal losses, burns, excessive diaphoresis
- Hypovolemia effects on pulse pressure:
  - Systolic decreases, diastolic maintains or elevates, NARROW pulse pressure
  - Example:
    - Baseline 130/80
    - Volume loss → 110/80, 100/80, 90/70
- Hemodynamics
  - ↓ B/P
  - ↓ Pulse pressure
  - ↓ Right atrial pressure (CVP)
  - ↓ Cardiac output, O_2 delivery
  - ↓ Left atrial (PAOP)
  - ↓ SvO_2
  - ↑ Systemic vascular resistance

Everything is decreased except SVR.

Treatment of Hypovolemic Shock

- Identify etiology and correct if possible
- Replace volume appropriately, "Fill up the tank!"
  - Rapid and vigorous volume loading
  - Requires at least 2 large bore IV sites (hemorrhagic), central line is not necessary but may assist fluid replacement
  - Use fluid warmer if > 2,000 mL in 1 hour (ALL fluids for trauma patients)
- Hemorrhagic vs. nonhemorrhagic
- Fluid resuscitation: goal is to maintain O_2 delivery (DO) and O_2 uptake (VO_2) into tissue and sustain aerobic metabolism

- Fluid resuscitate to clinical targets, e.g., decreased tachycardia, increased urine output
  - Use isotonic fluid, 0.9 normal saline or lactated Ringer's
  - Which is better? There are advantages and disadvantages to each (Table 7-1).

Table 7-1. Comparison of Normal Saline and Lactated Ringer's

Normal Saline	Lactated Ringer's
Isotonic crystalloid, effects last approximately 40 minutes, then leaves vascular space	Isotonic crystalloid, effects last approximately 40 minutes, then leaves vascular space
Disadvantage—large volumes may lead to hyperchloremic acidosis	Best mimics extracellular fluid (ECF) minus proteins, recommended resuscitation fluid by the ACS Committee on Trauma
Do not give to those with hypernatremia or renal failure	Has potential to correct lactic acidosis; yet in severe hypoperfusion, may promote lactic acidosis due to lactate accumulation
• Has 154 mmols Na^+, 154 of Cl^-, **NO** K^+, Ca^{++}, or lactate	Do not give to those who should not receive K^+ or lactate or through blood line
	• Has 130 mmols of Na^+; 109 Cl^-; 4 K^+; 2.7 Ca^{++}; 28 lactate

- Resuscitation end points
  - MAP ≥ 65 mmHg
  - CVP ~ 6 mmHg (not well defined)
  - Urine OP 0.5 mL/kg/hr
  - Heart rate decreased
  - Hgb > 7.0 g/dL and coagulation/platelet abnormalities corrected
    - Hemoglobin and hematocrit measurements are not accurate during active blood loss

NOTE

NO PRESSORS for hypovolemic shock! The SVR is already high due to compensatory mechanisms.

Hemorrhagic Shock

The severity of hemorrhagic shock is categorized into 4 classes (Table 7-2).

Table 7-2. Classification of Hemorrhagic Shock

	Class I	Class II	Class III	Class IV
Blood loss (mL)	Up to 750	750–1,500	1,500–2,000	> 2,000
Blood loss (% blood vol)	Up to 15%	15–30%	30–40%	> 40%
Heart rate	< 100	>100	>120	>140
Blood pressure	Normal	Normal	Decreased*	Decreased
Pulse pressure	Normal or ↓	Decreased	Decreased	Decreased
Capillary refill	Normal	Decreased	Decreased	Decreased
Respiratory rate	14–20	20–30	30–40	>35
Urine output (mL/hr)	>30	20–30	5–15	Scant
Mental status	Slightly anxious	Mildly anxious	Anxious, confused	Confused, lethargic

*Note that the blood pressure does not decrease in hemorrhagic shock until Class III, loss of 1,500–2,000 mL blood.

- Class I: treat with crystalloids
- Class II: treat with crystalloids
- Class III: treat with crystalloids + blood
- Class IV: treat with crystalloids + blood

Treatment of Hemorrhagic (Hypovolemic) Shock

- STOP the bleeding
- Blood transfusion

  - Optimal threshold remains controversial
  - 7.0 g/dL Hgb is fairly well established in the critically ill
  - Goal may be higher in the presence of

    - Active bleeding
    - Severe hypoxemia
    - Myocardial ischemia
    - Lactic acidosis

- Packed red blood cells (PRBCs), unlike whole blood, do not have plasma or platelets; therefore, the patient will need replacement of the coagulation components of blood with transfusion of multiple units of PRBCs

  - Fresh frozen plasma
  - Platelets
  - Cryoprecipitate

- Risks of blood product administration

  - Hemolytic and non-hemolytic reactions
  - Transfusion-mediated immunomodulation
  - Viral infection transmission
  - Transfusion-related acute lung injury (TRALI)
  - Hypothermia—WARM blood products to prevent this

    - Consequences of hypothermia:

      - ➤ Impairment of red cell deformability
      - ➤ Platelet dysfunction
      - ➤ Increase in affinity of hemoglobin to hold onto O_2

  - Coagulopathy: monitor coagulation status, provide plasma and platelets
  - Hypocalcemia, hypomagnesemia (citrate in transfused blood binds ionized Ca^{++} and Mg^{++})
  - Banked blood does not have adequate 2,3-DPG. What is the consequence?
    - Shifts oxyhemoglobin-dissociation curve to the LEFT (see Chapter 5), increases affinity of hemoglobin to hold onto O_2

Massive Transfusion Protocols

- Designed to provide rapid infusion of large quantities of blood products to restore oxygen delivery (DO_2), oxygen utilization (VO_2), and tissue perfusion (blood pressure)
- Indications include traumatic injuries, ruptured abdominal aortic or thoracic aneurysms, liver transplant, OB emergencies
- Definition: 10 units of RBCs in 24 hours, or 5 units in less than 3 hours

- Mortality > 50%
- Need to prevent the **triad of death**
  - Hypothermia
  - Acidosis
  - Coagulopathy

SEVERE SEPSIS/SEPTIC SHOCK

Most acute-care settings have developed protocols for the treatment of severe sepsis and septic shock based on a single-center trial (Rivers' study) that showed dramatic results over a decade ago. A recent study did not show a benefit of CVP and $ScvO_2$ monitoring, nor any improvement in outcomes, with the use of dobutamine, each of which has been included in most hospital protocols. Because use of CVP and $ScvO_2$ monitoring and dobutamine infusions for severe sepsis/septic shock are now coming into question, it is doubtful there will be questions on the CCRN exam related to these specific interventions for severe sepsis/septic shock. The test does not generally include controversial issues.

Overview

- #1 cause of death in the non-coronary ICUs
- Mortality rate of severe sepsis is same as AMI, ~ 215,000 deaths/year in U.S.
- Numbers are expected to increase due to high incidence of sepsis in the older adult
- For the Adult CCRN test, you will need to know the difference between the following:
  - Systemic inflammatory response syndrome (SIRS)
  - Sepsis
  - Severe sepsis
  - Septic shock
  - Multiple organ dysfunction syndrome (MODS)

Systemic Inflammatory Response Syndrome (SIRS)

- SIRS is a systemic response to a wide variety of severe clinical insults, manifested by 2 or more of the following:
  - Temp ≥ 38°C or < 36°C
  - Heart rate > 90 bpm
  - Resp rate > 20 or $PaCO_2$ < 32 mmHg
  - WBC > 12,000 or < 4,000 **or** bands >10% (shift to the left)
- **May have SIRS without sepsis**, i.e., traumatic injury, pancreatitis, burns

Sepsis

- Sepsis is the systemic inflammatory response to a documented infection.
- Clinical manifestations would include 2 or more of the SIRS criteria plus a documented infection (culture) **or** suspected infection.
- "Suspected infection" is the presence of one or more of the following:
  - Positive culture results from blood, sputum, urine, etc.
  - Receiving antibiotic, antifungal, or other anti-infective therapy

○ Altered mental status in elderly
  ○ Possible pneumonia (infiltrate on chest radiograph)
  ○ Nursing home patient with indwelling urinary catheter
  ○ Presence of pressure ulcers
  ○ Acute abdomen
  ○ Infected wounds, especially with history of diabetes
  ○ Immunosuppression

NOTE

Mortality is not especially high for sepsis. There is NO organ dysfunction in sepsis. Severe sepsis and septic shock have the higher mortality for which specialized, evidence-based protocols have been developed in order to decrease mortality.

Severe Sepsis

■ Severe sepsis is sepsis PLUS markers of organ dysfunction
■ Examples of organ dysfunction:
  ○ Hypotension
  ○ Acute hypoxemia
  ○ Acute drop in urine output (< 0.5 mL/kg)
  ○ Lactate greater than 2 mmol/kg
  ○ Abrupt mental status changes
  ○ Platelets below 100,000
  ○ Coagulopathy

Septic Shock

■ Septic shock is severe sepsis plus one or both of the following:
  ○ Systemic MAP < 65 mmHg despite adequate fluid resuscitation
  ○ Maintaining the systemic MAP > 65 mmHg **requires a pressor drug**, e.g., norepinephrine, dopamine, epinephrine

Differentiation of Sepsis, Severe Sepsis, Septic Shock

Match the condition in the left-hand column with the clinical signs of patients in the right-hand column, each of which has a documented infection.

A. Sepsis

B. Severe sepsis

C. Septic shock

1. _____ B/P 78/36 before fluids, 102/58 after a 500 mL fluid bolus, BE –5, pH 7.30, lactate 4 mmol/kg, acute abdomen

2. _____ B/P 110/80, BE –1, pH 7.32, lactate < 2 mmol/kg, temperature 39°C, WBC 15,000, acute abdomen

3. _____ B/P 78/40 before fluids, 88/49 after a 500 mL fluid bolus × 4, BE –5, pH 7.31, lactate 4 mmol/kg, acute abdomen

Check answers at the end of the "Severe Sepsis/Septic Shock" section on page 152.

Pathophysiology of Severe Sepsis/Septic Shock (Figure 7-4)

- Severe sepsis/septic shock is a process of malignant intravascular **inflammation**
- Activation of coagulation, inflammatory cytokines, complement, and kinin cascades with release of a variety of endogenous mediators
- Causative organisms include
  - Gram-negative bacteria
  - Gram-positive bacteria
  - Fungi, viruses, *Rickettsia*, parasites

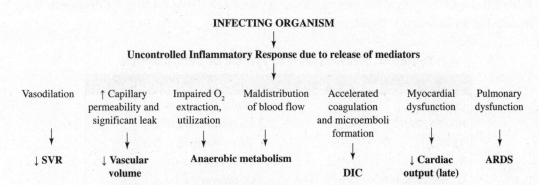

Figure 7-4. Pathophysiology of severe sepsis/septic shock

Risk Factors for Severe Sepsis, Septic Shock

- Extremes of age
- Chronic health problems
- Invasive procedures and devices
- Surgical wounds
- Genitourinary infections
- Prolonged hospitalizations
- Translocation of GI bacteria (NPO)
- Acquired immunodeficiency syndrome
- Use of cytotoxic and immunosuppressive agents
- Alcoholism
- Malignant neoplasms; bone marrow suppression
- Transplantation procedures
- History of splenectomy

Signs/Symptoms of Early Septic Shock

- Tachycardia, bounding pulse
- B/P normal or low
- Skin warm, flushed
- Respirations deep, somewhat fast
- Irritability, confusion → mental status change
- Oliguria
- Fever (temp > 38°C)

Signs/Symptoms of Progressive, Later, Septic Shock

- Hypotension
- Tachycardia, pulse weak and thready
- Skin cool, pale
- Resp fast . . . or may slow
- Lethargy, coma
- Anuria
- Hypothermia (temp < 36°C)

Table 7-3 shows the typical hemodynamics of septic shock. Table 7-4 lists the diagnostic test results that indicate septic shock.

MYTH

The patient with severe sepsis or septic shock always has a fever and elevated WBC.

Table 7-3. Hemodynamics Typical of Septic Shock

Early	Progressive, Late
CO/CI ↑	CO/CI ↓
RA, PA, PAOP ↓	RA, PA, PCWP ↑
SVR ↓	SVR (variable)
SvO$_2$ ↑	SvO$_2$ (variable)
O$_2$ delivery ↑	O$_2$ delivery ↓
O$_2$ consumption ↓	O$_2$ consumption ↓

Table 7-4. Diagnostic Test Results of Septic Shock

Early	Progressive, Late
ABGs → resp alkalosis, mild ↓ PaO$_2$, or may have a combined resp alkalosis and metabolic acidosis	ABGs → metabolic acidosis, ↓↓ PaO$_2$
PT, PTT ~ or ↑	PT, PTT ↑↑
Platelets ~ or ↓	Platelets ↓↓
WBC ↑~, or ↓	WBC ↓
Bands ↑	Bands ↑↑
Glucose ↑	Glucose ↓
Lactate ↑	BUN, creatinine ↑
Troponin ↑	Liver enzymes ↑
	Lactate ↑
	Troponin ↑

- Only 30–50% of patients presenting with severe sepsis/septic shock have positive blood cultures.

MYTH

The patient with severe sepsis or septic shock always has positive blood cultures.

Treatment

- Initial fluid challenge should be the administration of 30 mL/kg of crystalloid (2.1 L in a 70 kg or 154-pound person) in the first 3 hours to achieve goals listed below:
  - MAP ≥ 65 mmHg
  - UO ≥ 0.5 mL/kg/hr
  - Decrease in tachycardia

- If hypotension persists despite fluid resuscitation, start:
  - Vasopressor, pressor of choice is norepinephrine
    - **Norepinephrine (Levophed)** first line
    - **Epinephrine** (drip) is recommended when a second vasopressor agent is needed,
    - Vasopressin drip **IF** B/P does not respond to pressor, start vasopressin drip at 0.03 units/min
- Begin **antibiotic therapy as early as possible** after recognizing severe sepsis/ and septic shock, after blood cultures are drawn
  - In one study, every hour delay of antibiotic administration was associated with an approximately 12% decreased probability of survival compared with the previous hour over the entire observation period.
- Obtain two blood cultures drawn simultaneously from two different sites prior to antibiotic administration
- Inotropic therapy—**dobutamine** is recommended (by itself or in addition to a vasopressor) for patients with cardiac dysfunction as evidenced by high filling pressures and low cardiac output, or clinical signs of hypoperfusion after achievement of restoration of blood pressure with effective volume resuscitation
- Oxygenation goals for septic shock
  - Maintain SpO_2 95% or greater
  - Goal = $ScvO_2 \geq 70\%$, or $SvO_2 \geq 65\%$ (when CVP and MAP goals are met)
  - If $ScvO_2$ or SvO2 not achieved
    - Consider further fluids
    - Dobutamine infusion, max 20 mcg/kg/min
    - Consider transfusion PRBCs if Hgb 7.0 or less

Summary of Therapeutic Endpoints for Septic Shock

- CVP 8–12 mmHg
- MAP $\geq$ 65 mmHg
- UO $\geq$ 0.5 mL/kg/hr
- Central venous oxygen saturation ($ScvO_2$) $\geq$ 70% or $SvO_2 \geq 65\%$
- Normalization of heart rate
- Warm extremities
- Normal mental status
- Decreased lactate/improved base deficit

> **NOTE**
>
> **CVP and $ScvO_2$ monitoring and the use of dobutamine has become controversial as evidenced by newer, larger studies (see ProCESS trial reference) and will most likely not be included on the CCRN exam.**

Differentiation of Sepsis, Severe Sepsis, Septic Shock Answers

Match the condition in the left-hand column with the clinical signs in the right-hand column of patients, each of which has a documented infection.

A. Sepsis

B. Severe sepsis

C. Septic shock

1. __B__ B/P 78/36 before fluids, 102/58 after a 500 mL fluid bolus, BE –5, pH 7.30, lactate 4 mmol/kg, acute abdomen

2. __A__ B/P 110/80, BE –1, pH 7.32, lactate < 2 mmol/kg, temperature 39°C, WBC 15,000, acute abdomen

3. __C__ B/P 78/40 before fluids, 88/49 after a 500 mL fluid bolus × 4, BE –5, pH 7.31, lactate 4 mmol/kg, acute abdomen

ANAPHYLACTIC SHOCK

- Anaphylaxis is an allergic reaction, is rapid in onset, and may cause death.
- Usually occurs after previous exposure to the substance
- Hives, angioedema in 88% of cases
- Respiratory tract involvement 50%
- Shock in 30%

Etiology

- **IgE mediated** immediate hypersensitivity reaction to **protein** substances
  - Penicillin, dye, bee sting, food, dye, latex

Anaphylactoid response looks the same clinically but is NOT IgE mediated. Previous exposure is not necessary (Figure 7-5).

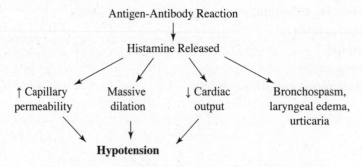

Figure 7-5. Pathophysiology of anaphylactic shock

Treatment

- Removal of offensive agent, if able
- O_2
- 0.3–0.5 mg of 1:1,000 epinephrine **IM** (more rapid absorption than subcutaneous) to decrease dilation, bronchospasm
- Aggressive fluid resuscitation (1–4 L) to treat the relative hypovolemia
- Antihistamine: diphenhydramine (Benadryl) 25–50 mg IV to decrease allergic response
- Inhaled B-adrenergic agents to decrease bronchospasm
- Steroids IV (high dose): peaks in 4–6 hrs, give ASAP to get "on board," to decrease inflammatory response

MULTIPLE ORGAN DYSFUNCTION SYNDROME (MODS)

- Progressive insufficiency of 2 or more organs in an acutely ill patient such that homeostasis cannot be maintained without intervention (Table 7-5)
- May be due to any type of shock
  - The greater the number of organs involved, the higher the mortality
  - Accounts for ~ 80% of all ICU deaths annually

Table 7-5. Markers of Acute Organ Dysfunction Syndrome (MODS)

Cardiovascular	Pulmonary	Renal
Hypotension	Tachypnea	Elevated creatinine
Tachycardia	Dyspnea	Decreased GFR
Dysrhythmias	Hypoxemia	Oliguria
Need for vasopressor support		Life-threatening electrolyte imbalances
Decreased systemic vascular resistance	**Neurologic**	**Endocrine**
Abnormal CVP (low or high)	Confusion	Hyper- or hypoglycemia
Positive troponin	Delirium	Adrenal insufficiency
	Disorientation	
	Lethargy, coma	
	Seizure	
Hepatic	**Hematologic**	**Metabolic**
Elevated liver enzymes	Thrombocytopenia	Metabolic acidosis
Hypoglycemia	Coagulopathy	Elevated lactate
Decreased albumin	Increased D-dimer levels	
Jaundice	Decreased protein C levels	

TRAUMA

- Trauma is included in the Adult CCRN blueprint. However, questions related to trauma are generally very straightforward.
- Ensure you know the trauma first-line and second-line assessment

Trauma First-Line Assessment (A, B, C, D, E)

- **A**irway: ensure patent airway—consider intubation
- **B**reathing: provide 100% oxygen and ventilation
- **C**irculation: two large-bore IV with warm isotonic lactated Ringer's
- **D**isability: perform quick neuro exam—LOC, motor, pupils
  - ○ Glasgow Coma Score is part of the neuro exam, not ALL of it
- **E**xpose/Environmental: remove clothes, provide warmth/cooling as needed

Trauma Second-Line Assessment (F, G, H, I)

- **F**ull set vital signs
  - ○ Focused adjuncts: ECG monitor, pulse oximeter, CO_2 detector, urinary catheter, gastric tube, radiography, FAST, CT, DPL, labs
  - ○ Family presence
- **G**ive comfort measures (pain management)
- **H**istory
- **I**nspect posterior: turn the patient over!

PROVIDING SEDATION TO THE CRITICALLY ILL

The Adult CCRN blueprint has included use of sedation agents in the multisystem section. Sedation is provided to prevent and treat anxiety and agitation.

Overview of Sedation

- The patient who is agitated (even the patient with a medical rather than a surgical diagnosis) should first receive an analgesic (**analgesia-first sedation**) before receiving anxiolytics. (Analgesic agents will be covered after anxiolytics.)
- The degree of sedation should be based on the needs of the patient. This sedation goal should be agreed upon and communicated to all members of the health care team.
- Maintaining **light levels** of sedation in adult ICU patients is associated with improved clinical outcomes (i.e., shorter duration of mechanical ventilation and a shorter ICU length of stay).
- When sedation is provided on an as-needed, PRN basis, there is less possibility of oversedation than when provided with a continuous infusion.
- Daily sedation interruption of continuous infusions of sedation agents allows assessment of further need of the sedation agent and neuro assessment of the patient.
- Nonpharmacological treatment should be considered before using an anxiolytic agent, especially for mild anxiety and agitation.

Assessment of Agitation and Sedation

- Rule out hypoxemia, hemodynamic instability, and pain as causes of agitation. If any of these is present, treat accordingly.
- Assess for additional etiologies (Table 7-6).
- Use a valid and reliable sedation assessment tool for measuring quality and depth of sedation before and after treatment.
  - The Richmond Agitation-Sedation Scale (RASS) and Sedation-Agitation Scale (SAS) are valid and reliable sedation assessment tools used for adult critical care patients.

Table 7-6. Causes of Agitation in Critically Ill Patients

Physiologic	Pharmacological	Emotional	Environmental
Hypoxemia	Anesthetics	Preexisting anxiety disorders	Noise, alarms
Hemodynamic instability (shock)	Sedatives	Preexisting psychoses	Lights
Pain	Analgesics	Dementia	Too cold or warm
DELIRIUM (hyperactive)	Steroids	Fear	Restraints
Withdrawal from ETOH, drugs	Bronchodilators	Anger	Tubes, lines
Dyspnea			Odors
Immobility			Isolation
Sleep deprivation			Sensory deprivation
			Sensory overload

Treatment with Select Sedation Agents

- The use of PRN dosing decreases the likelihood of oversedation.
- If using continuous sedation drips, provide daily sedation interruption or a light target level of sedation.
- See Table 7-7 for select sedation agents commonly used for the acute/critically ill patient.
- ☆ Note that memorization of exact dosing is not generally included on the test. You need to understand how to care for the patient who requires procedural and continuous sedation and how to deal with adverse effects.

Benzodiazepine Reversal with Flumazenil (Romazicon)

- Reverse effects of benzodiazepines with flumazenil (Romazicon) 0.2 mg IV over 15 seconds for moderate sedation or anesthesia, over 30 seconds for overdosage
- Repeat doses, 0.2 mg at 1-minute intervals, maximum of 4 doses, until patient awakens
- For re-sedation, give repeat doses at 20-minute intervals as needed, 0.2 mg per minute to a maximum of 1 mg total, and 3 mg total in 1 hour
- Onset of action of flumazenil is 1–2 minutes, 30% response within 3 minutes, peak effect in 6–10 minutes
- Re-sedation occurs after approximately 1 hour; duration of flumazenil is related to the dose given and benzodiazepine plasma concentrations
- ☆ Note that reversal effects of flumazenil may wear off before effects of benzodiazepine. Therefore monitor for return of sedation, respiratory depression, for at least 2 hours and until the patient is stable and re-sedation is unlikely.
- Use with caution for those with history of prolonged use. Seizure may occur with reversal.

Daily Sedation Withdrawal (Spontaneous Awakening Trial)

An evidence-based strategy for preventing oversedation and its complications is to withhold the sedation for patients who are receiving a continuous drip in order to perform a neurological assessment and determine whether the continuous sedation drip is still clinically beneficial. The daily spontaneous awakening trial (SAT), or sedation vacation, is best done in conjunction with the daily spontaneous breathing trial (SBT). Suggested guidelines for performing the daily SAT are listed below.

1. Screen the patient prior to the spontaneous awakening trial
   - No active seizures
   - No alcohol withdrawal
   - No paralytic drip
   - Stable intracranial pressure
   - No active titration up to maintain goal RASS or MAAS score

2. Turn off sedation drip
   - If the sedation agent is propofol, consider weaning down every 5 minutes to prevent sudden agitation

3. Monitor patient for awakening and tolerance to drug withdrawal
   - Assess neuro status, discomfort, and pain
   - Assess level of sedation/agitation with a sedation tool
   - Signs of SAT failure include:
     - Dangerous agitation
     - Sustained tachypnea, increased work of breathing
     - Sustained drop in SpO_2 to < 90%
     - Acute arrhythmia
     - Hypotension

4. Determine whether the sedation drip can be discontinued and replaced with PRN dosing, restarted at half the dose, or returned to pre-SAT dose

Table 7-7. Pharmacology of Select Sedatives[1]

Agent	Onset After IV Loading Dose	Elimination Half-life	Loading Dose	Maintenance Dosing (IV)	Unique Adverse Effects
Diazepam (Valium)	2–5 min	20–120 hr	5–10 mg	0.03–0.1 mg/kg q 0.5–6 hr prn[2]	Respiratory depression, hypotension, phlebitis (peripheral vein administration)
Lorazepam (Ativan)	15–20 min	8–15 hr	0.02–0.04 mg/kg (≤ 2 mg)	0.02–0.06 mg/kg q 2–6 hr prn or 0.01–0.1 mg/kg/hr (≤10 mg/hr); give loading dose before ↑ infusions rate*	Respiratory depression, hypotension; propylene glycol-related acidosis/renal failure
Midazolam (Versed)	2–5 min	3–11 hr	0.01–0.05 mg/kg over several minutes	0.024–0.1 mg/kg/hr; give loading dose before ↑ infusion rate*	Respiratory depression, hypotension
Propofol (Diprivan)	1–2 min	Short-term use = 3–12 hr Long-term use = 50 ± 18.6 hr	5 mcg/kg/min over 5 min* *Administer loading dose only to patient in whom hypotension is unlikely to occur	5–50 mcg/kg/min, allow 5 minutes between increase of dose	Pain on injection, hypotension, respiratory depression, hypertriglyceridemia, pancreatitis, allergic reactions, propofol-related infusion syndrome; Deep sedation with propofol is associated with significantly longer emergence times than with light sedation
Dexmedetomidine (Precedex)	5–10 min	1.8–3.1 hr	1 mcg/kg over 10 min* *Avoid loading dose if hemodynamically unstable	0.2–0.7 mcg/kg/hr; may increase to 1.5 mcg/kg/hr	Bradycardia, hypotension; hypertension with loading dose; loss of airway reflexes

[1]Barr J, Fraser GL, Puntillo K, Ely EW, Gelinas C, Dasta JF, et. al. Clinical practice guidelines for the management of pain, agitation, and delirium in adult patients in the intensive care unit. *Crit Care Med* 2013; 41:263–306.
[2]There is NO ABSOLUTE maximum dose for benzodiazepines.

Assessment and management of pain is included in the multisystem section of the Adult CCRN test blueprint.

Overview of Pain

- Pain has adverse physiological and psychological effects including activation of the physiologic stress response, depression, and delirium.
- Etiologies of pain in the acute and critically ill include the obvious sources and the not-so-obvious sources (Table 7-8).

Table 7-8. Causes of Pain/Discomfort in the Critically Ill Patient

Incisions Invasive procedures Trauma, fractures Prolonged immobility	Monitoring and therapeutic devices (catheters, drains, endotracheal tubes, noninvasive ventilating devices) Routine nursing care (airway suctioning, dressing changes, physical therapy)

Pain Assessment

- It is recommended that pain be routinely assessed in all adult ICU patients.
- Attempt to obtain the patient's self-report of pain using numerical rating scales, pointing, and head nodding.
- The behavioral pain scale (BPS) is recommended for the patient receiving mechanical ventilation and unable to self-report pain. The critical-care pain observation tool (CPOT) is recommended for assessing the pain of patients unable to self-report pain, with or without mechanical ventilation.
- Vital signs alone should not be used for pain assessment, but they can be used as a cue to assess pain further.
- Consider asking a family or friend who knows the patient well whether patient behavior may indicate the presence of pain.

Pain Management

- Intravenous (IV) opioids are the first-line choice to treat non-neuropathic pain in critically ill patients. All available IV opioids, when titrated to similar pain intensity endpoints, are equally effective (Table 7-9).
- **Prevent** pain as able by use of:
  - Preemptive analgesia prior to procedures likely to cause pain.
  - Nonpharmacological interventions (distraction, relaxation therapy)
- If the patient is agitated, treat pain first and then sedate.

Opioid Reversal with Naloxone

- Give 0.4 to 2 mg IV every 2 minutes until effect to a maximum of 10 mg
- Duration of naloxone action is 1 to 2 hours, repeated doses may be needed for a long-acting opioid

Table 7-9. Pharmacology of Select Opiate Analgesics[1]

Drug	Equian-algesic Dose (mg)	Onset	Elimination Half-Life	Intermittent Dose	Infusion Dose Range (Usual)	Comments
Fentanyl (Sublimaze)	0.1	1–2 min	2–4 hr	0.35–0.5 mcg/kg IV q 0.5–1 hr	0.7–10 mcg/kg/hr ↑ continuous infusion by ↑ing rate 25–30% q 30 minutes	Less hypotension than with morphine Accumulation with hepatic impairment
Hydromorphone (Dilaudid)	1.5	5–15 min	2–3 hr	0.2–0.6 mg IV q 1–2 hrs	0.5–3 mg/hr ↑ continuous infusion by ↑ing rate 25–30% q 30 minutes	Therapeutic option in patients tolerant to morphine/fentanyl Accumulation with hepatic/renal impairment
Morphine	10	5–10 min	3–4 hr	2–4 mg IV q 1–2 hrs	2–30 mg/hr If goal pain score not achieved, give 1–5 mg IVP, then ↑ infusion by 1–2 mg/hr q 30 minutes	Histamine release, potential hypotension Accumulation with hepatic/renal impairment
Remifentanil (Ultiva)	N/A	1–3 min	3–10 min	N/A	Loading dose: 1.5 mcg/kg IV Maintenance dose: 0.5–15 mcg/kg/hr IV	Use IBW if body weight > 130% IBW No accumulation in hepatic/renal failure

[1]Barr J, Fraser GL, Puntillo K, Ely EW, Gelinas C, Dasta JF, et. al. Clinical practice guidelines for the management of pain, agitation, and delirium in adult patients in the intensive care unit. *Crit Care Med* 2013; 41:263–306.

Overview

- Therapeutic hypothermia (TH) is a treatment that lowers the patient's core body temperature in order to prevent the neurological effects of ischemic injury to the brain of survivors of sudden cardiac death.
- The treatment was initially endorsed by the American Heart Association in 2005 and re-endorsed in 2010.
- Assess patients after cardiac arrest for inclusion and exclusion criteria (Table 7-10).

Table 7-10. Inclusion and Exclusion Criteria for Use of Therapeutic Hypothermia

Inclusion Criteria	Exclusion Criteria
Cardiac arrest with return of spontaneous circulation Unresponsive or not following commands after cardiac arrest Witnessed arrest with downtime of less than 60 minutes	Pregnancy Core temperature of less than 35°C Age < 18 or > 85 Existing DNR status or terminal disease Chronic renal failure Sustained refractory ventricular arrhythmias Active bleeding Shock Hemodynamic instability Drug intoxication

The therapy involves 3 phases.

1. Induction, 33°C, **start ASAP**

    ○ Should initiate within 90 minutes of arrest, may go out to 6 hours of arrest

2. Maintenance, 24 hours at 33°C

3. Rewarming, slowly increasing to 36.5°C

NOTE

The target temperature of 32–34°C has come into question. Therefore, it most likely will not be specifically included on the test.

Induction Phase

- Set goal time to target temperature
- Monitor core temp (bladder, rectal)
- Application of device (external pads or internal central venous catheter)
- Goal systolic B/P > 90 mmHg and goal MAP > 70 mmHg
- Obtain baseline labs, generally complete metabolic profile, complete blood count, coagulation panel, magnesium, phosphorous, arterial blood gas
- Get baseline bedside glucose
- 12-lead ECG
- Sedation (deep)
- Paralytic agent for shivering not controlled with meperidine
- Monitor/manage systemic effects of hypothermia

Systemic Effects of Hypothermia

- Insulin resistance → hyperglycemia
- Electrolyte and fluid shifts

- Shivering
- Skin breakdown
- Decreased cardiac output
  - Up to 25%
- Alteration in coagulation
  - Platelet dysfunction
- Increase risk for infection
  - Neutrophil and macrophage functions decrease at temperatures less than 35°C

Maintenance Phase (duration, 24 hours)

- Continuous temp, no lower than goal, 33°C
- Monitor vital signs, at least hourly
- Bedside blood glucose, insulin drip as needed
- Monitor train-of-4 (TOF) every hour if paralytic used with goal twitch 1–2 to prevent prolonged paralyzation
- Labs (same as baseline) every 8 hours until rewarmed

Rewarming Phase

- Passive rewarming to 36.5°C
- Program cooling unit to increase target temp by 1 degree per hour
- Stop all potassium administration 8 hours prior to rewarming
  - Rewarming causes rebound hyperkalemia
- Discontinue paralytics (if used) after patient is warmed to 36.5°C
- Repeat labs (same as baseline) when patient is rewarmed
- Close neurological assessment

TOXIC INGESTION

The exam may include one question related to toxic ingestions.

General Points

- May be accidental or intentional
  - ☆ Initial management—always ABCs (airway, breathing, circulation)
- If comatose, be prepared to give 50% dextrose 50 mL, thiamine 50–100 mg, naloxone 2 mg IV
- Activated charcoal 1 gm/kg via gastric lavage
  - Contraindicated with hydrocarbon or corrosive ingestions
  - Not necessary—iron, lithium, alcohols
- Facilitate removal of drug—urine alkalization, hemodialysis
- Administer antidote, if indicated, e.g., naloxone
- Monitor for arrhythmias
- Monitor urine output

Management of Toxic Ingestion

■ See Table 7-11 for management of specific toxic substances.

Table 7-11. Signs, Symptoms, and Treatment of Specific Toxic Agents

Drug	Signs/Symptoms	Treatment
Acetaminophen (Tylenol)	Nausea, vomiting, perhaps none early on	N-acetylcysteine, dosing effective for 8 hours after ingestion • 140 mg/kg loading dose, then • 70 mg/kg every 4 hrs for 17 doses
	Later RUQ pain, abnormal liver function tests, mental status changes	GI lavage with activated charcoal within 4 hours after ingestion
Benzodiazepines	Drowsiness, confusion, slurred speech, respiratory depression, hypotension, aspiration	Support airway
		Flumazenil (Romazicon) 0.2 mg IV slow, then 0.3 mg IV, then 0.5 mg IV at one minute intervals, total 3 mg
		Short half-life, watch for reoccurrence of symptoms
		Gastric lavage with activated charcoal
		Fluid resuscitation
Beta blockers	Bradycardia	Glucagon, epinephrine, insulin plus dextrose, sodium bicarb
	Hypotension	
	CV collapse	
Calcium-channel blockers	Bradycardia	Calcium gluconate, epinephrine, insulin plus dextrose, sodium bicarb
	Hypotension	
	CV collapse	
Cocaine	Seizure activity, agitation, hyperthermia, rhabdomyolysis	Activated charcoal
		Fluids, glucose, thiamine IV
		Benzodiazepines for sedation, seizures
		Vasopressin preferred over epinephrine in full arrest
		Vasodilators for hypertension
		Nitrates, calcium blockers for ischemia, NO beta blockers
		Cooling for hyperthermia
Ethylene glycol	Intoxication behavior	Gastric lavage
	Vomiting	Sodium bicarb
	Metabolic acidosis, anion gap	Antidotes: ethanol or fomepizole
	Renal failure	Dialysis

Drug	Signs/Symptoms	Treatment
ETOH	Stupor, respiratory depression, aspiration risk	Support, protect airway
		Fluid resuscitation
		MVI, thiamine 100 mg IV
		Electrolyte replacement PRN (Mg^{++}, Ph^{++}, K$^+$)
	Intermittent agitation	DT prevention: benzodiazepines, CIWA protocol
Methamphetamine	Fever, tachycardia, hypertension, seizure, agitation, renal failure	Fluids, cooling
		Benzodiazepines, haloperidol
		Physical restraint, protect self and others
Opioids	Drowsiness, hypoventilation, hypotension, hypothermia, deep sedation, pinpoint pupils	Support airway
		Naloxone (Narcan), 0.4–2 mg IV every 2 minutes until effect to a maximum of 10 mg
		Gastric lavage with activated charcoal
Phencyclidine (PCP)	Blank stare, rapid involuntary eye movement, hallucinations, severe mood disorder, flushing, sweating, hypertension, tachycardia, seizure, coma	Support airway
		Provide calm environment, do not leave alone due to high possibility of harm to self and others
		Benzodiazepines for agitation
		Fluids, cooling, monitor renal function
Salicylates	Vomiting, tinnitus, confusion, hyperthermia, respiratory alkalosis, metabolic acidosis, and multiple organ failure	Activated charcoal
		Urine alkalization
		Dialysis
Tricyclic antidepressants	CV signs: arrhythmias, shock	Sodium bicarb, activated charcoal, fluids, cardiac monitoring
	Neuro signs: drowsiness, delirium, seizures, coma	
	Anticholinergic signs: blurred vision, fever, twitching	

Now that you have reviewed key multisystem concepts, go to the Multisystem Practice Questions. Answer the questions, and then check your answers. Continue to review the information until you get at least 80% on the practice questions.

MULTISYSTEM PRACTICE QUESTIONS

1. Which medications are most often prescribed for anaphylaxis after initial therapy with IM epinephrine?

   (A) antihistamines and corticosteroids
   (B) vasopressors and inotropes
   (C) antihistamines and antibiotics
   (D) corticosteroids and vasopressors

2. Which of the following would most likely result in an SvO_2 of 82%?

   (A) hypovolemic shock
   (B) anaphylactic shock
   (C) septic shock
   (D) cardiogenic shock

3. The initial management of any drug intoxication is to:

   (A) prevent further absorption of the drug.
   (B) increase excretion of the drug.
   (C) administer an antidote when appropriate.
   (D) ensure a patent airway and adequate breathing.

4. The patient is being treated for severe sepsis with fluid resuscitation, but the MAP is 55 mmHg and norepinephrine is ordered. What primary beneficial effect will norepinephrine provide for this patient?

   (A) maintain renal blood flow
   (B) increase coronary blood flow
   (C) increase venous return and preload
   (D) restore vascular tone and afterload

5. Which of the following would be an indicator that fluid resuscitation is adequate?

   (A) CVP of 2 mmHg
   (B) heart rate decreasing
   (C) narrowing of pulse pressure
   (D) serum bicarbonate 16 mEq/L

6. Which of the following is TRUE related to shock?

   (A) The MAP is adequate in the compensatory phase of shock.
   (B) The blood pressure is maintained in Class III hemorrhagic shock.
   (C) Elevated lactate level occurs late in septic shock.
   (D) Serum bicarbonate is elevated in shock.

7. The patient with upper GI bleeding received procedural sedation with midazolam during his endoscopy procedure. He required higher doses to maintain sedation and screened positive for obstructive sleep apnea (OSA). Which of the following is TRUE related to this patient's plan of care?

    (A) Respiratory depression will generally precede sedation.
    (B) Pulse oximetry will detect early hypoventilation.
    (C) Waveform capnography monitoring is indicated for this patient post procedure.
    (D) Maximum dose of flumazenil (Romazicon) for midazolam reversal is 0.2 mg IV.

8. The patient is receiving a continuous sedation infusion of propofol (Diprivan) at 30 mcg/kg/min. Which of the following is an appropriate intervention?

    (A) Reverse the side effects with flumazenil (Romazicon).
    (B) Provide a daily spontaneous awakening trial.
    (C) Avoid administration of analgesia.
    (D) Monitor closely for hypertension.

9. Which of the following statements is TRUE related to the differentiation of terms related to sepsis?

    (A) Special protocols, "bundles" of interventions, are intended for severe sepsis or septic shock, not sepsis.
    (B) Administration of pressors is required for severe sepsis.
    (C) By definition, the patient with systemic inflammatory response syndrome (SIRS) has an infection.
    (D) Positive cultures are required in order to make the diagnosis of septic shock.

10. Which of the following statements related to therapeutic hypothermia is CORRECT?

    (A) Therapeutic hypothermia should be provided for all patients status post ventricular fibrillation.
    (B) Potassium infusions will most likely be required during rewarming.
    (C) Shivering is expected and is generally self-limiting.
    (D) Insulin infusions are often required during the maintenance phase.

11. The patient who has sustained traumatic injuries, including a pelvic fracture and soft tissue injuries, has required transfusion of 7 units of packed red blood cells (PRBCs). Which of the following is TRUE related to the care of this patient?

    (A) Pressors will most likely be required.
    (B) The patient will need to be monitored for hypercalcemia.
    (C) Blood products and crystalloids should be warmed.
    (D) Platelets will need to be given if the platelet count drops.

12. The patient is receiving mechanical ventilation and is able to write notes to communicate. Which of the following is TRUE related to the management of pain for this patient?

(A) Coach the patient in the use of self-reporting with the numerical rating scale (NRS).

(B) Initiate pain medication during procedures when the patient first demonstrates pain behaviors.

(C) Disregard use of non-pharmacological interventions for pain since the patient is receiving mechanical ventilation.

(D) Ensure the mean arterial pressure (MAP) is greater than 60 mmHg before providing intravenous opiates.

ANSWER KEY

| 1. **A** | 3. **D** | 5. **B** | 7. **C** | 9. **A** | 11. **C** |
| 2. **C** | 4. **D** | 6. **A** | 8. **B** | 10. **D** | 12. **A** |

ANSWERS EXPLAINED

1. **(A)** An antihistamine will help halt the allergic response, and a corticosteroid will help halt the inflammatory response. Vasopressors, inotropes, and antibiotics are not helpful for anaphylactic shock.

2. **(C)** The normal SvO_2 is 60% to 75%. In septic shock, oxygen delivery (DO_2) is adequate, but oxygen utilization (VO_2) at the cellular level is low. A sign of poor oxygen utilization is an elevated SvO_2. Oxygen is not being used, and blood is returning to the pulmonary artery with more oxygen than expected. The other 3 types of shock result in poor oxygen delivery, which causes low oxygen utilization and a low SvO_2.

3. **(D)** If the intoxication affects airway and breathing, the other 3 interventions listed will be of no use as the patient will not survive.

4. **(D)** The problem in septic shock is massive dilation (low SVR) and capillary leak (resulting in a relative hypovolemia). Pressors (norepinephrine is the first-line pressor) cause vasoconstriction and increase SVR (afterload). Although pressors may also increase preload and renal blood flow, these are secondary effects. The primary effect of pressors is on afterload. Although septic shock may result in ventricular damage with resultant elevated troponin, myocardial damage is not due to a drop in coronary artery blood flow but to endotoxin effects on cardiac muscle.

5. **(B)** As vascular volume is restored and preload is increased, there is less need for compensatory mechanisms (increase in heart rate). A CVP of 2 mmHg, narrowing of pulse pressure, and metabolic acidosis are all signs that filling pressures have not been optimized.

6. **(A)** Because compensatory mechanisms are working, the MAP is maintained in the compensatory phase. If these mechanisms fail, the MAP drops and hypotension results (progressive phase). In Class III hemorrhagic shock, the blood pressure decreases

and is no longer maintained. In septic shock, lactate rises early on, during the severe sepsis, not late. Serum bicarbonate is decreased (not elevated) in shock due to the lactic acidosis.

7. **(C)** Waveform capnography is indicated during and after procedural sedation in order to identify EARLY hypoventilation. Longer monitoring may be required for the patient with a history of obstructive sleep apnea (OSA). Sedation usually precedes respiratory depression. SpO_2 will not decrease until the $PaCO_2$ is very high. Flumazenil reverses benzodiazepines. However, re-sedation may occur, and subsequent doses of flumazenil may be necessary.

8. **(B)** Studies have shown improved patient outcomes, shorter ventilator times, and less risk of oversedation when "awakening trials" are done for the patient on a continuous sedation infusion. Propofol is not reversed with flumazenil. Analgesia should be used for agitation, not avoided. Propofol is more likely to cause hypotension, not hypertension.

9. **(A)** "Sepsis bundles" are indicated for severe sepsis or septic shock since these 2 problems result in organ dysfunction and increased mortality. These "bundles" are not intended for sepsis (which does not include organ dysfunction and increased mortality). Severe sepsis, by definition, does not require pressor administration. SIRS may be present without an infection, e.g., trauma and pancreatitis. In addition, only 30–50% of patients with severe sepsis/septic shock present with positive cultures.

10. **(D)** Hypothermia may result in hyperglycemia, which will necessitate insulin infusions to maintain normoglycemia during the maintenance phase of TH. Therapeutic hypothermia is indicated for only the unresponsive patient s/p cardiac arrest not for ALL patients. Potassium is required during the maintenance phase of TH to correct hypokalemia. However, during rewarming, potassium replacement needs to be stopped. Shivering will prevent temperature reduction, is not self-limiting, and will need to be treated with either meperidine or neuromuscular blocking agents.

11. **(C)** It is important to prevent hypothermia and its resultant adverse consequences during fluid/transfusion resuscitation. Therefore, fluids and blood products need to be warmed. Pressors are not indicated in hypovolemic shock since the afterload in hypovolemic shock is already abnormally high due to compensation for volume loss. The problem needs to be addressed by "filling up the tank" to restore circulation volume. HYPOCALCEMIA (not hypercalcemia) secondary to calcium binding to citrate in stored blood is a potential problem related to transfusion of PRBCs. Platelets are not in PRBCs and should be replaced regardless of platelet count when large volume of PRBCs are administered. Replacing platelets will prevent thrombocytopenia and coagulation problems.

12. **(A)** Self-reporting of pain is always preferred. In the scenario described, the patient is capable of providing a pain intensity number. Preemptive analgesia is preferred for procedures likely to be painful rather than waiting until pain is experienced. Nonpharmacological interventions are always appropriate. Hypotensive patients still require pain management. Pain should not be used to "keep up the B/P." An opiate may be needed because it is less likely to cause a drop in blood pressure, e.g., fentanyl, and can treat the hypotension as needed.

Gastrointestinal Concepts

8

Luck is what happens when preparation meets opportunity.

—Darrel Royal

GASTROINTESTINAL TEST BLUEPRINT

Gastrointestinal 6% of total test   **9 Questions**

→ Acute abdominal trauma
→ Acute GI hemorrhage
→ Bowel infarction/obstruction/perforation (e.g., mesenteric ischemia, adhesions)
→ GI surgeries
→ Hepatic failure/coma (e.g., portal hypertension, cirrhosis, esophageal varices)
→ Malnutrition and malabsorption
→ Pancreatitis

GASTROINTESTINAL TESTABLE NURSING ACTIONS

☐ Identify and monitor normal and abnormal physical assessment findings
☐ Recognize and monitor normal and abnormal gastrointestinal diagnostic test results
☐ Recognize indications for and manage patients requiring gastrointestinal:

　○ Monitoring devices (e.g., intra-abdominal compartment pressure)
　○ Drains

☐ Manage patients receiving gastrointestinal medications and monitor response
☐ Monitor patient and follow protocols, pre-, intra- and post-procedure (e.g., EGD, PEG placement)
☐ Recognize indications for and complications of enteral and parenteral nutrition
☐ Monitor patients and follow protocols for gastrointestinal surgery
☐ Recognize signs and symptoms of emergencies (e.g., GI bleed, ischemic bowel), initiate interventions, and seek assistance as needed

OVERVIEW OF ABDOMINAL ANATOMY

Although there will not be questions on abdominal anatomy, the Adult CCRN exam may have questions on physical assessment findings. The GI concepts are easier to understand if you have a good idea of abdominal structures (Figure 8-1).

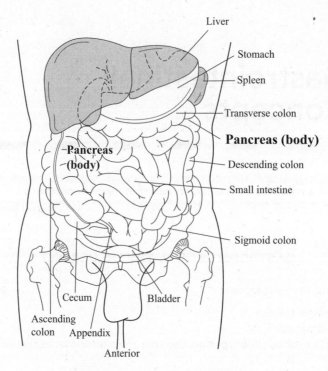

Liver
Stomach
Spleen
Transverse colon
Pancreas (body)
Descending colon
Small intestine
Sigmoid colon
Bladder
Pancreas (body)
Cecum
Ascending colon
Appendix
Anterior

Figure 8-1. Anatomy of the abdomen

Midline
Urinary bladder
Urethra (female)

Right Upper Quadrant	Left Upper Quadrant
Pylorous	Stomach
Duodenum	Spleen
Liver	Left kidney and adrenal gland
Right kidney and adrenal gland	Splenic flexure of the colon
Hepatic flexure of the colon	Body of the pancreas
Head of the pancreas	
Right Lower Quadrant	**Left Lower Quadrant**
Cecum	Sigmoid colon
Appendix	Left ovary and fallopian tube (female)
Right ovary and fallopian tube (female)	Left ureter and lower kidney pole
Right ureter and lower kidney pole	Left spermatic cord (male)
Right spermatic cord (male)	

GASTROINTESTINAL BLEEDING

- Acute GI hemorrhage may be divided into 2 broad categories, upper and lower
  - Upper GI bleeding accounts for approximately 80% of acute GI bleeding
    - Peptic ulcer disease (gastric, duodenal) ~50%
    - Esophageal ~10–20%
    - Stress ulcers
    - Mallory-Weiss tear
    - Cancer

- Lower GI bleeding accounts for approximately 20% of acute GI bleeding
  - Diverticulosis
  - Angiodysplasia (AVMs)
  - Tumor
  - Radiation
  - Colitis
  - Inflammatory
    - Crohn's
  - Infectious
    - *Clostridium difficile*
    - *E. Coli*
- Which has higher mortality? **UPPER**
  - Seldom do patients with lower GI bleeding require ICU admission

General Management of Upper GI Bleeding

- ADDRESS the CAUSE
- Isotonic fluid resuscitation as for hypovolemic shock
- PRBCs
- Replace clotting factors, (fresh frozen plasma, platelets)
- Medications
  - Vasopressin constricts splanchnic arteriolar bed, decreases portal venous pressure, watch for chest pain, ST elevation
  - Octreotide (Sandostatin) reduces splanchnic blood flow, gastric acid secretion, GI mobility
  - Osmotic laxatives (sorbitol) removes nitrogenous materials (blood) out of gut to prevent ammonia conversion; important in the presence of liver disease
  - Beta blockers constrict mesenteric arterioles reducing portal venous flow

Esophageal Varices

- Common cause is portal hypertension secondary to liver disease
- Venous drainage of GI tract (Figure 8-2)

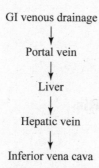

GI venous drainage

↓

Portal vein

↓

Liver

↓

Hepatic vein

↓

Inferior vena cava

Figure 8-2. Venous drainage of the GI tract

Liver cirrhosis prevents normal drainage through the liver. Pressure backs up into esophageal vein, like "hemorrhoids of the esophagus."

Treatment of Esophageal Varices

- General management as described previously
- Endoscopy procedure with banding or sclerosing of varices
- Esophageal balloon tamponade (Sengstaken-Blakemore tube)
    - Gastric balloon, 200–500 mL, attached to suction, empty stomach
    - Esophageal balloon, 20 mmHg or up to 40 mmHg (prescribed by physician) to control bleeding
    - If esophageal balloon displaced up, the inflated balloon may occlude the airway
    - ☆ Cut esophageal balloon if respiratory distress

ACUTE PANCREATITIS

- The pancreas has both exocrine and endocrine functions (Table 8-1).

Table 8-1. Exocrine and Endocrine Functions of the Pancreas

Exocrine Functions	Endocrine Functions
Secretion of: • Bicarbonate to neutralize stomach acid • H_2O • Na^+, K^+ • Digestive enzymes → trypsin, amylase, lipase Secretion ↑ by: • Parasympathetic stimulation • Food (secretin and choleycystokinin)	Alpha cells → secrete **glucagon** Beta cells → secrete **insulin** Delta cells → **inhibit** secretion of above

Acute pancreatitis is diffuse inflammation, destruction, and auto-digestion of the pancreas from premature activation of exocrine enzymes. It is NOT always caused by an infection!

- Up to 6 L of fluid may be secreted into interstitial spaces
- Activation of inflammatory mediators (cytokines, kinins, histamine, clotting factors)
- Results in systemic inflammatory response syndrome (SIRS)
    - ↑ Vascular permeability
    - Vasodilatation
    - Vascular stasis
    - Microthrombosis

Etiology of Acute Pancreatitis

- Alcoholism
- Obstruction (gall stones)
- Abdominal surgery
- Drugs
- Hyperlipidemia
- Trauma
- Infection (although it is seldom an infection)

☆ Pulmonary Complications of Acute Pancreatitis

- Atelectasis, left lower lobe
- Left pleural effusion
- Bilateral crackles
- ARDS

Signs and Symptoms of Acute Pancreatitis

- Abdominal pain—boring
- Pain radiates to all quadrants and lumbar area
- N/V, rigid abdomen, no rebound tenderness
- ↓ or absent bowel sounds
- Low-grade fever
- ↑WBC
- ↑Amylase—peaks in 4–24 hrs, returns to normal in 4 days
- ↑Lipase, stays elevated longer than amylase
- ↓Calcium
- ↑Blood sugar

RATIONALE FOR SIGNS AND SYMPTOMS OF ACUTE PANCREATITIS

- Calcium used up for autodigestion, precipitates hypocalcemia → Trousseau's sign, prolonged QT, seizures
  - Trousseau's sign: during inflation of the blood pressure cuff, the brachial artery is occluded. The absence of blood flow, the patient's hypocalcemia, and subsequent neuromuscular irritability will induce **spasm of the muscles of the hand and forearm**.
- Beta cell injury → hyperglycemia, hyperglycemic hypertonic syndrome
- Phospholipase A released → "kills" Type II alveolar cells → ↓ surfactant → ARDS
- Left diaphragm lifted, left atelectasis, left pleural effusion

☆ Signs of Hemorrhagic Pancreatitis

- Cullen's sign—bluish discoloration and ecchymosis of periumbilical area (Cullen . . . umbilicus)
  - In acute pancreatitis, **methemalbumin** forms from digested blood and tracks around the abdomen from the inflamed pancreas
- Grey Turner's sign—bluish discoloration of flanks (turn . . . flank)
  - Hemorrhagic pancreatitis

Ranson's Criteria of Severity of Acute Pancreatitis

- The more criteria present, the more severe the acute pancreatitis and increased morbidity (Table 8-2)

Table 8-2. Ranson's Criteria of Acute Pancreatitis Severity

At Admission	During Next 48 Hrs
Age > 55 years WBC > 16,000/mm^3 Glucose > 200 mg/dl LDH > 350 IU/L AST > 250 U/L	Hct decrease of > 10 BUN increase of > 5 mg/dl Fluid sequestration > 6 L Ca^{++} < 8 mg/dl PaO$_2$ < 60 mmHg Base deficit > 4 mEq/L

☆ Treatment of Acute Pancreatitis

- Fluid replacement
- Calcium, K$^+$, and Mg^{++} replacement
- H$_2$ blockers or proton pump inhibitors (PPIs) to decrease gastric pH
- NG suction to decrease gastric secretion
- Pain management, morphine
- Glucose control
- Enteral feeding below duodenum
- ☆ Monitor for pulmonary complications:
  - ARDS
  - Elevation of diaphragm and bilateral basilar crackles
  - Atelectasis especially left base

LIVER FAILURE

- Most common cause of **acute** liver failure → acetaminophen (Tylenol) OD
- Most common cause of **chronic** liver failure → alcohol abuse

Liver Failure Lab Abnormalities

- ↓ Serum protein
- ↓ Serum albumin and ascites
- Pancytopenia (↓ WBC, RBC, platelets)
- Coagulopathies (↑ PT, PTT)
- ↑ AST, ALT, alkaline phosphatase, GGT
- ↑ Serum bilirubin
- ↓ Blood sugar
- Hyperventilation, respiratory alkalosis → ↑ lactate—metabolic acidosis
- ↑ NH$_3$
- ↑ Serum creatinine, BUN—late

Clinical Findings of Liver Failure

- Mental status change due to hepatic encephalopathy, secondary to elevated NH$_3$
- **Asterixis** (flappy hand tremor seen in liver failure) due to elevated NH$_3$
- Ascites due to low albumin and protein, risk of spontaneous bacterial peritonitis
- Jaundice due to elevated bilirubin

- Renal failure (hepatorenal syndrome), not fully understood, but high mortality (~80%), usually due to bleeding or infection
- Sepsis, bacterial or fungal due to decreased immune function
- Liver becomes enlarged, tender during **acute inflammatory** state
- Liver becomes non-palpable as hepatocellular necrosis progresses .

Stages of Hepatic Encephalopathy

- Stage I: Mild confusion, forgetfulness, irritability, change in sleep patterns, EEG normal
- Stage II: Lethargy, confusion, apathy, aberrant behavior, asterixis, EEG normal
- Stage III: Severe confusion, semi-stupor to stupor, hyperactive deep tendon reflexes, hyperventilation, EEG abnormal
- Stage IV: No response to stimuli, posturing, positive Babinski, areflexia except for pathologic reflexes, EEG abnormal

☆ Factors That Increase Serum NH_3 (which worsens encephalopathy)

- Hypokalemia: triggers ammonia genesis in the kidneys (mechanism entirely unclear)
- ↑ BUN: breakdown of nitrogen
- ↑ Protein: breakdown of nitrogen
- ↑ Lactic acidosis: may be precipitated by administration of Ringer's lactate—normally it is converted into bicarb by healthy liver (not in liver failure)

NOTE

Anything that increases ammonia level causes hepatic encephalopathy, may ↑ ICP.

Management of Liver Failure

- Prevent anything that will increase serum NH_3; attempt to decrease serum NH_3
  - Prevent low K^+ level, causes worse NH_3, use aldactone (potassium-sparing diuretic) to treat ascites
  - Prevent ↑ BUN, increases NH_3
  - Prevent GI bleeding, breakdown of protein in gut increases NH_3
  - Prevent acid buildup (lactic acidosis due to low B/P, no lactated Ringer's), increases NH_3
- Restrict protein **only** if hepatic encephalopathy is present
- Administer clotting factors
- Lactulose—for increased serum ammonia
- Neomycin—kills bacteria in gut that produce NH_3
  - Complication of neomycin therapy—vitamin K deficiency
  - Bacteria (*E. coli*) in gut help produce folic acid, riboflavin, and vitamin K
- Adjust doses of medication metabolized by liver
- Monitor glucose
- Administer acetylcysteine (Mucomyst) or Acetadote, for **all** suspected acetaminophen OD
  - Give all doses if confirmed, not related to acetaminophen levels
- Close neuro assessment

- Transjugular intrahepatic porto-systemic shunt (TIPS procedure)
  - Procedure for select patients with cirrhosis to relieve esophageal varices or ascites
  - Complication of procedure is hepatic encephalopathy, why?
    - The stent inserted during the procedure allows shunting of blood directly from hepatic veins into the portal vein, **bypassing the liver** (which decreases portal hypertension) but decreases detoxification of blood
- Manage medically with neomycin and lactulose
- May need to decrease diameter of stent

SPLEEN

Remember 2 concepts related to the spleen:

- The patient with a history of a splenectomy has reduced immune function since the spleen is thought to "filter" the blood
- Signs of splenic rupture
  - Sharp pain, left shoulder—**Kehr's sign** (diaphragmatic irritation causes referred pain)
  - Abdominal distention with absent bowel sounds

ABDOMINAL TRAUMA

Clinical Signs

- Ecchymosis over upper left quadrant → soft tissue trauma or splenic injury
- Ecchymosis around umbilicus (**Cullen's**) → intraperitoneal bleeding
- Ecchymosis of flank (**Grey Turner's**) → retroperitoneal bleeding
- Left shoulder pain (**Kehr's sign**) → ruptured spleen (referred pain due to diaphragmatic irritation)
- Absence of bowel sounds with abdominal distention and guarding → visceral injury
- Bowel sounds in chest → diaphragmatic rupture
- Free air in abdomen by X-ray → disruption of GI tract
- Diagnostic peritoneal lavage positive for blood → intra-abdominal bleeding

Intra-abdominal Hypertension and Abdominal Compartment Syndrome

ETIOLOGY

- Massive fluid resuscitation
- Trauma
- Emergent abdominal surgery

PATHOPHYSIOLOGY

- If pressure in the abdominal cavity becomes greater than the pressure in the capillaries that perfuse the abdominal organs, ischemia and infarction may result.
- Increased intra-abdominal pressure may result in reduced cardiac output, increased systemic vascular resistance, reduced venous return, and decreased renal perfusion.
- Affects multiple organ systems: cardiovascular, pulmonary, renal, liver, GI
- May occur without obvious clinical abdominal distention

DEFINITIONS

- Intra-abdominal hypertension (**IAH**) = intra-abdominal pressure (IAP) > 12–15 mmHg
- Abdominal perfusion pressure (**APP**) = difference between MAP and IAP
  - APP 60 mmHg or > associated with improved survival
  - APP 50 mmHg or < associated with increased mortality
- Abdominal compartment syndrome (**ACS**) is a sustained IAP of > 20 mmHg, with or without an APP of 60 mmHg, and associated with new organ dysfunction or failure

ASSESSMENT

- Measure bladder pressure; it most closely approximates intraperitoneal pressure
- Level transducer to symphysis pubis
  - Physiologic compromise begins at pressure 12–15 mmHg
  - Decompression laparotomy should be considered if pressure exceeds 20 mmHg

TREATMENT

- For IAP 12 mmHg or greater:
  - Optimize patient position by placing in reverse Trendelenburg, maintain head of bed elevation 20 degrees or less
  - Loosen constrictive clothing, dressings, binders
  - Manage pain and agitation
  - Prevent overhydration
  - Place nasogastric tube to low intermittent suction to decompress abdomen
  - Optimize stool management, assess for impaction and treat, consider rectal tube or enema
  - Discuss with physician whether gastro/colo prokinetic agents are appropriate for the patient
- Intra-abdominal pressures ≥ 20 mmHg
  - Considered abdominal compartment syndrome
  - Decompression surgery may be indicated

Complications of Bariatric Surgery

- Malabsorption—vitamin supplements needed
  - ○ Vitamin deficiencies: protein, calcium, iron, B12, folate
  - ○ Symptoms include vomiting, headache, diplopia, memory loss
- Wound related
- Enteric leakage from anastomosis
- Gallstones—52% within 1 year
- Bowel obstruction secondary to scar tissue or kink

BOWEL INFARCTION

Etiology

NOTE

The superior mesenteric artery provides arterial perfusion to the small intestine.

- Thrombus
- Hypercoagulability
- Arteriosclerosis
- Surgical procedure (aortic clamping)
- Vasopressors (endogenous or exogenous)
- Intra-abdominal infection

Pathophysiology

↓ Blood flow to mesenteric vessels → prolonged ischemia → edema of intestinal wall → full thickness necrosis → perforation, peritonitis

Clinical Presentation

- Abdominal pain (severe cramping—periumbilical or diffuse)
- Abdominal distention, vomiting
- Hypoactive or absent bowel sounds
- Fever, tachycardia, hypotension

Treatment of Bowel Infarction

- Airway, breathing, circulation (ABCs)
- Fluids
- Gastric decompression (nasogastric tube)
- Treat pain
- Bowel resection with debridement of necrotic tissue
- Monitor for sepsis

Tables 8-3 and 8-4 describe the types, etiologies, and clinical presentations of bowel obstructions.

Table 8-3. Types and Etiologies of Bowel Obstruction

Paralytic Ileus	Small Bowel	Large Bowel
Hypokalemia	Adhesions	Neoplasm
Abdominal surgery	Hernia	Stricture
Peritonitis	Volvulus	Diverticulitis
Intestinal distention	Neoplasm	Fecal or barium impaction
Pneumonia	(May be partial or complete, simple or strangulated)	
Pancreatitis		
Opiates		
Sepsis		
(Paralytic ileus is usually transient)		

Table 8-4. Clinical Presentation of Bowel Obstruction

Small Bowel	Large Bowel
Sharp, episodic pain	Dull pain
Vomiting **early** (projectile and/or fecal)	Change in bowel habits
Hypokalemia	Vomiting **late**
High-pitched bowel sounds (↑ early, ↓ late)	Abdominal distention
KUB, dilated loops of gas-filled bowel	Low-pitched bowel sounds (↑ early, ↓ late)
	KUB, dilated loops of gas-filled bowel

Treatment of Bowel Obstruction

- ABCs
- Prevent perforation (N/G tube)
- Fluids/electrolytes
- Treat pain
- Monitor for infection, complications
- Appropriate nutritional support: if use gut, must feed distal to obstruction
- Surgery
  - May or may not be needed
  - For complete or strangulated SBO, surgery will be done; if perforation has occurred, surgery will be done
    - Lysis of adhesion, herniorrhaphy, reduction of volvulus
    - Bowel resection with debridement of necrotic tissue

Table 8-5 lists the etiology and clinical presentation of bowel perforations.

Table 8-5. Bowel Perforations

Etiology	Clinical Presentation
Peptic ulcer Bowel obstruction Appendicitis Penetrating wound Ulcerative colitis	Nausea Vomiting Fever, tachypnea, tachycardia Abdominal pain, tenderness that increases with coughing or with hip flexion Rigid abdomen, "boardlike" Rebound tenderness Bowel sounds diminished, absent KUB, free air in peritoneum may be seen
Pathophysiology	
Leakage of GI content into peritoneal cavity → leakage of bacteria causes infection, and chemical irritation causes inflammation of the peritoneum (peritonitis)	

Treatment of Bowel Perforation

- ABCs
- Gastric decompression (N/G tube)
- Fluids/electrolytes
- Treat pain
- Antibiotics, blood cultures
- Monitor for infection, complications
- Appropriate nutritional support
- **Surgery**
  - Repair of perforation, may require temporary bowel diversion to allow anastomosis to heal
  - Antibiotic lavage during surgery

See Table 8-6 for the differentiation of abdominal pain of select disorders.

Table 8-6. Differentiation of Abdominal Pain

Condition	Location of Pain	Quality of Pain	Associated Symptoms
Gastritis	Epigastric or slightly left	Indigestion	Nausea, vomiting May have hematemesis Abdominal tenderness
Peptic ulcer	Epigastric or RUQ	Gnawing, burning	Abdominal tenderness Hematemesis (gastric) or melena (duodenal)

Pancreatitis	Epigastric or LUQ
	May radiate to back,
	   flanks, left shoulder
		Boring
		Worsened by
		   lying down
			Nausea, vomiting
			Mild fever
			Abdominal tenderness

Cholecystitis	Epigastric or RUQ
	May be referred to below
	   right scapula
		Cramping	Nausea, vomiting
			Abdominal tenderness in
			   RUQ

Appendicitis	Epigastric or periumbilical pain, later localizes to RUQ	Dull to sharp	Anorexia, nausea, vomiting Fever, leukocytosis Diarrhea Rebound tenderness
Small bowel obstruction	Across abdomen, in waves, tender to palpation	Cramping, severe, sharp	Distention, vomiting, hypokalemia, hyperactive to hypoactive BS
Ruptured spleen	Left shoulder (Kehr's sign)	Sharp	Abdominal distention, no bowel sounds

Peritonitis "acute abdomen"	Generalized, may become
	localized later
		Dull initially,
		then intensifies
		and worse with
		movement
			Rigid abdomen,
			   "boardlike"
			Rebound tenderness
			Bowel sounds diminished,
			   absent

NUTRITIONAL THERAPY

Indications for Enteral Nutrition

- Use enteral nutrition (EN) in the critically ill patient who is unable to maintain volitional intake.
- EN is the preferred route of feeding over parenteral nutrition (PN).
- EN should be started early within the first 24–48 hrs following admission.
- Feeding should be advanced toward goal over the next 48–72 hrs.
- If patient is hemodynamically unstable, EN should be withheld until the patient is fully resuscitated.
- In the ICU patient population, neither the presence nor absence of bowel sounds and passage of flatus/stool is required for the initiation of enteral feeding.
- In the ICU setting, evidence of resolution of clinical ileus is not required to initiate EN.

Advantages of Enteral Nutrition vs. Parenteral Nutrition

- Provides adequate metabolic support
- Maintains gut structure and function
- Prevents translocation of bacteria, gut toxins
- Associated with fewer complications (infection, problems with catheter placement)
- Less costly, less monitoring required

Complications of Enteral Nutritional Therapy

- Inappropriate tube placement during insertion or maintenance
  - Esophageal placement: increased aspiration
  - Lung placement: pneumothorax, pneumonia
- Pulmonary aspiration
- Digestive intolerance
  - High gastric residual volume, the definition of "high" has increased (see gastric residual volume information later in this section)
  - Diarrhea
  - Constipation
- Tube obstruction

Enteral Nutritional Therapy Nursing Considerations

- Maintain head of bed elevation of 30 degrees
- Use a variety of bedside methods to predict tube location **during** the insertion procedure:
  - Observe for signs of respiratory distress
  - Use capnography if available
  - Measure pH of aspirate from tube if pH strips are available
  - Observe visual characteristics of aspirate from the tube
  - Recognize that auscultatory (air bolus) and water-bubbling methods are unreliable.
- Obtain radiographic confirmation of correct placement of any blindly inserted tube prior to its initial use for feedings or medication administration
  - The radiograph should visualize the entire course of the feeding tube in the gastrointestinal tract
  - Mark and document the tube's exit site from the nose or mouth immediately after radiographic confirmation of correct tube placement
- Check tube location at 4-hour intervals after feedings are started
  - Observe for a change in length of the external portion of the feeding tube (as determined by movement of the marked portion of the tube)
  - Review routine chest and abdominal X-ray reports to look for notations about tube location
  - Observe changes in volume of aspirate from feeding tube
  - Obtain an X-ray to confirm tube position if there is doubt about the tube's location
- The benefit of measuring gastric residual volume (GRV) has now come into question, and the definition of "high" is changing

- Current accepted practice (Bankhead):
  - If the GRV is greater than 250 mL after a second gastric residual check, consider a promotility agent
  - A GRV greater than 500 mL should result in holding the feeding and reassessing the patient tolerance by use of an established algorithm including physical assessment, GI assessment, evaluation of glycemic control, minimization of sedation, and consideration of promotility agent use if not already prescribed
- Use promotility agents to assist in timely gastric emptying, withhold for diarrhea
- Dye should **not** be added to enteral feeding as a method for identifying aspiration of gastric contents.

Indications for Parenteral Nutrition (PN)

- If EN is not feasible or available over the first 7 days following admission to the ICU, no nutritional support therapy should be provided.
- In the patient who was previously healthy before critical illness with no evidence of protein-calorie malnutrition, use of PN should be reserved and initiated only after the first 7 days.
- If there is protein-calorie malnutrition at admission and EN is not feasible, initiate PN ASAP after adequate resuscitation.

NOTE

PN meets total nutritional needs but does not enhance anabolism as well as enteral nutrition support.

Now that you have reviewed key gastrointestinal concepts, go to the Gastrointestinal Practice Questions. Answer the questions, and then check your answers. Continue to review the information until you get at least 80% on the practice questions.

GASTROINTESTINAL PRACTICE QUESTIONS

1. A patient is admitted after an assault with a tire iron. You notice that the patient has a bluish discoloration to her left flank when turned to the side. The patient most likely has:

   (A) retroperitoneal bleeding.
   (B) hemorrhagic pancreatitis.
   (C) ruptured spleen.
   (D) hypocalcemia.

2. A patient is admitted with acute epigastric pain that radiates to his back. He says he has been continuously vomiting for 12 hours and pain has been worsening. He reports drinking 2 six packs of beer a night. His lips are cracked, poor skin turgor, abdomen distended and tender. He is restless and agitated. Vitals are B/P 90/50, HR 135/min, respirations 28/minute. When assessing the B/P, the nurse notices spasms of the patient's hand. This is indicative of:

   (A) hyponatremia due to overhydration.
   (B) metabolic acidosis due to hypoperfusion.
   (C) hypoalbuminemia due to protein loss.
   (D) hypocalcemia due to fat necrosis and calcium precipitation.

3. Which is the most critical concern during the acute phase of care of the patient with an intestinal obstruction?

   (A) aspiration
   (B) hyperkalemia
   (C) hypovolemia
   (D) metabolic alkalosis

4. The following are complications related to the pathophysiologic changes in acute pancreatitis EXCEPT for:

   (A) hyperglycemia related to beta cell injury.
   (B) hypercalcemia due to pancreatic autodigestion.
   (C) ARDS related to Type II alveolar cell injury.
   (D) left atelectasis related to left diaphragm lift.

5. The patient with abdominal trauma and hypovolemic shock was stabilized. However, now hypotension has recurred, urine output has dropped, and BUN and creatinine have increased. You suspect intra-abdominal hypertension. Which of the following interventions would you anticipate?

   (A) Elevate the head of the bed to 45 degrees.
   (B) Remove the nasogastric tube.
   (C) Measure the bladder pressure.
   (D) Withhold opiates.

6. Which of the following is an appropriate intervention related to the patient receiving enteral nutrition via a small-bore feeding tube?

(A) Maintain the head of bed elevation less than 20 degrees.
(B) Hold feeding if diarrhea develops.
(C) Assess placement with air insufflation.
(D) Mark the tube exit site with an indelible marker.

7. The following statements are true regarding liver failure EXCEPT for:

(A) Alcohol abuse is the leading cause of acute liver failure.
(B) Pancytopenia may be a manifestation of the disease.
(C) GI hemorrhage will increase serum NH_3.
(D) Development of hepatic-renal syndrome has high mortality.

8. The patient was admitted with generalized abdominal pain, dull in quality, and diminished bowel sounds, low-grade fever. The patient now complains of more severe pain, worse with movement. On examination, bowel sounds are absent, abdomen is rigid to palpation, and pain is less with palpation down than when released. Which of the following is a priority for the patient at this time?

(A) increase dose of opiate
(B) surgery
(C) insertion of nasogastric tube
(D) antibiotic therapy

9. The patient with esophageal varices was admitted with hypovolemic shock secondary to upper GI bleed. The following interventions related to the care of this patient are appropriate EXCEPT for:

(A) prepare for emergent surgery.
(B) ensure scissors are at the bedside if the patient has an esophageal balloon (Sengstaken-Blakemore tube) in place.
(C) administer sorbitol if the patient has a history of cirrhosis.
(D) closely monitor respiratory and neuro status.

ANSWER KEY

1. **A**	3. **C**	5. **C**	7. **A**	9. **A**
2. **D**	4. **B**	6. **D**	8. **B**	

ANSWERS EXPLAINED

1. **(A)** The flank discoloration is indicative of Grey Turner's sign. The patient's history of trauma may lead to retroperitoneal bleeding. Although Grey Turner's may be due to acute hemorrhagic pancreatitis, choice (B), the history indicates a traumatic etiology rather than pancreatitis. Grey Turner's is not a sign for choices (C) or (D).

2. **(D)** The clinical picture is one of acute pancreatitis. Hand spasms seen in the patient population indicate low calcium due to precipitation of calcium secondary to auto-digestion. The other 3 choices would not result in hand spasm in the setting of acute pancreatitis.

3. **(C)** Sequestration of fluid from the vasculature to third spaces is a life-threatening phenomenon of bowel obstruction, generally worse with small-bowel obstruction. Although aspiration may occur if there is secondary abdominal distention, hyperkalemia and metabolic alkalosis are not associated with bowel obstruction.

4. **(B)** Hypocalcemia (not hypercalcemia) is a complication of acute pancreatitis. The other 3 choices are often a result of acute pancreatitis.

5. **(C)** The patient history of trauma and requirement for fluid resuscitation along with the cardiovascular and renal organ dysfunction points to intra-abdominal pressure elevation. Measurement of bladder pressure and comparison to MAP will help direct therapy. The other 3 choices are not appropriate interventions for increased intra-abdominal pressure.

6. **(D)** The marking can be used as a reference for correct placement. Choices (A), (B), and (C) are not evidence-based practices related to enteral nutritional support.

7. **(A)** The leading cause of acute liver failure is acetaminophen overdose; alcohol abuse is the leading cause of chronic liver failure. Choices (B), (C), and (D) are all signs of liver failure.

8. **(B)** The clinical picture is one of peritonitis. Addressing the problem surgically will prevent increased morbidity. Although the patient may need the other 3 choices, these will not definitively treat the urgent problem.

9. **(A)** Surgery is not indicated for esophageal varices. Rather, endoscopic procedures (banding, sclerosing) will address the cause more effectively. Esophageal balloon therapy may be used. If so, scissors should be at the bedside in order to cut the esophageal balloon in the event it displaces upward and occludes the airway. Sorbitol may be needed to move blood quickly from the bowel and decrease ammonia, choice (C). Choice (D) is indicated since aspiration and encephalopathy are possible complications.

Renal Concepts

9

A dream doesn't become reality through magic; it takes sweat, determination, and hard work.

—Colin Powell

RENAL TEST BLUEPRINT

Renal 6% of total test   **9 Questions**

→ Acute renal failure
→ Chronic renal failure
→ Life-threatening electrolyte imbalances

RENAL TESTABLE NURSING ACTIONS

☐ Recognize normal and abnormal physical assessment findings
☐ Identify and monitor normal and abnormal diagnostic test results
☐ Manage patients receiving renal medications, and monitor response
☐ Recognize indications for and manage patients requiring renal therapeutic intervention (e.g., CRRT, peritoneal dialysis)
☐ Monitor patients and follow protocols for:

  ○ Renal surgery
  ○ Pre-, intra- and post-procedure (e.g., renal biopsy, ultrasound)

☐ Recognize signs and symptoms of renal emergencies
☐ Initiate interventions, and seek assistance as needed

RENAL ANATOMIC CONCEPTS

- The nephron is the functional unit of the kidneys, whose structure is complex
- Each kidney has approximately 1 million nephrons, and each nephron has a vascular system and a tubular system (Table 9-1).

NOTE

The vascular
system of the
kidney, unlike
other organs,
has 2 arterioles,
an afferent and
efferent.

Table 9-1. Vascular and Tubular Systems of the Nephron

Vascular System	Tubular System
Artery	Bowman's capsule
Afferent arteriole	Proximal tubule
Capillary (glomerulus)	Loop of Henle
Efferent arteriole	Distal tubule
Vein	Collecting duct

- If the blood pressure falls and renal perfusion is decreased, the compensatory response at the level of the nephron occurs (Figure 9-1)
  - Afferent arteriole DILATES, increasing flow to the glomerular capillaries AND efferent arteriole CONSTRICTS, decreasing flow from the glomerular capillaries
  - These two mechanisms above result in an increased pressure gradient within the capillary bed.
- Any condition that prevents afferent arteriolar dilation or efferent arteriolar constriction interferes with this compensatory mechanism

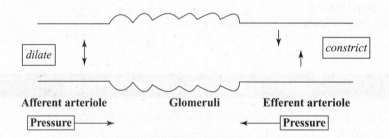

Figure 9-1. Renal arterioles

PREVENTION OF ACUTE RENAL FAILURE

Prevention is of vital importance in the critically ill!

- Identify patient comorbidities that put them at increased risk
  - Diabetes
  - Heart failure
  - Hypertension
- Avoid potentially nephrotoxic substances as able, or monitor renal function more closely if administered
  - Antibiotics
  - NSAIDs
  - ACE inhibitors, ARBs
  - Antineoplastics
  - Contrast media
  - Diuretics, if overused and result in vascular volume depletion

- Careful assessment and monitoring of:
  - Fluid balance (especially in patients presenting with signs of hypovolemia or who are being treated with diuretics)
  - Hemodynamics, hypotension
  - Renal function, labs
  - Urine output (decreased urine OP and use of appropriate types and doses of meds)

Assessment of Fluid, Electrolyte, and Renal Status

LAB VALUES

- Blood urea nitrogen (BUN)
  - Measures the amount of nitrogen in the blood that comes from the waste product urea (formed in liver)
  - Dehydration and shock may elevate BUN, not the best parameter for monitoring renal function or glomerular filtration rate (GFR)
  - Normal 10–23 mg/dL
- Creatinine
  - A non-protein waste product of creatinine phosphate metabolism by skeletal muscle tissue
  - Better indicator of renal function (GFR) than BUN
  - Normal: males 0.8–1.4 mg/dL; females 0.6–1.1 mg/dL
- 24-hour urine for creatinine clearance **is the best indicator of the glomerular filtration rate (GFR)**
  - Variables needed to calculate include urine creatinine, serum creatinine, and volume of urine

Glomerular Filtration Rate (GFR)

- GFR is the **volume** of plasma filtered from the glomerular capillaries into Bowman's capsule per minute
- Normal GFR = 125 mL/minute, total blood volume filtered ~ 60 times per day!
- Normal urine volume is ~ 1,000 mL/day, > 99% reabsorption of filtrate
- $Cr.Cl. = \dfrac{(140 - age) \times (IBW) \times (0.85 \text{ if female})}{72 \times serum\ creatinine}$
- The GFR is inversely related to the **serum creatinine** (NOT the BUN).
- Only small molecules are filtered; the presence of large molecules (protein) in urine indicates glomerular damage.
- Urinalysis, spot urine electrolytes, culture
  - Visual exam
  - Proteinuria
    - Normoalbuminuria, less than 20 mg/day albumin
    - Microalbuminuria, persistent excretion 30–300 mg/day
    - Important in detecting **EARLY** diabetic nephropathy
    - Proteinuria, albumin excretion of > 300 mg/day

> **NOTE**
>
> **Do not memorize the formula for the test. However, be aware of the importance of patient's age, sex, size, and serum creatinine when calculating the GFR.**

NOTE

The patient may
have edema
yet have
intravascular
dehydration.

- ○ Specific gravity (1.010–1.020)
- ○ Casts
- ○ Spot urine Na$^+$; normal 40–220, see further information below
- ○ Culture/sensitivities for select patients
- Electrolytes: see Table 9-7 later in this section
- Serum albumin: if low, there may be a decrease in oncotic pressure, increased third spacing, decreased vascular volume
- Serum CK: extremely high is indicative of rhabdomyolysis (see below)
- ABGs: metabolic acidosis if in intrarenal failure with renal injury due to abnormal excretion of acids

Renal Assessment—Clinical

- Flank pain: possible infection
- Bladder distension: obstruction
- Ultrasound: kidney size, stones, urine retention

Definitions Related to Types of Renal Failure

NOTE

Do not memorize
the RIFLE
criteria for the
test. However,
familiarize
yourself with the
categories.

- Acute renal failure or, now often referred to as acute kidney injury **(AKI),** is an increase in serum creatinine by ≥ 1.5 of baseline within 7 days
- Stages of acute kidney injury are defined according to serum creatinine and urine output (Table 9-2)

Table 9-2. RIFLE Criteria for Renal Failure

Stage	Serum Creatinine Criteria	Urine Output Criteria
Risk	Increase in serum creatinine by 1.5 to < 2 times baseline	UO < 0.5 mL/kg/h x 6 hours
Injury	Increase in SCr by 2.0 to < 3.0 times baseline	UO < 0.5 mL/kg/h x 12 hours
Failure	Increase in SCr by ≥ 3.0 times baseline	UO < 0.5 mL/kg/h x 12 hours or anuria x 12 hours
Loss	Persistent acute kidney injury for > 4 weeks	
End-stage kidney disease	Persistent acute kidney injury for > 3 months	

- In addition to the stages of the RIFLE criteria, acute renal failure can be categorized as prerenal, intrarenal, and postrenal.

PRERENAL FAILURE

- Prerenal failure: perfusion is reduced to the kidneys (Figure 9-2 and Table 9-3), but there is no destruction of the tubular basement membranes
- Most common type of acute renal failure, seldom requires hemodialysis

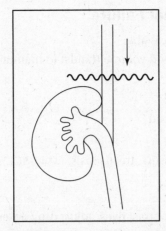

Figure 9-2. Illustration of prerenal failure

Table 9-3. Etiologies of Prerenal Failure

Impaired Cardiac Performance	Vasodilation	Intravascular Volume Depletion
Heart failure Myocardial infarction Cardiogenic shock Pericardial tamponade Dysrhythmias with low CO Acute pulmonary embolism	Sepsis Anaphylaxis Drugs (ACE inhibitors)	Volume depletion • Hemorrhage • GI losses Renal losses • Osmotic diuresis • Diuretic drugs Volume shifts • Burns • Pancreatitis • Ileus Inadequate volume replacement
	Vasoconstriction	
	Pressors Compensatory response	

Drugs That May Contribute to Prerenal Failure

- NSAIDs
  - Block production of prostaglandins in afferent arteriole → results in afferent arteriole constriction, ↓ inflow of blood into glomerulus → GFR is ↓
  - Can result with normal doses, especially when associated with other renal risks, e.g., heart failure, sepsis, pre-existing renal insufficiency

- ACE inhibitors
  - Prevent production of angiotensin II, efferent arteriole will remain in a **dilated** state
  - Prevents the maintenance of adequate glomeruli pressure
  - May cause problems for patients dependent upon efferent arteriole constriction to maintain adequate pressure within the glomeruli, e.g., heart failure and hypovolemia

Prerenal failure _can_ **progress to intrarenal failure if not corrected!**

Management of Prerenal Failure

- Correct underlying problem as able
- Restore effective arterial blood volume (fluids) to maintain MAP > 70 mmHg in order to improve renal perfusion
- Improve cardiac performance
  - Decrease preload/afterload
  - Improve contractility
- Control vasodilatation: pressors, treat sepsis, avoid ACEIs, NSAIDs in high risk populations
- I&O with weight correlation
- Avoid nephrotoxic agents, contrast dyes, adjust drug doses
- Wean pressors as able

INTRARENAL FAILURE

- Intrarenal failure: destruction of the tubular basement membrane occurs (Figure 9-3 and Table 9-4)

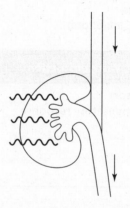

Figure 9-3. Illustration of intrarenal failure

Table 9-4. Etiologies of Intrarenal Failure

| Cortical | Medullary (ATN)* | |
	Nephrotoxic (Often Non-oliguric, Better Prognosis)	Ischemic (Often Oliguric, Worse Prognosis)
Post-infectious (strep, hepatitis, varicella) Systemic lupus erythematosus (SLE) Vasculitis	Contrast dye Drugs (antibiotics, NSAIDs) Rhabdomyolysis Organic solvents	All causes of prerenal, postrenal failure Surgery (CABG, vascular, valve) Cardiopulmonary bypass Hypotension (sepsis, hypovolemia)

*ATN is the most common type of hospital-acquired intrarenal failure and is usually caused by **prolonged** hypoperfusion of the kidneys.

Contrast Medium Nephropathy

RISKS

- Pre-existing renal insufficiency
- Diabetes
- Dehydration
- Heart failure
- Elderly
- Large doses of contrast material
- Use of NSAIDs
- Use of ACEIs
- Use of metformin

SIGNS

- Anuria
- Elevated BUN
- Creatinine, fluid overload

INITIAL TREATMENT

- Diuretics if no response
- Treat as intrarenal failure

Prevention of Contrast Medium Nephropathy

- Evaluate risks, weigh risks/benefits
- Hydrate (0.9 NS) before procedure (1 mL/kg/hr) for 6–12 hrs prior and 4 hrs or > afterward
  - Hydration ↑ renal prostaglandins → improves renal medullary blood flow
- **OR**, hydrate with D5W with sodium bicarb before procedure (3 mL/kg) for 1 hour and after (1 mL/kg)
  - Alkaline urine may reduce free radicals
- Avoid offending drugs
- Use iso-osmolar rather than low-osmolar contrast media; may help, conflicting data
- Decrease volume of dye given
- Use of acetylcysteine (before or after procedure) is not shown to be effective in studies; this will most likely not be seen on the exam

Rhabdomyolysis (Table 9-5)

- Causes include crush injuries, prolonged immobility, compartment syndrome, hyperthermia, delirium tremens (DTs)
- Release of myoglobin, creatinine phosphokinase (CK), potassium into the extracellular and intravascular spaces due to damaged muscles
- Creatinine kinase and myoglobin obstruct renal tubules
- Clinical sequelae:
  - Hypovolemia
  - Hyperkalemia
  - Metabolic acidosis
  - Acute renal failure

Table 9-5. Rhabdomyolysis

Signs/Symptoms	Treatment
Dark, tea-colored urine	Fluids (0.9 NS) to maintain urine flow of
Low urine output	~ 300 mL/hr, may need up to
Positive on dipstick for hemoglobin but no	500 mL/hour to do so
RBC on UA	Bicarbonate infusion to alkalinize urine
Myoglobin in urine	Mannitol
Elevated CK > 10,000 U/L	Monitor for and treat hyperkalemia
Muscle cramping	Therapy should continue until myoglobin
Arrhythmias	clears from urine

Management of Acute Intrarenal Failure

- Maintain fluid volume: monitor for fluid overload
  - Administer loop diuretics, furosemide acts on the ascending limb of the loop of Henle to decrease sodium and water reabsorption
  - Often used to attempt to "convert" non-oliguric to oliguric renal failure
- Maintain normal electrolyte balance: treat life-threatening electrolyte imbalances, especially hyperkalemia
- Maintain acid-base: dialyze for extreme metabolic acidosis
- Prevent uremia: dialyze early
- Prevent infection: highest cause of mortality, poorer immune function
- Address anemia: use packed red blood cells for extreme anemia; epogen is used for chronic patients
- Prevent bleeding: platelet counts are normal, but platelet function is affected by renal failure
- Adjust drug doses: lower
- Prevent malnutrition: do not restrict protein
- Dialysis as needed

> Who is most likely a candidate for dialysis? If the patient has any of the "AEIOU" criteria:
>
> Acidemia
> Electrolyte disorders (hyperkalemia)
> Intoxication (methanol, ethylene glycol, aspirin, lithium, theophylline)
> Overload (heart failure)
> Uremia (elevated BUN with associated mental status changes)

Types of Dialysis Therapy

- Hemodialysis
  - Double-lumen central line access (temporary or permanent catheter)
  - Fistula access
  - A-V graft access

- Peritoneal is not often used for acutely/critically ill but may be admitted with peritoneal dialysis access
- Continuous renal replacement therapy (CRRT)
  - Considered in certain patients with ARF
    - Hemodynamically unstable patients who cannot tolerate rapid fluid shifts that occur with intermittent hemodialysis
    - During CRRT, after insertion of a double-lumen central venous line, the blood is continually passed through a filtration circuit via a machine to a filter where waste products and water are removed; replacement fluid is added, and the filtered blood is returned to the patient

Differentiation of Prerenal and Intrarenal Failure

- Occasionally, the patient history, clinical presentation, and labs do not clearly put the patient in either the prerenal (risk) or intrarenal (injury) categories and additional labs will be examined (Table 9-6)

☆ **Table 9-6. Differentiation of Prerenal (Risk) and Intrarenal (Injury)**

Laboratory Values	Prerenal	Intrarenal
BUN:creatinine ratio	20–40:1	10–15:1
Urine sodium	<20 mEq/L	> 20 mEq/L
Urine concentration	Concentrated	Dilute
Urine osmolality	High (> 500)	Low (< 300)
Specific gravity	High (< 1.020)	Low (< 1.010)
Urinary sediment	Normal (Hyaline casts)	Abnormal (Cellular casts and debris)
Fractional excretion of sodium	≤ 1%	> 1%
Response to Lasix	> 40 mL/hr	No response

- When the BUN is elevated, look at the BUN:creatinine ratio
  - Wide ratio, 20–40:1 is usually associated with prerenal failure
  - Narrower ratio, 10–15:1 ratio is usually associated with intrarenal failure

- BUN:creatinine ratio examples:
  - BUN 90, creatinine 2.8: prerenal
  - BUN 50, creatinine 11: intrarenal
  - BUN 90, creatinine 9.5: intrarenal
  - BUN 70, creatinine 3.1: prerenal
  - BUN 108, creatinine 4.8: prerenal

- In general, when the renal tubules are still able to function, the urine sodium may be low (able to hold onto sodium) and the osmolality is high (able to concentrate urine)

- Accounts for 5–10% of the cases of ARF
- Caused by any obstruction in the flow of urine from the collecting ducts in the kidney to the external urethral orifice (Figure 9-4)
  - Examples: ureteral blockage (bilateral renal stones), urethral blockage (prostate stricture or BPH), neurogenic bladder, or extrinsic source (tumor)

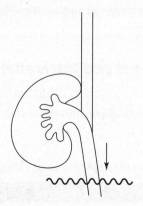

Figure 9-4. Illustration of postrenal failure

NOTE

Postrenal renal failure may progress to intrarenal renal failure if not corrected!

Treatment of Postrenal Failure

- Identify and correct obstruction
- Recovery of renal function is directly proportional to the duration of the obstruction
- Generally, easiest renal failure to treat

Life-Threatening Electrolyte Abnormalities (Table 9-7)

The Adult CCRN Test blueprint includes life-threatening electrolyte abnormalities. If you become familiar with the information in the following table, you will be ready for these questions!

Table 9-7. Electrolyte Abnormalities

Electrolyte Problem	Signs/Symptoms	Causes	Treatment
Calcium (Ca^{++}): Normal 8.5–10.5 mg/dL			
Hypocalcemia	Anxiety, irritability Twitching around mouth Laryngospasm Seizures **Chvostek** sign (below) **Trousseau** sign (below) Torsades VT	Acute pancreatitis Massive infection of subcutaneous tissues Hypoparathyroidism Chronic renal failure Vitamin D deficiency Hypoalbuminemia Alkalotic states: hyperventilation, prolonged vomiting	IV fluids, normal saline Calcium gluconate or calcium chloride, vitamin D Correct respiratory alkalosis
Positive Chvostek sign (spasm of lip and cheek)		Positive Trousseau sign (carpopedal spasm)	

Positive Chvostek sign (spasm of lip and cheek)

Positive Trousseau sign (carpopedal spasm)

Electrolyte Problem	Signs/Symptoms	Causes	Treatment
Hypercalcemia	Lethargy, fatigue, altered mental status DTRs decreased to absent Abdominal pain, constipation Muscle weakness N/V, "metallic" taste Anorexia, weight loss Kidney stones	Renal disease Hyperparathyroidism Prolonged immobilization, bed rest Malignancies	IV 0.9 NS to promote diuresis Promote renal excretion with furosemide; note, first rule out hypokalemia Glucocorticoids, decrease GI absorption of Ca^{++} Mithracin IV, calcitonin, or etidronate; decrease Ca^{++} release from bones
Potassium (K$^+$): Normal 3.5–5.0 mEq/L			
Hyperkalemia	Muscle weakness; irritability Nausea, diarrhea Muscle cramps, pain ECG changes • Peaked T-waves • Widening of QRS • Loss of P-waves • Bradycardia • PEA	Renal failure Burns (early) Massive crush injuries Excessive potassium intake Acidosis, relative Adrenal cortical insufficiency	Calcium chloride (or gluconate), sodium bicarbonate, insulin/glucose, albuterol Elimination of potassium intake Correct acidosis Kayexalate Dialysis
Hypokalemia	Muscles weakness, ↓ reflexes Nausea, vomiting Paralytic ileus or abdominal distention/gas Shallow respirations Mental depression ECG changes; fast, irritable (VT/VF)	Diuretics Metabolic alkalosis Acute alcoholism Uncontrolled diabetes Excessive perspiration Excess production of aldosterone Cirrhosis	KCl Correct alkalosis IV lactated Ringer's Correct hypomagnesemia

Table 9-7. Electrolyte Abnormalities (continued)

Electrolyte Problem	Signs/Symptoms	Causes	Treatment
Sodium (Na$^+$): Normal 135–145 mEq/L			
Hypernatremia	Classic signs of hypovolemic hypernatremia (thirst, tachycardia, orthostasis, and hypotension) may be present, as can dry, sticky mucous membranes Restlessness and irritability to obtundation, stupor, coma	Insensible losses, dehydration Osmotic diuresis, mannitol Diabetic ketoacidosis (DKA) Hyperglycemic hyperosmotic syndrome (HHS) Diabetes insipidus (DI)	Identify cause, evaluate urine Na$^+$ (will be > 20 if hypervolemic, variable with the other 2 causes) Correct slowly to prevent cerebral edema D5W, 0.45 NS Sodium restriction Vasopressin for DI
Hyponatremia	Edema Fatigue, muscle cramps, weakness Abdominal cramps, diarrhea Lethargy, confusion, ↓DTRs Seizures, coma, brain herniation	Fluid overload: heart failure, cirrhosis Excessive water ingestion Excessive infusion of D5W SIADH	If hypervolemic or euvolemic, water restriction Loop diuretics Dehydration with Na$^+$ deficits, 0.9 NS Water intoxication: water restriction, avoid hypotonic fluids Acute, severe: 3% saline, small amounts
Magnesium (Mg^{++}): Normal 1.5–2.5 mEq/L			
Hypermagnesemia	Decreased DTRs, respiratory depression, arrest Bradyarrhythmias, hypotension Lethargy, coma N/V Flushing	Renal failure Mag-containing laxative abuse Mag-containing antacid abuse Iatrogenic OD	Stop magnesium substances Give calcium as for hyperkalemia Furosemide as for hypercalcemia if renal function OK May need dialysis
Hypomagnesemia	Hyperreflexia (Chvostek sign, Trousseau sign) Ventricular arrhythmias, PSVT Sensitivity to digoxin Insulin resistance, hypokalemia, hypocalcemia, hypophosphatemia Agitation, confusion Impedes correction of low K$^+$	Chronic alcoholism (most common cause!) Vomiting, diarrhea, NG suction malabsorption Post-CABG or AMI DKA, HHS, hyperthyroidism Nephrotic syndrome Drugs: aminoglycosides, diuretics, ETOH, dig, cisplatin Malnutrition, enteral or parenteral feedings	MgSO$_4$, generally max of 1 gram/minute
Phosphate (Ph^{++}): Normal: 3–4.5 mEq/L			
Hypophosphatemia	Same as hypercalcemia Lethargy, fatigue, altered mental status DTRs decreased to absent Abdominal pain, peptic ulcers, constipation Muscle weakness, hypoventilation	Due to ↑cellular uptake of phosphorous with TPN admin ↑glucose admin (TPN) Alcoholism	Replace
Hyperphosphatemia	Same as hypocalcemia Anxiety, irritability Twitching around mouth Laryngospasm Seizures	Due to ↓ renal excretion, renal failure	Phosphate binders (Amphogel), calcium carbonate (Caltrate)

Now that you have reviewed key renal concepts, go to the Renal Practice Questions. Answer the questions, and then check your answers. Continue to review the information until you get at least 80% on the practice questions.

RENAL PRACTICE QUESTIONS

1. A patient with renal failure has the following blood gas: pH 7.32, $PaCO_2$ 35, HCO_3 18. This acid-base abnormality is the result of the kidney's inability to:

   (A) excrete acid by-products of metabolism.
   (B) excrete carbon dioxide.
   (C) excrete bicarbonate ions.
   (D) excrete calcium ions.

2. The action of furosemide (Lasix) includes which of the following?

   (A) acts as an osmotic agent pulling fluid into the renal tubule
   (B) acts on the ascending limb of the loop of Henle to decrease sodium and water reabsorption
   (C) acts as an ADH antagonist
   (D) acts as an aldosterone antagonist

3. What is the best lab test to evaluate the patient's glomerular filtration rate?

   (A) blood urea nitrogen (BUN)
   (B) serum creatinine
   (C) urine creatinine clearance
   (D) serum amylase

4. After CT scan with contrast infusion, which of the following nursing interventions is most important?

   (A) ensuring adequate fluid intake
   (B) maintaining fluid restriction
   (C) providing extra doses of sodium
   (D) administering antibiotics

5. A 35-year-old man developed ARF after upper GI bleeding secondary to esophageal varices in which he lost a great deal of blood. Which of the following lab results would he be expected to have?

   (A) low urine osmolality, high urine sodium concentration
   (B) high urine osmolality, high urine sodium concentration
   (C) low urine osmolality, low urine sodium concentration
   (D) high urine osmolality, low urine sodium concentration

6. A patient has a serum K$^+$ of 8.8 mEq/L and has slowing of the heart rate with widening of the QRS. Which of the following would be an appropriate treatment?

   (A) Kayexalate enema
   (B) calcium gluconate, glucose, and insulin intravenously
   (C) sorbitol by mouth
   (D) hemodialysis

For questions 7 and 8

A female patient, brought in after having fallen on the kitchen floor and unable to move for approximately 48 hours, has dark tea-colored urine, urine positive for myoglobin, BUN 52 mEq/L, serum creatinine 4.2 mEq/L, and serum potassium 5.6 mEq/L.

7. Which of the following is a priority treatment for the patient?

   (A) Administer a loop diuretic.
   (B) Administer an amp of sodium bicarbonate.
   (C) Administer 0.9 normal saline at a rate to maintain a urine output of 300 mL/hour.
   (D) Dialyze the patient as soon as possible.

8. Which of the lab values below would be an expected finding of the patient described?

   (A) CK 30,000
   (B) amylase 500
   (C) troponin 12
   (D) bilirubin 4.2

   _____

9. A 17-year-old male patient who sustained multiple trauma and subsequent multisystem organ dysfunction has a BUN of 60 mEq/L, serum creatinine of 6.1 mEq/L, fluid overload, and blood pressure 98/50 mmHg. Which of the following is the most appropriate treatment for this patient?

   (A) loop diuretics
   (B) hemodialysis
   (C) peritoneal dialysis
   (D) continuous renal replacement therapy (CRRT)

ANSWER KEY

1. **A**   3. **C**   5. **D**   7. **C**   9. **D**
2. **B**   4. **A**   6. **B**   8. **A**

ANSWERS EXPLAINED

1. **(A)** When the body accumulates H^+, bicarbonate drops (HCO_3 of 18) in an attempt to neutralize the acid. Excretion of carbon dioxide is not a problem as evidenced by the normal $PaCO_2$. Excretion of bicarbonate ions is not the problem; this would be evidenced by elevated bicarbonate level. The example does not address calcium ions.

2. **(B)** Furosemide acts in the ascending Loop of Henle (remember Lasix, loop). A decrease in sodium and water reabsorption leads to a diuresis. Furosemide is not an osmotic agent. Instead, mannitol acts in this manner. It does not act as an ADH antagonist or as an aldosterone-antagonist.

3. **(C)** Urine creatinine clearance best reflects the glomerular filtration (GFR) or tubular function. BUN may be altered by volume depletion, and serum amylase does not reflect renal function. Although serum creatinine is needed to calculate GFR and is a better reflection of tubular function than BUN, it does not take into account the variables that urine creatinine clearance includes.

4. **(A)** Exposure to contrast used for the test can cause contrast nephropathy in at-risk patients. An increase in fluid (especially prior to the procedure) has been shown to prevent renal damage. The other 3 choices either increase the chance of nephropathy or do not prevent it.

5. **(D)** Initially, volume depletion will result in acute prerenal failure, yet the basement membranes of the renal tubules are not affected (intrarenal failure). The tubules can still concentrate urine and hold onto sodium. Choice (A) is seen in intrarenal failure. The other 2 choices are not typical of any renal problem.

6. **(B)** Calcium will stabilize cell membranes. Insulin will drive potassium into the intracellular space, thereby decreasing serum potassium. Kayexalate and hemodialysis will decrease total body potassium but will take hours. Sorbitol does not decrease potassium.

7. **(C)** The clinical scenario describes rhabdomyolysis (tea-colored urine, urine positive for myoglobin). Administration of large volumes of fluid in order to maintain "flushing" of the kidneys is needed to prevent permanent renal tubular damage. Diuretics and hemodialysis have not been shown to prevent permanent damage. Alkalization of urine is beneficial. However, it is done by placing sodium bicarbonate into large-volume IV bags and infusing it over several hours. The patient should not be given undiluted IV.

8. **(A)** Rhabdomyolysis is due to crush injury of skeletal muscle cells, which releases myoglobin and CK into the blood that may "clog" renal tubules. The other 3 lab results are not typical of rhabdomyolysis.

9. **(D)** The patient has acute renal failure with hemodynamic instability. CRRT is less likely than hemodialysis to worsen hemodynamic status. The other 2 choices have not been shown to improve the outcome of acute renal failure.

Endocrine Concepts

10

*You've got to do your own growing no matter how tall your
grandfather was.*

—Irish saying

ENDOCRINE TEST BLUEPRINT

Endocrine 4% of total test   **6 Questions**

→ Acute hypoglycemia
→ Diabetes insipidus (DI)
→ Diabetic ketoacidosis (DKA)
→ Hyperglycemic hyperosmolar nonketotic syndrome (HHNK)*
→ Syndrome of inappropriate secretion of antidiuretic hormone (SIADH)

*Now more commonly referred to as hyperosmolar hyperglycemic syndrome (HHS)

ENDOCRINE TESTABLE NURSING ACTIONS

☐ Recognize normal and abnormal physical assessment findings
☐ Recognize signs and symptoms of endocrine emergencies, initiate interventions, and
seek assistance as needed
☐ Identify and monitor normal and abnormal diagnostic test results
☐ Implement treatment modalities for acute hypoglycemia/hyperglycemia (e.g., insulin
therapy)
☐ Monitor patient and follow protocols for surgery related to the endocrine system
☐ Manage patients receiving medications and monitor response

ASSESSMENT OVERVIEW OF ENDOCRINE EMERGENCIES

Serum Osmolality

- Endocrine problems often result in abnormalities of serum osmolality (osmo), therefore
a general knowledge of the regulation of serum osmolality is needed
- Osmolality of body fluids: the measure of the number of particles in a solution
  - Expressed as milliosmoles
  - Normal osmolality of body fluids is 275–295 mOsm/kg

- Hypo-osmolar < 275
- Hyperosmolar > 295

- Cell membranes are permeable to water, therefore serum osmo will affect the intracellular fluid (ICF) osmo
- On examination of the equation for determination of calculated serum osmolality, note that serum sodium, BUN and glucose each play a role:

$$2(Na^+) + \frac{BUN}{5} + \frac{Glucose}{20} = 275\text{–}295 \text{ mOsm/kg}$$

- According to the formula above, an increase in serum sodium, BUN, and/or glucose will affect the serum osmo, **increasing** the serum osmolality

TIP

Do not memorize the formula for the test, but be aware of the variables that affect osmolality.

Hypothalamus

- The hypothalamus (via pituitary gland) is the endocrine "monitoring central" and regulates:
  - Temperature
  - Intake drives
  - Autonomic nervous system (sympathetic/ parasympathetic)
- Only the pancreas and parathyroid release hormones that are not controlled by hypothalamus

Antidiuretic Hormone (ADH) Imbalances

- ADH is formed in hypothalamus
- Stored in posterior pituitary
- Works on distal convoluted and collecting tubule of kidney to **reabsorb water** (prevents diuresis)
- Concentrates urine
  - Normal urine osmolality (1.010–1.020)

SYNDROME OF INAPPROPRIATE ADH (SIADH)

The pathophysiology of SIADH is shown in Figure 10-1.

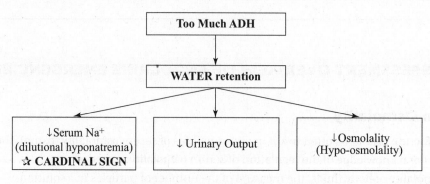

Figure 10-1. Pathophysiology of SIADH

Etiology of SIADH

- Oat cell carcinoma
- Viral pneumonia — Most Common
- Head problems
- Increased osmolality, anesthesia, analgesia, stress
- Thiazide diuretics (especially elderly)
- ☆ What is the biggest danger of hyponatremia? **SEIZURE!**

Treatment of SIADH

- Address etiology:
  - Oat cell carcinoma
  - Viral pneumonia
  - Head problems
- Fluid restriction
- 3% saline (generally reserved for serum Na$^+$ less than 120 mEq/L)
- Administer phenytoin (Dilantin) → inhibits ADH secretion
- NO hypotonic solutions or free water

DIABETES INSIPIDUS (DI)

The pathophysiology of diabetes insipidus is described in Figure 10-2.

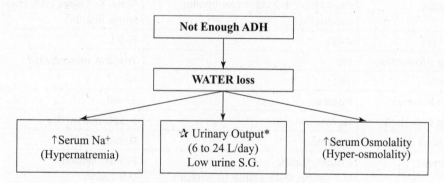

Figure 10-2. Pathophysiology of DI

☆ *DILUTE** urine (specific gravity 1.001–1.005)

Etiology of DI

- Head problems (surgery, trauma)
- Phenytoin (Dilantin)

Complication of DI

- Hypovolemia, hypovolemic shock

Treatment of DI

- Give ADH (pitressin, DDAVP), use cautiously in those with heart disease, may cause coronary artery ischemia
- Give fluids to replenish intravascular volume
- Monitor urinary output/specific gravity

DIABETIC KETOACIDOSIS (DKA) AND HYPEROSMOLAR HYPERGLYCEMIC STATE (HHS)

- Diabetic ketoacidosis (DKA) and hyperosmolar hyperglycemic state or HHS (a.k.a. hyperglycemic hyperosmolar nonketotic syndrome or HHNK) are included in the test blueprint. The best way to prepare for questions related to these 2 problems is to compare and contrast them (Table 10-1).

☆ Table 10-1. Comparison of DKA and HHS

	DKA	HHS
Etiologies	Younger Type I diabetes New onset Type I Infection Stress Noncompliance	Older Type II diabetes Pancreatitis Total parenteral nutrition (TPN) Steroid use
Blood sugar	> 250 mg/dL	> 600 mg/dL
Develops	Rapid over 1–2 days (no insulin production)	Slow, 5–7 days (still making some insulin)
Fluid loss	4–6 L	6–9 L
Insulin production	No	Yes, but inadequate
Acidosis	Yes	No
Serum ketones	Positive	Small
Serum osmolality	Normal or high	> 320 mOsm/kg
Breathing pattern	Kussmaul	Rapid, shallow
Treatment	Insulin, fluids 0.9 saline, 0.45 saline (if sodium high and B/P normal or high) Decrease blood sugar by 50–100 mg/dL/hour Add dextrose to IV fluids after serum glucose reaches ~ 250 mg/dL Continue insulin infusion until acidosis is resolved	Fluids, insulin 0.9 saline Decrease blood sugar by 50–100 mg/dL/hour Add dextrose to IV fluids after serum glucose reaches ~ 300 mg/dL
Serum K^+	Elevated K^+ in the presence of acidosis, although total body potassium is low (see Table 10-2); it decreases as acidosis is corrected	Often elevated due to insulin deficiency

- In a state of metabolic acidosis, hydrogen ions (H^+) move into the intracellular space. In exchange, potassium leaves the intracellular space. The movement of K^+ into the extracellular space results in hyperkalemia, yet total body K^+ has not increased.
- For every 0.1 decrease in pH, the serum K^+ will increase by 0.6 mEq/L (Table 10-2).

Table 10-2. Arterial pH and K^+ Relationship in the Presence of Acidosis

pH	K^+
7.40	4.0
7.30	4.6
7.20	5.2
7.10	5.8
7.0	6.4

- If pH is 7.2 and K^+ is 4.0, total body (ICF and serum), relative, hypokalemia!
- With DKA, there may be total body hypokalemia due to diuresis that occurred due to elevated blood sugar.

ACUTE HYPOGLYCEMIA

Etiology of Acute Hypoglycemia (Table 10-3)

- Insulin if dose more than body requirements
- Oral hypoglycemic agents if dose more than body requires
- Increase in physical activity of diabetics . . . ↑ in utilization of glucose
- Septic shock in late stages, not well understood
- Beta blockers mask early signs of hypoglycemia (for Type I diabetics)

Table 10-3. Signs and Symptoms of Hypoglycemia

Initial Signs/Symptoms (Due to sympathetic effects of adrenaline release in an attempt to raise glucose)	Later Signs/Symptoms (Due to lack of glucose on the brain)
Tachycardia	Confusion
Palpitations	Lethargy
Diaphoresis	Slurred speech
Irritability	Seizure
Restlessness	Coma

☆ **Note:** If the diabetic patient becomes hypoglycemic and is receiving beta-adrenergic blocking agents, the initial signs of hypoglycemia may be masked. The patient's first signs of hypoglycemia will be the later signs. You need to be aware of this, especially for patients with Type I diabetes.

Treatment of Hypoglycemia

- Complex carbohydrates by mouth
- 50% dextrose if unable to take oral carbohydrates (irritates vein)
- 10% dextrose infusion for refractory hypoglycemia
- Glucagon 1 mg
  - ↓ GI motility, monitor for nausea/vomiting

Now that you have reviewed key endocrine concepts, go to the Endocrine Practice Questions. Answer the questions, and then check your answers. Continue to review the information until you get at least 80% on the practice questions.

ENDOCRINE PRACTICE QUESTIONS

1. A patient was admitted with blood sugar 450, potassium of 4.5 mEq/L, and initial pH of 7.15. She received an insulin loading dose and infusion, 2 L normal saline. Now the blood sugar is 215 and the pH is 7.32. Which of the following would be appropriate at this time?

   (A) change the IV solution to lactated Ringer's
   (B) add potassium to the IV solution
   (C) administer sodium bicarbonate
   (D) increase the insulin infusion

For questions 2 and 3

A post-op craniotomy patient began having hourly urine output of 400–500 mL/hour, serum glucose 100, B/P 100/68, HR 102/min, RR 22/min.

2. Which of the following lab results would you expect for this patient?

   (A) serum osmolality 265 mOsm/kg
   (B) specific gravity 1.030, Na^+ 120 mEq/L
   (C) serum osmolality 280 mOsm/kg
   (D) specific gravity 1.001, Na^+ 151 mEq/L

3. The IV solution most appropriate at this time for the patient described would be:

   (A) lactated Ringer's
   (B) 5% dextrose in water
   (C) normal saline
   (D) 10% dextrose in water

4. A 64-year-old female patient was admitted with new onset seizure she had at home. She has a history of oat cell carcinoma of the lung for which she had treatment over the past 6 months. CT of the head was negative; additional findings included Na^+ 116 mEq/L, K^+ 3.9 mEq/L, urine output 25 mL/hour, serum osmolality 260 mOsm/kg, urine specific gravity 1.030. Which of the following interventions is indicated for this patient?

   (A) restrict free water
   (B) administer NSAIDs
   (C) 0.45 normal saline fluid boluses
   (D) administer pitressin

5. A 25-year-old male with Type I diabetes developed weakness, palpitations, diaphoresis, and confusion after completing a 10K race. His wife stated his diabetes had been controlled on the same dose of insulin for greater than 1 year. This patient will most likely need:

(A) insulin
(B) Dilantin
(C) 50% dextrose
(D) beta blocker

6. Which of the following findings would be expected for a patient with HHS?

(A) pH 7.15
(B) specific gravity 1.030
(C) K^+ 6.1 mEq/L
(D) serum osmolality 270 mOsm/kg

7. The diabetic patient with hypoglycemia is most likely to present with coma if the patient is also receiving which of the following?

(A) glipizide
(B) phenytoin
(C) hydrochlorothiazide
(D) metoprolol

ANSWER KEY

1. **B**   3. **A**   5. **C**   7. **D**
2. **D**   4. **A**   6. **B**

ANSWERS EXPLAINED

1. **(B)** If the potassium was normal (4.5 mEq/L) when the pH was 7.15, it would have decreased as the pH was corrected, unmasking a deficit in total body potassium. The intravenous solution should be changed to include dextrose, not lactated Ringer's. The pH is now close to normal, so there is no need for sodium bicarbonate administration. The insulin infusion needs to be decreased, not increased.

2. **(D)** The clinical scenario describes diabetes insipidus (DI) secondary to head injury. Insufficient ADH is produced (low ADH), resulting in large-volume diuresis with dilute urine. The serum osmolality would be expected to be high, not low or normal. Serum sodium will increase, not drop.

3. **(A)** The patient requires an isotonic cryst lloid, one with lower amounts of sodium (normal saline has higher levels of sodiu   notonic solution, a solution high in sodium, or one high in dextrose will not   lemic shock.

4. **(A)** The patient scenario describes SIADH with dilutional hyponatremia secondary to oat cell carcinoma. Free water will further decrease the serum sodium. Therefore, restriction of free water is crucial. No evidence is provided to indicate that NSAID administration will be useful. A solution containing 0.45 normal saline is a hypotonic solution. Therefore, administering this solution will worsen the hypotonicity already present. Pitressin administration (choice D) will further increase ADH and worsen the SIADH.

5. **(C)** The symptoms describe hypoglycemia. Therefore, administration of 50% dextrose is appropriate. The other 3 choices will either worsen the hypoglycemia or not be of any benefit.

6. **(B)** The person with HHS has an extremely high blood sugar that progresses over several days. During this time, the patient has extreme diuresis with fluid loss. Of the 4 available choices, only an elevated urine specific gravity would be the result of this hypovolemia. Acidosis and hyperkalemia are seen with DKA. Low serum osmolality is seen with fluid overload, not volume loss.

7. **(D)** Metoprolol, a beta-adrenergic blocker, will prevent the early signs of hypoglycemia (irritability, shakiness, increased heart rate) that are due to sympathetic nervous system activation precipitated by the low blood sugar. The first signs may be lethargy and coma. The other 3 choices will not result in sudden lethargy and coma.

Hematology Concepts

11

"Believe you can and you're halfway there."

—Theodore Roosevelt

HEMATOLOGY TEST BLUEPRINT

Hematology 2% of total test   **3 Questions**

→ **Coagulopathies (e.g., ITP, DIC, HIT)**

HEMATOLOGY TESTABLE NURSING ACTIONS

- ☐ Recognize normal and abnormal physical assessment findings of patients with:
  - ○ Hematologic problems
  - ○ Immunologic problems
- ☐ Identify and monitor normal and abnormal diagnostic test results (e.g., PT/INR, PTT, fibrinogen, CBC)
- ☐ Manage patients receiving medications (e.g., IVIG, steroids, chemotherapy) and monitor response
- ☐ Recognize and manage complications associated with transfusion of blood products
- ☐ Monitor patient and follow protocols pre-, intra- and post-procedure (e.g., plasmapheresis, exchange transfusion, autotransfusion)
- ☐ Recognize signs and symptoms of hematologic/immunologic emergencies, initiate interventions, and seek assistance as needed

The test includes only 3 questions on hematology. Therefore, 3 hours of studying this topic is generally adequate in order to do well. Most test versions include DIC and HIT questions.

- Blood is a river of living tissue and needs to know when to be liquid and when to be solid (clot).
- Blood has several "jobs," one of which is to clot in the presence of an injury.

Platelet Phase of Clot Formation (Figure 11-1)

- Smallest of blood cells, made in bone marrow
- 200 billion produced per day, greater than 1 trillion circulating at all times
- White, live 7–10 days
- Platelet plug (white clot) is effective for small injuries
- Ordinarily, platelets do not react with endothelium; **but** in the presence of injury, platelets become activated and actually change shape and appearance

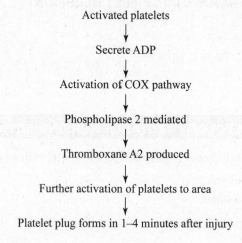

Activated platelets

↓

Secrete ADP

↓

Activation of COX pathway

↓

Phospholipase 2 mediated

↓

Thromboxane A2 produced

↓

Further activation of platelets to area

↓

Platelet plug forms in 1–4 minutes after injury

Figure 11-1. Physiology of platelet "white" clot formation

- Platelet count measures platelet quantity
- Bleeding time measures platelet function, how well platelets work

Coagulation Pathway Phase of Coagulation

- Various physiological problems may trigger either the intrinsic or the extrinsic coagulation pathways, followed by clotting (Figure 11-2).
- **Intrinsic coagulation pathway** stimulated by vascular endothelium injury
  - Cell trauma (valve, IABP)
  - Sepsis
  - Shock
  - ARDS
  - Hypoxemia, acidemia
  - Cardiopulmonary arrest

NOTE

Specific coagulation factors do not need to be memorized for the CCRN test.

- **Extrinsic coagulation pathway** stimulated by tissue injury, releases "tissue thromboplastin"

  - ○ Extensive trauma
  - ○ OB emergencies
  - ○ Malignancies
  - ○ Dissecting aortic aneurysm
  - ○ Extensive MI

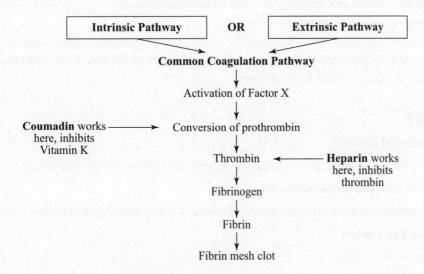

Figure 11-2. Coagulation Pathways

Inhibition of Clot Formation

- As we are making clots, we are also dissolving clots (Figure 11-3).

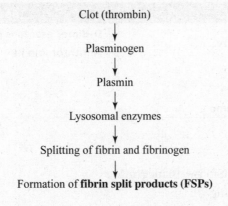

Figure 11-3. Inhibition of clot formation

Anticoagulant Reversal

- What reverses heparin? Protamine
- What reverses warfarin (Coumadin)? Vitamin K

COAGULOPATHIES: DISSEMINATED INTRAVASCULAR COAGULOPATHY (DIC)

- DIC is a complex condition caused by activation of clotting (fibrinolytic system) with resultant consumption of clotting factors (Table 11-1)
- Results in deposition of thrombi in microvasculature (**microembolism**) and consumption of clotting factors (**hemorrhage**)
- DIC is primarily a clotting problem, **not** a bleeding problem
- **Always** secondary to another problem
- Fortunately, massive bleeding from multiple sites is now rare since there is a better understanding of etiology; massive bleeding is screened for DIC in its early stages and treatment occurs earlier in most cases

Etiology

- **Endothelial damage**
  - ○ Sepsis, hypoxemia, shock, ARDS, AAA, acidemia, cardiopulmonary arrest
- **Release of tissue thromboplastin**
  - ○ Extensive trauma, malignancies, OB emergencies, dissecting aortic aneurysm
- **Factor X activation**
  - ○ Acute pancreatitis
  - ○ Liver disease
- **Miscellaneous**
  - ○ Massive transfusions, PE, hemolytic anemia, fresh H_2O drowning, ASA poisoning

☆ **Table 11-1. Lab Values of DIC**

Primary	Secondary
↓ Platelets	↑ **D-dimer** assesses presence of clotting
↓ Fibrinogen	↑ Antithrombin III
↓ Hematocrit	
↑ **FSP (D/T ↑ fibrinolysis)**	
↑ PT, PTT, INR, bleeding time	

Normals:

- Fibrin split products (FSP) is < 10 mcg/mL
- Fibrinogen is 200–400 mg/dL
- ☆ Elevated FSP is the definitive lab test for the presence of DIC.
- ☆ D-dimer must be elevated; however it is not a definitive test for DIC.

Treatment of DIC

- Identify and eliminate underlying cause, as able
- Vitamin K
- Blood component therapy
    - Fresh frozen plasma (FFP)
    - Cryoprecipitate
    - Platelets
- Heparin (low dose) is controversial but may be used for patients with chronic, low-grade DIC who have predominantly thrombotic manifestations
- Maintain hemodynamic stability

COAGULOPATHIES: HEPARIN-INDUCED THROMBOCYTOPENIA (HIT)

- ~ 50% of patients exposed to heparin are heparin antibody positive
    - Most are asymptomatic
    - ~ 5% develop HIT or "white clot syndrome"

Etiology of HIT

- Due to an immune (IgG) response
- Results in thrombosis (white clots) that consumes platelets

Signs/Symptoms of HIT

- Platelets decrease to < 150,000 **or** precipitously drop 30% to 50%
- Early sign—petechiae
- Clots may lead to PE, MI, stroke, amputation
- Frequently unrecognized

Treatment of HIT

- Stop heparin (fractionated as well as unfractionated)
- Test for presence of heparin antibodies, enzyme-linked immunosorbent assay (ELISA), but do not wait for test results to stop heparin and start treatment
- Start direct thrombin inhibitor and continue until platelets stabilize, monitor PTTs
    - Argatroban
- Start warfarin
- Platelets < 10,000, monitor for changes in LOC (intracranial bleed)

COAGULOPATHIES: IMMUNE (IDIOPATHIC) THROMBOCYTOPENIA PURPURA (ITP)

☆ This coagulopathy is seldom on the test but is included in the test blueprint.

ITP is an acquired disorder with 2 criteria for diagnosis:

- Only a decrease in platelets is present. The rest of the complete blood count is normal.
- Drugs that lead to thrombocytopenia and other clinical conditions, e.g., lupus and chronic lymphocytic leukemia, are not present.

Signs and Symptoms of ITP

- Expected: petechiae, purpura, and easy bruising
- Common: epistaxis, gingival bleeding, and menorrhagia
- Rare: GI bleeding, hematuria, intracranial hemorrhage
- Numerous differential diagnoses need to be ruled out
- Life-threatening bleeding is rarely seen

PLASMAPHERESIS

- The filtering and separation of plasma from whole blood via semipermeable membranes; done via a central line similar to the catheters used for hemodialysis
- Therapeutic plasmapheresis is indicated for disorders thought to be due to an abnormal immunologic response:
  - Guillain-Barré syndrome
  - Myasthenia gravis
  - Thrombotic thrombocytopenic purpura
- Contraindications include:
  - Patients who cannot tolerate central line placement
  - Patients who are actively septic or are hemodynamically unstable
  - Patients who have allergies to fresh frozen plasma or albumin depending on the type of plasma exchange
  - Patients with heparin allergies should not receive heparin as an anticoagulant during plasmapheresis.
  - Patients with hypocalcemia are at risk for worsening of their condition because citrate is commonly used to prevent clotting and can potentiate hypocalcemia.

RECOGNITION AND MANAGEMENT OF TRANSFUSION REACTIONS

- Although included in the test blueprint, transfusion reactions are less likely to be included on the test than DIC-related or HIT-related questions.

Signs of Transfusion Reactions

- **Acute transfusion reaction**: Occurs within 24 hours of blood product administration (Table 11-2)
- **Delayed transfusion reaction**: Occurs after 24 hours of blood product administration (Table 11-2)

Table 11-2. Blood Product Transfusion Reactions

Body System	Acute Reaction: Signs and Symptoms
Respiratory	Tachypnea, dyspnea, wheezing, rales, stridor, hypoxia
Cardiovascular	Tachycardia, bradycardia, hypertension, hypotension, jugular venous distention, arrhythmia
Immune	Fever (temperature increase > 1°C), chills, rigors
Cutaneous	Pruritus, uticaria, erythema, flushing, petechiae, cyanosis
Gastrointestinal	Nausea, vomiting
Pain	Headache, chest, abdominal, back/flank, infusion site
Renal	Red-colored urine (hemolytic, non-antibody mediated)

Management of Transfusion Reaction

- General interventions for ALL suspected reactions
  - Stop the transfusion.
  - Disconnect the blood tubing at the intravenous catheter hub, and begin a new normal saline and new tubing to keep the vein open.
  - Assess the patient.
  - Monitor the patient's vital signs until stable.
  - Perform a clerical check on the blood product and the patient's identification.
- Acute hemolytic reactions (antibody mediated)
  - Anticipate hypotension, renal failure, and DIC.
  - Prophylactic measures to reduce the risk of renal failure may include vigorous hydration with crystalloid solutions (3,000 mL/m^2/24 hr), and osmotic diuresis with 20% mannitol (100 mL/m^2/bolus, followed by 30 mL/m^2/hr for 12 hr).
  - If DIC is documented and bleeding requires treatment, transfusions of frozen plasma, pooled cryoprecipitate, and/or platelet concentrates may be indicated.
- Acute hemolytic reactions (non-antibody mediated)
  - The transfusion of serologically compatible, although damaged, RBCs usually does not require rigorous management.
  - Diuresis induced by an infusion of 500 mL of 0.9% sodium chloride per hour, or as tolerated by the patient, until the intense red color of urine subsides.

- Febrile, non-hemolytic reactions
  - Acetaminophen
- Allergic reactions
  - Diphenhydramine (Benadryl) is usually effective for relieving pruritus that is associated with hives or a rash.
- Anaphylactic reactions
  - A subcutaneous injection of epinephrine (0.3–0.5 mL of a 1:1,000 aqueous solution) is standard treatment. If the patient is sufficiently hypotensive to raise the question of the efficacy of the subcutaneous route, epinephrine (0.5 mL of a 1:10,000 aqueous solution) may be administered intravenously.
  - Steroids if epinephrine does not relieve symptoms
- Transfusion-related acute lung injury (TRALI)
  - Oxygen, mechanical ventilation if necessary
  - Diuretics (only if there is also volume overload or cardiogenic pulmonary edema)
- Circulatory (volume) overload
  - Oxygen
  - If practical, the unit of blood component being transfused may be lowered
  - Diuretics
- Bacterial contamination (sepsis)
  - Blood cultures
  - Antibiotics

Now that you have reviewed key hematology concepts, go to the Hematology Practice Questions. Answer the questions, and then check your answers. Continue to review the information until you get at least 80% on the practice questions.

HEMATOLOGY PRACTICE QUESTIONS

For questions 1 and 2

A 54-year-old woman was admitted with deep-vein thrombosis and pulmonary emboli. She received a heparin bolus and a continuous heparin infusion. The next day, heparin-induced thrombocytopenia (HIT) was suspected, and the heparin infusion was discontinued.

1. Which of the following would be most indicative of HIT?

   (A) surface bleeding from IV sites, PTT 50 seconds
   (B) loss of pulses, INR 5
   (C) petechiae, platelet count 50,000/mm³
   (D) change in level of consciousness

2. Two days later, the patient is scheduled for insertion of a Greenfield filter to protect her lungs from future emboli. The preoperative laboratory results show a platelet count of 20,000/mm³. Which nursing action is most appropriate?

   (A) Notify the surgeon.
   (B) Start an extra IV line with a large-gauge catheter.
   (C) Monitor neurological status carefully.
   (D) Discontinue argatroban.

3. A patient with septic shock is thought to be developing DIC. Which of the following lab results would be most indicative for DIC?

   (A) prolonged PT, PTT, bleeding time
   (B) decreased platelet count
   (C) positive ELISA
   (D) elevated fibrin split products and D-dimer

ANSWER KEY

1. **C**   2. **A**   3. **D**

ANSWERS EXPLAINED

1. **(C)** Petechiae are a sign of HIT (although not present in all cases). The platelet count of 50,000/mm^3 would meet the criteria for HIT (decrease to < 150,000 **or** precipitously drop 30–50%). Surface bleeding from IV sites and/or a prolonged PTT is not an indication of HIT. Although loss of pulses may be seen, a prolonged INR is not a sign of HIT. Even though a change in level of consciousness may be due to a stroke secondary to HIT, petechiae and a drop in platelet count are more specific.

2. **(A)** The surgeon needs to know of the extreme drop in platelet count as he/she may want to transfuse platelets prior to the procedure. The other interventions are not a priority. (An intracranial bleed would be more likely with a platelet count less than 20,000 /mm^3.)

3. **(D)** Elevated fibrin split products (FSP) is due to breakdown of the massive amount of clots that occur with DIC. The other lab values are not specific to DIC.

Hemodynamics Concepts

12

One of the most important keys to Success is having the discipline to do what you know you should do, even when you don't feel like doing it.

—Unknown

Hemodynamics is included in the cardiovascular section of the adult CCRN blueprint. However, it has been placed at the end of the clinical content of the book since hemodynamics summarizes problems other than cardiovascular (multisystem, pulmonary).

Although most critically ill patients do not receive invasive hemodynamic monitoring, ALL patients have hemodynamics that reflect their specific problems. These determine, to a degree, the plan of care. Hemodynamics and invasive hemodynamic monitoring are included in numerous CCRN exam questions.

☆ The equation in Figure 12-1 is the foundation of hemodynamics. The cardiac output (CO) is equal to the heart rate (HR) times the stroke volume (SV). The SV is dependent on the preload, afterload, and contractility of the ventricles of the heart.

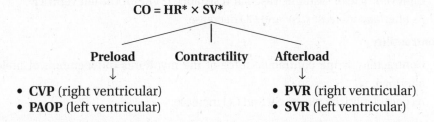

CO = HR* × SV*

Preload   Contractility   Afterload
   ↓   ↓
• **CVP** (right ventricular)   • **PVR** (right ventricular)
• **PAOP** (left ventricular)   • **SVR** (left ventricular)

*Heart rate (HR); stroke volume (SV); central venous pressure (CVP); pulmonary artery occlusive pressure (PAOP); pulmonary vascular resistance (PVR); systemic vascular resistance (SVR)

Figure 12-1. Regulation of hemodynamics

CRITICAL POINTS

■ The normal cardiac output (CO) is 4 L to 8 L per minute. If it becomes critically low, the blood pressure will decrease.

○ Cardiac index (CI) takes into account the body surface area (BSA) and is **a more meaningful value than CO**.

○ The normal CI is 2.5 to 4.0 L/min/m^2.

■ As **heart rate** (HR) increases, CO increases up to a point. The point is determined by age and condition of the ventricles. Generally, 130–170 beats per minute is the maximal heart rate attainable for most people.

- Extreme bradycardia results in low CO and hypotension.
- An increase in HR is the first sign of compensation for a low CO. This will occur before the B/P drops. Patients on beta blocker drugs, or any drug that decreases heart rate, may not be able to compensate as well for a problem that is decreasing cardiac output.
- Conversely, extreme tachycardia will also decrease CO no matter the age or condition of the ventricles. Why? Loss of diastolic filling time occurs. If diastolic filling time is decreased, the ventricles do not have time to fill, ventricular preload drops, and ultimately the ventricle cannot put out what is not delivered.

- As **stroke volume** increases, CO increases. The stroke volume (SV) is how many mL per beat the left ventricle ejects. It is determined by the preload, afterload, and contractility. The normal SV is 50–100 mL per beat.
- **Preload**
  - Preload is the volume/pressure in the ventricle at the end of diastole after the AV valves close, just prior to ejection. The right atrial (RA) pressure or central venous pressure (CVP) reflects the right ventricular preload. The PAOP reflects the left ventricular preload.
  - As preload increases, SV and CO increase up to a point.
  - Too high of a preload may lead to heart failure.
  - In general, preload will seldom be elevated if the heart is without disease and there are no metabolic abnormalities.

- **Afterload**
  - Afterload is the pressure (resistance) against which the ventricle must pump to open the valve (pulmonic or aortic).
  - Afterload is clinically measured by the pulmonary vascular resistance (PVR) for the right ventricle or systemic vascular resistance (SVR) for the left ventricle.
  - As afterload increases, SV and CO decrease.

- **Contractility**
  - Contractility is the contractile force of the myofibrils independent of preload and afterload.
  - As contractility increases, SV and CO increase.

☆ For the test, you need to know normal hemodynamic values and how various drugs and therapies affect preload, afterload, and contractility. Therefore, you need to know how these drugs and therapies affect stroke volume and, ultimately, cardiac output.

Table 12-1 summarizes normal hemodynamics, and Table 12-2 outlines how various clinical problems affect hemodynamics. Table 12-3 lists the hemodynamic effects of various cardiovascular agents. You **must** have an understanding of this information as it is the foundation for patient management.

⭐ **Table 12-1. Normal Hemodynamic and Oxygenation Parameters**

Parameter	Normal	Formula
Heart rate (HR)	60–100 beats/minute	Direct measurement
Blood pressure (B/P)	90/60–140/90 mmHg	Direct measurement
Mean arterial pressure (MAP)	70–110 mmHg	SBP – DBP ÷ 3 + DBP
Cardiac output (CO)	4–8 L/min	Direct measurement
Cardiac index (CI)	2.5–4.0 L/min/m^2	CO ÷ BSA
Stroke volume (SV)	50–100 ml/beat	CO ÷ HR × 1000
Stroke index (SI)	25–45 ml/beat/m^2	CI ÷ HR × 1000
Right atrial pressure (RAP)	2–6 mmHg 3–8 cm H_2O	Direct measurement
Pulmonary artery pressure (PAP)	20/8–30/15 mmHg Mean: < 20 mmHg	Direct measurement
Pulmonary artery occlusive (wedge) pressure (PAOP)	8–12 mmHg (although varies depending on the LV function)	Direct measurement
Systemic vascular resistance (SVR)	800–1200 dynes/s/cm^{-5}	MAP – CVP ÷ CO × 80
Pulmonary vascular resistance (PVR)	50–250 dynes/s/cm^{-5}	MPAP – PAOP ÷ CO × 80
Coronary artery perfusion pressure (CAPP)	60–80 mmHg	DBP – PAOP
Mixed venous oxygen saturation (SvO_2)	60–75%	Direct measurement (pulmonary artery)
Central venous oxygen saturation ($ScvO_2$)	> 70%	Direct measurement (superior vena cava)
Arterial oxygen saturation (SaO_2)	95–99% on room air	Direct measurement
Arterial oxygen content (CaO_2)	12–16 mL/dl	(Hgb x 1.39 × SaO_2) + (PaO_2 × 0.003)
Oxygen delivery (DO_2)	900–1,100 mL/min	CaO_2 x CO x 10
Oxygen consumption (VO_2)	250–350 mL/min	(SaO_2 – SvO_2) × Hgb × 13.9 × CO

■ "Normal" differs somewhat from resource to resource. Those values listed in Table 12-1 are generally accepted.

■ You do not need to memorize formulas for the test.

★ Table 12-2. Hemodynamic Profiles for Select Abnormal Conditions

Condition	B/P	RAP (CVP)	PAP	PAOP	CO/CI	SV/SI*	SVR	PVR	SvO$_2$**	Comments
Shock States										
Cardiogenic	↓	↑	↑	↑	↓	↓	↑	~ or ↑	↓	
Hypovolemic	↓	↓	↓	↓	↓	↓	↑	~	↓	
Septic	↓	↓	↓	↓	↑	↑	↓	~	↑	Lactate may ↑ before B/P ↓
Septic, late	↓	↓	↑	~ or ↑	↓	↓	↑	~	↓	
Cardiogenic pulmonary edema	~ or ↑	↑	↑	↑	↓	↓	~	~ or ↑	↓	
Noncardiogenic pulmonary edema (ARDS)	~ or ↓	~ or ↑	↑	~ or ↓	~	~	~	↑	~ or ↓	PAP↑ due to hypoxemia
Pulmonary hypertension (PE, COPD, hypoxemia)	~	↑	↑	~	~	~	~	↑	↓	B/P, CO may ↓ if PE
Cardiac tamponade	↓	↑	↑	↑	↓	↓	↑	~ or ↑	↓	Pressures equalize

*May decrease before CO/CI or B/P if compensation is adequate, e.g., increase in heart rate

**May decrease or increase before CO/CI or B/P change since it represents change at the tissue level

Key: ↓ = decrease; ↑ = increase; ~ = no change

⭐ **Table 12-3. Hemodynamic Effects of Various Cardiovascular Agents**

Drug	B/P	RAP (CVP)	PAP	PAOP	CO/CI	SV/SI	SVR	PVR	Heart Rate
Dopamine									
• Low dose (1–3 mcg/kg/m)	~	~	~	~	~	~	~	~	~
• Medium dose (4–10 mcg/kg/m)	~ or ↑	~	~ or ↑	~ or ↑	↑↑	↑	~	~	↑
• High dose (11–20 mcg/kg/m)	↑	~ or ↑	↑	↑	↑	↑	↑	↑	↑↑
Norepinephrine (Levophed)	↑	↑ or ~	↑	↑	↑	↑	↑↑	~ or ↑	~
Phenylephrine (Neosynephrine)	↑	~	↑	~ or ↑	~	↑	↑	↑	~
Epinephrine drip	↑	↑ or ~	↑	↑	↑	↑	↑↑	~ or ↑	↑
Nitroglycerin									
• Doses up to 1 mcg/kg	~ or ↓	↓	↓	↓↓	~	~ or ↑	~	~ or ↓	~ or ↑
• Doses >1 mcg/kg*	↓	↓	↓	↓	~ or ↑	~ or ↑	↓	↓	~ or ↑
Nesiritide (Natrecor)*	~ or ↓	↓	↓	↓	~ or ↑	~ or ↑	↓	↓	~
Nitroprusside (Nipride)*	↓↓	↓	↓	↓↓	~ or ↑	~ or ↑	↓↓	↓	~ or ↑
ACE inhibitors	↓	~	~ or ↓	~ or ↓	~ or ↑	~ or ↑	↓	~	~
Dobutamine (Dobutrex)	~, ↑ or ↓	~	~	↓	↑	↑	~ or ↓	~	↑
Milrinone (Primacor)	~ or ↓	~ or ↓	~ or ↓	↓	↑	↑	↓	~	~
Labetalol (Normadyne)	↓	~	~	~	↓	~	~ or ↓	~	↓
Morphine	↓	↓	↓	↓	~	~	~	↓	↓

Key: ↓ = decrease; ↑ = increase; ~ = no change

*High dose NTG, nesiritide, and nitroprusside are afterload reducers, not positive inotropes, but may increase CO indirectly by decreasing afterload.

There will be questions that test your knowledge on appropriate interventions for various abnormal hemodynamics and the significance of various oxygenation parameters. Table 12-4 summarizes therapies for alteration in hemodynamics and Table 12-5 outlines oxygenation parameters.

⭐ Table 12-4. Therapies for Alterations in Hemodynamics*

PRELOAD Therapies	
Increases	**Decreases**

Volume expanders
 • Crystalloids
 • Colloids
 Pressors
	Diuretics
	 Dilators
	   • Nitrates
	   • Nitroprusside
	   • Nesiritide
	 Morphine

AFTERLOAD Therapies	
Increases	**Decreases**
Norepinephrine Phenylephrine High-dose dopamine Epinephrine drip	Nitroprusside ACE inhibitors Hydralazine Calcium-channel blockers IABP Nitroglycerin (high doses)
CONTRACTILITY Therapies	
Increases	**Decreases**
Positive inotropes • Dobutamine • Dopamine 5–10 mcg/kg/min • Primacor • Epinephrine drip	Negative inotropes • Beta blockers • Calcium-channel blockers Metabolic problems, i.e., metabolic acidosis, endotoxins of sepsis

*For all abnormalities, attempt to identify the underlying cause(s) and, if able, correct them.

Table 12-5. Hemodynamic Oxygenation Parameters

Parameter	Normal	How Calculated/ Measured	Clinical Relevance
Mixed venous oxygen saturation (SvO_2)	60–75%	Direct measurement, intermittent or continuous (pulmonary artery)	Most sensitive indicator of cellular oxygenation
Central venous oxygen saturation ($ScvO_2$)	> 70%	Direct measurement, intermittent or continuous (superior vena cava)	Used to monitor therapy for septic shock
Oxygen delivery (DO_2)	900–1,100 mL/min	$CaO_2 \times CO \times 10$	Pump problems (heart) will decrease DO_2
Oxygen consumption (VO_2)	250–350 mL/min	$(SaO_2 - SvO_2) \times Hgb \times 13.9 \times CO$	Low with septic shock
Oxygen extraction	~ 50% of O_2 delivery	$(CaO_2 - CvO_2)$	Myocardial oxygen extraction is > than any other muscle; increases with a drop in CO

- You do not need to memorize formulas for the test but should know the normal values and their clinical relevance.

SvO_2: normal is 60% to 75% (too low or too high is **BAD**)

- Sustained changes, not brief changes (e.g. during position change), are significant (Table 12-6).

Table 12-6. SvO₂ Changes

Increased	Decreased
Septic shock Hypothermia Paralysis	Low cardiac output Decreased PaO_2 Increased O_2 demand (fever, shivering, seizures, increased WOB)
If SvO_2 is increased: • Assess for severe sepsis, septic shock • Assess for hypothermia	If SvO_2 is decreased: • Assess for hypoxemia, increased WOB • Assess for hypotension • Assess for hypovolemia • Assess hemoglobin (drop) • Assess temperature (fever) • Assess for arrhythmias

☆ For the test, concentrate on studying the normal and abnormal hemodynamic ranges. Also study the therapies that affect hemodynamics. Note that printed waveform strips are seldom included (Figure 12-2).

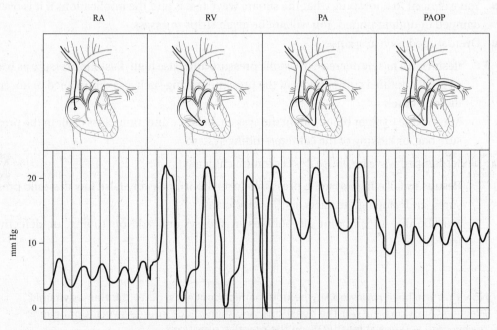

Figure 12-2. Normal pulmonary artery waves

Acute Mitral Valve Insufficiency: In the presence of mitral valve insufficiency, the PAOP waveform changes appearance. When the PA catheter balloon is inflated, **"giant V-waves"** appear on the PAOP tracing (see Figure 12-3).

- The PAOP is read at the A-wave, not at the V-wave.

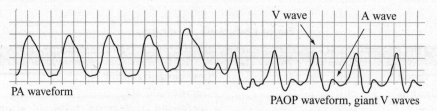

Figure 12-3. Giant V-waves on the PAOP waveform

If you see the term "giant V-waves" on the test, the problem is mitral valve insufficiency (regurgitation). As you should recall from the CV section, this is often associated with acute inferior wall myocardial infarction/papillary muscle dysfunction/rupture.

Square Wave Test (Dynamic Response Test)

- The **dynamic response test,** also called the "square wave test," is performed to assess the accuracy of the hemodynamic monitoring system. This is done immediately after catheter insertion, at the beginning of each shift, after zeroing the system, and whenever values are questionable. The strip recorder is started. Then the flush device is squeezed and immediately released. The dynamic response documented on the strip is then examined.

- You will need to know only what the square wave test is and the implications if it is overdamped or underdamped. You will not be given strips to assess.

- Overdamped wave response:

  - Results in a falsely decreased systolic pressure and false high diastolic pressure as well as poorly defined components of the pressure tracing such as a diminished or absent dicrotic notch

  - May be due to air or blood clot in the system, loose connections, loss of air in the pressure bag, or kinking of the catheter/tubing system

- Underdamped wave response (less common clinically):

  - Results in false high systolic pressures (overshoot), possibly false low diastolic pressures, and "ringing" artifacts on the waveform

  - May be due to pinpoint air bubbles in the system, add-on tubing, or defective transducer

> Now that you have reviewed key hemodynamics concepts, go to the Hemodynamic Practice Questions, answer the questions, and then check your answers. Continue to review until you get at least 80% on the practice questions.

HEMODYNAMICS PRACTICE QUESTIONS

<u>For questions 1–3</u>

The following hemodynamic profile has been obtained for a patient.

B/P	112/60 mmHg	RA	3 mmHg
PA	44/24 mmHg	PAOP	22 mmHg
SVR	1,600 dynes/s/cm^{-5}	CI	1.9 L/min/m^2
SVI	23 mL/m^2	SvO$_2$	0.58

1. What conclusion is correct?

    (A) The patient is hypovolemic.
    (B) The patient has evidence of left ventricular failure.
    (C) The patient seems to have severe sepsis.
    (D) The patient has developed ARDS.

2. Shortly after obtaining the values above, you inflated (wedged) the catheter balloon and observed giant V-waves on the PAOP tracing. What is the most likely problem?

    (A) The patient has evidence of mitral valve regurgitation.
    (B) The PA catheter has fallen back into the RV.
    (C) The PA catheter needs to be advanced.
    (D) The PAOP seems to be 40 mmHg.

3. What would be the most appropriate intervention related to the waveform above?

    (A) Call the physician for possible catheter repositioning.
    (B) Document the strip, administer the PRN order for furosemide (Lasix) for PAOP > 16 mmHg, and reassess in 1 hour.
    (C) Label the balloon "do not wedge."
    (D) Document the strip, interpret the pressure, and notify the physician.

---

4. The patient with continuous SvO$_2$ monitoring has a sustained decrease in SvO$_2$ to 0.50. Priority interventions would include each of the following EXCEPT:

    (A) check urine output.
    (B) check B/P and CO/CI.
    (C) check O$_2$ sat with pulse oximeter (SpO$_2$).
    (D) check temperature.

For questions 5–8

It is important to integrate hemodynamic parameters with each other and not evaluate parameters individually in isolation. Assess the following hemodynamic profiles. Match each profile with the clinical problem most likely associated with it and listed below.

(B/P = blood pressure; HR = heart rate; CVP = central venous pressure; PAOP = pulmonary artery occlusive pressure; SVR = systemic vascular resistance; CI = cardiac index; SV = stroke volume)

	Profile 5	Profile 6	Profile 7	Profile 8
B/P	78/40	78/40	78/40	78/40
HR	120	120	120	120
CVP	5	2	15	1
PAOP	19	4	5	4
SVR	1697	453	1300	1387
CI	2.0	5.5	2.5	3.0
SV	29	75	27	25
	5._____	6._____	7._____	8._____

(A) Hypovolemic shock.
(B) Cardiogenic shock
(C) Acute right ventricular failure
(D) Septic shock

For questions 9–20

Match the drug with its **primary** hemodynamic effect. Consult Table 12-3.

9. _E_ Dopamine 5–10 mcg/kg/min

10. _C_ Dopamine > 10 mcg/kg/min

11. _E_ Dobutamine

12. _B_ Nitroglycerin 20 mcg/min

13. _C_ Norepinephrine

14. _F_ Beta blockers

15. _B, D_ Nitroprusside (choose 2)

16. _D_ ACE inhibitors

17. _B_ Furosemide

18. _A_ Fluid bolus

19. _E_ Milrinone

20. _B_ Morphine

(A) Increase preload
(B) Decrease preload
(C) Increase afterload
(D) Decrease afterload
(E) Increase contractility
(F) Decrease contractility

For questions 21 and 22

Mr. A, 66-year-old male, presents S/P colectomy for colon cancer. He has the following upon examination:

MAP 58 mmHg ($\downarrow$ from 70) after 1L of 0.9 normal saline; heart rate 112/minute; respiratory rate 34/minute; temperature 38.9°C; Urine output < 0.5 mL/kg for the past 2 hrs; lungs clear; skin warm and dry; WBC 20,000; 66% segs; 24% bands; 7% lymphs; blood cultures positive for gram-negative organisms

21. The patient does not have a pulmonary artery catheter. If he did and his systemic vascular resistance was measured, what SVR do you anticipate the patient would have?

   (A)   2,550 dynes/s/cm^{-5}

   (B)   1,550 dynes/s/cm^{-5}

   (C)   550 dynes/s/cm^{-5}

   (D)   900 dynes/s/cm^{-5}

22. What hemodynamic changes are consistent with the patient's clinical status?

   (A)   increase in preload and decrease in afterload

   (B)   decrease in preload and increase in afterload

   (C)   decrease in preload and decrease in afterload

   (D)   decrease in CO due to impaired contractility

---

23. Ms. B, a 78-year-old female, is admitted with the following clinical findings:

- Chief complaint of SOB and fatigue
- Bibasilar crackles noted with S3 gallop
- Chest radiograph shows venous congestion and cardiomegaly
- Weight increase of 20 pounds over the last two weeks

Which of the following hemodynamic alterations is found with her presenting problems, and what treatment and rationale for treatment is indicated?

   (A)   increased afterload, decreased contractility, and decreased preload; nesiritide to increase contractility

   (B)   decreased afterload, decreased contractility, and increased preload; furosemide (Lasix) to increase afterload

   (C)   decreased afterload, increased contractility, and increased preload; amiodarone to decrease preload

   (D)   increased afterload, decreased contractility, and increased preload; dobutamine to increase contractility

For questions 24 and 25

Mr. C, a 54-year-old male, presents with near syncope. He has no significant past medical history. He sought medical help today after almost fainting in the shower. Clinical findings include:

- Blood pressure 98/58 mmHg; heart rate 108/minute with S1 and S2; respiratory rate 18/minute; temperature 37.1°C
- Alert and orientated × 3, lungs clear, skin cool and dry, neck veins flat
- Thirsty with dry oral mucous membranes; abdomen soft/non-tender with hyperactive bowel sounds

24. The next vital sign assessment revealed a blood pressure of 88/60 mmHg. Which of the following does Mr. C seem to need?

(A) Volume expansion is needed to increase preload and myocardial stretch.
(B) Pressors are needed to increase afterload and increase myocardial stretch.
(C) Volume expansion is needed to decrease afterload and increase myocardial stretch.
(D) Pressors are needed to decrease preload and myocardial stretch.

25. The nurse suspects that the arterial line waveform appearance has changed. The recommended method for assessing the adequacy of the tubing catheter set is to:

(A) perform a square wave test.
(B) zero balance.
(C) check a cuff pressure.
(D) calibrate the monitor.

ANSWER KEY

1. **B**	6. **D**	11. **E**	16. **D**	21. **C**
2. **A**	7. **C**	12. **B**	17. **B**	22. **C**
3. **D**	8. **A**	13. **C**	18. **A**	23. **D**
4. **A**	9. **E**	14. **F**	19. **E**	24. **A**
5. **B**	10. **C**	15. **B, D**	20. **B**	25. **A**

ANSWERS EXPLAINED

1. **(B)** Although there are several hemodynamic abnormalities, the key here is the PAOP of 22 mmHg. Left heart failure is the only problem of those listed that would result in an elevated PAOP. Because the LV is in failure and not emptying normally, there is a backup of volume, reflected as a higher pressure on the left side of the heart. This, in turn, causes the pulmonary capillary pressures to exceed 18 mmHg and cause pulmonary edema. The low CI causes the elevated PAOP. However, other problems such as hypovolemia may also result in a low CI. The SVR is high due to compensatory vasoconstriction, which in this case seems to be maintaining the blood pressure.

2. **(A)** The giant V-waves are due to mitral valve insufficiency or regurgitation, which may be acute or chronic. The PAOP is measured, however, at the A-wave.

3. **(D)** If the patient develops acute mitral valve insufficiency, the physician needs to be notified. There is no problem with the PA catheter. It does not automatically require a diuretic (but it might). The balloon is OK, so it doesn't need to be labeled.

4. **(A)** The SvO_2 is low, therefore, the reason needs to be determined. A drop in blood pressure or cardiac output, a decrease in the arterial oxygen saturation, or a fever are possible causes. Urine output is not directly associated with a decrease in the SvO_2.

5. **(B)** The key indicator is the elevated PAOP with the low CI. The SVR is elevated as a compensatory response.

6. **(D)** The key indicator is the low SVR (massive dilation) with higher-than-normal CI.

7. **(C)** The key indicator is the high CVP with low PAOP due to poor RV output. Since volume is not getting to the left heart, the left heart pressure (PAOP) is low and the CI is low.

8. **(A)** The key indicator is the low CVP and PAOP with the elevated SVR as a compensatory response to the hypovolemia.

9. **(E)** "Midrange" dopamine stimulates the beta-1 receptors in the heart to increase contractility.

10. **(C)** High-dose dopamine stimulates the alpha receptors in the arteries to cause vasoconstriction and to increase afterload.

11. **(E)** Dobutamine stimulates the beta-1 receptors in the heart and increases contractility.

12. **(B)** Nitroglycerin at lower doses causes venodilatation and results in a decrease in preload. Only at higher doses does it dilate the arterial vessels.

13. **(C)** Norepinephrine is a potent vasoconstrictor as it stimulates the alpha receptors of the arteries and increases afterload.

14. **(F)** Beta blockers block the beta-1 receptors of the heart, blocking the adrenergic effects of the autonomic nervous system from affecting the heart. This results in decreased contractility as well as a decrease in heart rate.

15. **(B, D)** Nitroprusside dilates both the venous and arterial sides of the vascular system, resulting in a decrease in preload and afterload.

16. **(D)** ACE inhibitors or angiotensin-converting enzyme inhibitors block the conversion of angiotensin 1 to angiotensin 2. Angiotensin 2 is a potent constrictor. By blocking its formation, the arterial vessels dilate more, resulting in a decrease in afterload.

17. **(B)** Furosemide is a potent loop diuretic and venodilator. The resulting diuresis and venodilation cause a reduction in preload.

18. **(A)** A fluid bolus increases volume in the vasculature, thereby increasing the preload.

19. **(E)** Milrinone, in the class of phosphodiesterase inhibitors, stimulates cardiac muscle contraction and increases contractility.

20. **(B)** Morphine mildly dilates the venous bed, thereby reducing preload. It may be used in low doses to treat heart failure.

21. **(C)** The scenario describes a patient with septic shock as evidenced by an infection and hypotension despite 1 L of fluid. The endotoxins cause massive vasodilation, which results in loss of vascular tone, a low SVR.

22. **(C)** Septic shock causes massive vasodilation that decreases primarily afterload. It also causes capillary leakage with loss of volume in the vasculature, resulting in a decrease in preload.

23. **(D)** The patient scenario reflects heart failure. To compensate for the reduced cardiac output, the patient with heart failure vasoconstricts. Therefore, afterload is high. The heart muscle loses contractility. So contractility is decreased. Due to low ejection fraction, the left heart pressure increases, resulting in lung crackles, S3, and increased preload. A positive inotropic drug such as dobutamine (as well as other drugs) may be indicated.

24. **(A)** The patient scenario is one of hypovolemia. Fluid administration will increase preload (fill up the tank), which will in turn improve myocardial stretch. This increase in stretch to increase output is the Frank-Starling law of the heart. Because the patient is volume depleted, the systemic vascular resistance (SVR) is most likely high because vasoconstriction occurs as a compensatory response to maintain the arterial blood pressure. Pressors should not be used in the presence of hypovolemia.

25. **(A)** The square wave (or dynamic response) test provides information as to whether the catheter/tubing system is optimally damped, overdamped, or underdamped. Then troubleshooting needs to be done accordingly. Cuff pressures should not be used to verify accuracy of intra-arterial pressures.

Behavioral Concepts

13

A year from now, you may have wished that you started today.

—Karen Lamb

BEHAVIORAL TEST BLUEPRINT

Behavioral 4% of total test **6 Questions**

→ Abuse/neglect
→ Antisocial behaviors, aggression, violence
→ Delirium and dementia
→ Developmental delays
→ Failure to thrive
→ Mood disorders and depression
→ Substance dependence (e.g., withdrawal, drug-seeking behavior, chronic alcohol or drug dependence)
→ Suicidal behavior

BEHAVIORAL TESTABLE NURSING ACTIONS

☐ Recognize normal and abnormal:
   ○ Physical and psychosocial assessment findings
   ○ Developmental assessment findings and provide developmentally appropriate care

☐ Recognize the need for restraints and manage patients requiring them
☐ Recognize indications for and manage patients requiring behavioral therapeutic interventions
☐ Identify and monitor normal and abnormal diagnostic test results
☐ Manage patients receiving medications (e.g., antipsychotics, antidepressants) and monitor response
☐ Recognize signs and symptoms of behavioral/psychosocial emergencies, initiate interventions, and seek assistance as needed

- Delirium may cause agitation. However, not all delirious patients are agitated and not all agitated patients are delirious!
- Delirium is an acute organic mental syndrome with potentially reversible impairment of consciousness and cognitive function that fluctuates in severity.
- Types of delirium:
  - **Mixed** delirium (hyperactive and hypoactive type in the same patient) is the most common, seen in approximately 55% of delirium cases.
  - **Hypoactive** delirium is the second most common type, seen in approximately 43% of patients with delirium.
  - Purely **hyperactive** delirium is the least common, seen in approximately 2% of patients with delirium.
- Another possibility, often unrecognized, is the patient with dementia who develops delirium in the hospital, **superimposed on dementia**.
- Since delirium may result in agitation, risk factors for both delirium and agitation are similar (Table 13-1).
- Consider delirium as a medical emergency.
- Studies have shown that delirium results in increased length of stay. The more severe the delirium is, the longer the stay.
- Studies have also shown that patients who develop delirium have an increase in 6-month mortality and the severity of the delirium episode predicts mortality rate.
- Prevention, or appropriate treatment that decreases severity, may **improve patient outcome**.

Table 13-1. Risks for Delirium

Significant Risk for Delirium	Less Risk for Delirium
Preexisting dementia	Age
History of hypertension	Pain
History of alcoholism	Restraints
• Defined as 2–3 drinks or more per day	Tubes and lines
High severity of illness at admission	Sensory deprivation or overload
Coma—primary neurological, sedative induced, multifactorial	
Benzodiazepine drugs	

Assessment of Delirium—Overview

- Delirium identification is important due to delirium's effect on morbidity and mortality; use of an assessment tool to determine the presence of delirium (any type) increases identification of patients with delirium
- 2 valid/reliable tools can be used to assess for delirium for the critically ill:
  - The confusion assessment method for the ICU (CAM-ICU)
  - The intensive care delirium screening checklist (ICDSC)
- Studies have shown that nurses' ability to recognize delirium is low, especially identification of hypoactive delirium, even when assessment tools are available

STEPS TO ASSESS DELIRIUM (FIGURE 13-1)

☆ **Do not assess for delirium if the patient is not responsive or is heavily sedated**

1. Must have **acute onset, fluctuating course**

   ■ Is the patient different than his/her baseline mental status?
   Alternatively, has the patient had any fluctuation in mental status in the past 24 hours as evidenced by fluctuation on the sedation scale (MAAS or RASS) or Glasgow Coma Scale (GCS)?

   If negative for fluctuating course or mental status, patient is negative for delirium. STOP the assessment. If positive, continue the assessment.

   and

2. Patient must also exhibit **inattention,** i.e., administer "Letters Attention Test."

   ■ Say to the patient, "I am going to read you a series of 10 letters. Whenever you hear the letter 'A,' indicate by squeezing my hand." Read letters from the following letter list in a normal tone and 3 seconds apart.

   S A V E A H A A R T or **C A S A B L A N C A**

   ○ Errors are counted when the patient fails to squeeze on the letter "A" and when the patient squeezes on any letter other than "A."

   ■ Positive for inattention if > 2 errors are made

   If negative for inattention, the patient is negative for delirium. STOP the assessment. If positive for inattention, continue the assessment.

   Patient needs to exhibit **EITHER feature 3 or 4:**

3. Altered level of consciousness . . . anything other than calm and cooperative (RASS of 0 or MAAS of +3)

   or

4. Disorganized thinking . . . assess by either asking a question or the patient's ability to follow a specific command

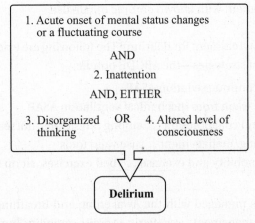

Figure 13-1. Summary of delirium assessment

Prevention and Treatment of Delirium

- Interventions that prevent delirium may also be used to treat delirium and perhaps make it less severe and prolonged.
- These measures should be done for ALL critically ill patients since delirium is quite common in the critically ill population and PREVENTION is key.
- **Remember that hypoactive delirium (often not diagnosed) also adversely affects outcome.**
- Suggested interventions include:
  - Strategies to promote patient orientation
    - Provide visual and hearing aids
    - Encourage communication and reorient patient repetitively
    - Have familiar objects from patient's home in the room
    - Attempt consistency in nursing staff
    - Allow television during day with daily news
    - Music (instrumental, without words)
  - Assess/manage environment
    - Sleep hygiene: lights off at night, on during day
    - Control excess noise (staff, equipment, visitors) at night
    - Avoid restraints as able
    - Remove/camouflage tubes
  - Control clinical parameters
    - Maintain systolic blood pressure > 90 mmHg
    - Maintain oxygen saturation > 90%
    - Treat underlying metabolic derangements and infections
  - Prevent/treat delirium secondary to substance abuse (alcohol, opiates, benzodiazepines, nicotine)
    - Assess for chronic substance abuse, adjust medication doses accordingly (tolerance)
    - Provide benzodiazepines to prevent/minimize alcohol withdrawal; provide opiates to the patient with known chronic opiate use

PREVENTION is the best treatment for delirium! The following are evidence-based measures, referred to as a bundle of strategies—the ABCDE bundle:

A: Awakening . . . discontinue sedation ASAP
B: Breathing trials . . . wean from mechanical ventilation ASAP
C: Communication and collaboration . . . among physicians, nurses, respiratory care, PT
D: Delirium monitoring/management . . . use valid tools
E: Early progressive mobility and exercise . . . bed exercises, sit on side of bed, stand, and walk to chair

- Critically ill patients managed with the Awakening and Breathing, Coordination, Delirium monitoring/management, and Early exercise/mobility bundle spent three more days breathing without assistance, experienced less delirium, and were more likely to be mobilized during their ICU stay than patients treated with usual care (Balas reference).

Pharmacological Management of Delirium

The use of drugs to treat delirium is generally utilized for **hyperactive** delirium not responsive to non-pharmacological measures. As mentioned earlier, there is no pharmacological "magic bullet" for the treatment of delirium. Paradoxically, sedation agents can cause delirium in some patients. The following recommendations are from the "2013 Clinical Practice Guidelines for the Management of Pain, Agitation, Delirium."

- Treat pain with analgesics if pain is thought to be the cause of delirium.
- In mechanically ventilated adult ICU patients at risk for delirium, dexmedetomidine infusions may be associated with a lower prevalence of delirium compared with benzodiazepine infusions.
- For delirium related to alcohol or benzodiazepine withdrawal, use benzodiazepines for delirium.
- For delirium unrelated to alcohol or benzodiazepine withdrawal, use dexmedetomidine rather than benzodiazepine infusions to reduce the duration of delirium.
- Avoid antipsychotics if there is a risk for torsades de pointes ventricular tachycardia.

HALOPERIDOL

- Antipsychotic medications such as haloperidol may be used for patients with delirium.
- **Haloperidol** may be useful for the treatment of agitation in patients who cannot tolerate respiratory depression that is possible with benzodiazepines or in those who paradoxically become more agitated when given benzodiazepines for agitation.
- Onset: IV, 3–20 minutes
- Duration: 4–6 hours
- Initial dose, 2 mg, followed by repeated doses (double the previous dose) every 15–20 minutes while agitation persists
  - Maintenance dose usually 25% of loading dose every 4–6 hours
- ☆ Prolongs QT interval, may cause torsades de pointes ventricular tachycardia.
  - Obtain baseline QTc interval measurement and monitor QTc regularly throughout therapy
  - Monitor for addition of other drugs that may prolong the QT interval

DEMENTIA

- Dementia (neurocognitive disorder) affects the brain's ability to think, reason, and remember clearly.
- The most common affected areas include memory, visual-spatial, language, attention, and problem solving.
- Unlike delirium, which is acute and temporary, most types of dementia are slow and progressive in onset and are permanent (Table 13-2).
- The most common form of dementia is Alzheimer's disease (75%); vascular brain disease/stroke is another cause, among others.
- Symptoms vary depending on whether the dementia is in early, mid, or late stages.
- If the patient with dementia requires care in an ICU, there is a higher incidence of delirium.
- Patient safety is a priority; inclusion of the family/significant others in the plan of care is required.

☆ Table 13-2. Delirium and Dementia Comparison

Delirium	Dementia
Acute, fluctuating	Chronic
Rapid progression	Slow progression
Reversible	Irreversible
Strategies available for prevention Organic brain changes	No known prevention Organic brain changes
May include agitation, not all cases	May include agitation, not always

VIOLENT BEHAVIOR

- Be aware and alert.
- Maintain a calm, quiet manner.
- Maintain a quiet environment.
- Stand at a slight angle to the patient.
- Do not provide care alone.
- Activate an emergency response as needed.

DEPRESSION

- Affects all age groups
- Affects all social classes
- Twice as frequent in women
- 18.8 million in U.S. (9.5% of population)

Cause of Depression

- No single known cause
- MRIs of the brain show changes
- Imbalance of brain neurotransmitters
  - Hereditary
  - Environmental
  - Psychological

Diagnosis of Depression

1. Depressed mood (feeling sad or low) **or**
2. Loss of interest or pleasure in nearly all activities

Plus 4 additional signs/symptoms from the following:
- Significant loss of appetite or weight loss or gain
- Insomnia or hypersomnia
- Psychomotor agitation or retardation
- Fatigue or loss of energy

- Feelings of worthlessness or guilt
- Impaired thinking or concentration; indecisiveness
- Suicidal thoughts/thoughts of death

Therapeutic Interventions for Depression

- Do NOT isolate
- Provide safety
- Avoid excessive environmental stimulation
- Do not force decision making
- Encourage expressions of feelings
- Explore sources of emotional support
- Involve family members, personal support system
- Ensure continuation of home medications as condition permits
- Assess suicide risk
- Psychiatric referral

Pharmacological Management of Depression

TRICYCLIC ANTIDEPRESSANTS

- Use has declined with availability of SSRIs
  - Amitriptyline
  - Nortriptyline
  - Imipramine
  - Clomipramine
  - Desipramine
- Adverse Effects
  - Highly lethal in overdose (tachycardia, hypotension, fatal arrhythmias)
  - Vertigo
  - Dry mouth, dental caries
  - Urinary retention
  - Constipation
  - Orthostatic hypotension
  - Prolonged QT

SELECTIVE SEROTONIN REUPTAKE INHIBITORS (SSRIs)

- First-line pharmacological therapy for depression (Table 13-3)
- Abnormalities in brain serotonin activity have been implicated in many emotional and behavioral disorders, including mood disorders, obsessive-compulsive disorder, aggressive behaviors.
- SSRIs block the action of the presynaptic serotonin reuptake pump, thereby increasing the amount of serotonin available in the synapse and increasing postsynaptic serotonin receptor occupancy.
- Well tolerated, once a day administration, fewer adverse effects than tricyclic antidepressants

Table 13-3. Types of SSRIs (New-Generation Antidepressants)

Generic Name	Brand Name
Fluoxetine	Prozac
Citalopram	Celexa
Escitalopram	Lexapro
Sertaline	Zoloft
Paroxetine	Paxil
Fluvoxamine	Luvox
Buproprion	Wellbutrin
Mirtazapine	Remeron
Venlafaxine	Effexor
Duloxetine	Cymbalta
Desvenlafaxine	Pristiq

Adverse Effects of SSRIs

- Generally well tolerated, adverse effects dose dependent, most subside after 1–2 weeks or dose reduction
- Headache, abdominal pain, nausea, diarrhea, sleep changes, jitteriness, or agitation
- Less common—diaphoresis, akathisia (restlessness and inability to sit still), bruising, changes in sexual functioning
- Can induce a manic or hypomanic episode
- Potential for increased suicidality
- Inhibit metabolism of meds—antiarrhythmics, benzodiazepines, warfarin, tricyclics, neuroleptics

SUICIDE

- Nearly 500,000 patients per year are admitted for suicide-related injuries
- Over 33,000 suicides annually
- 11th leading cause of death
- Over 60% suffer from major depression
- Alcoholism is a factor in 30%
- By gender

  - Four men succeed for every woman
  - Women attempt **twice** as often as men
  - Men over 65 years of age at greater risk

- Suicide behavior continuum

  - Ideation—contemplation without action
  - Gesture—nonlethal action
  - Attempt—potentially lethal
  - Suicide—30% successful on 1st try

Assessment for Suicide Intent

Evaluate Intent, Plan, and Ability

- Are you feeling depressed, sad, or discouraged?
- How long have you felt like this?
- Do you feel that your life is no longer worth living?
- Are you thinking of acting on that feeling by hurting yourself or taking your own life?
- Do you have a suicide plan?
- Can you tell me about your plan?

Nursing Interventions for the Patient With Suicide Intent/Attempt

- Establish a **safe** environment
- One-on-one observation
- Explain precautions to patient
- Comprehensive documentation

Safety Measures

- Remove hazards from room
  - Sharp or hazardous objects (plastic bags, cords, metal coat hangers)
  - Personal items (shoelaces, belts, lighters)
- Contraband check on personal belongings
- Paper/plastic food service
- Do not allow visitors to leave anything with the patient unless the nurse approves
- Make sure the patient swallows medications
- Move the patient near the nurses' station

ABUSE

Unfortunately, various types of abuse occur. Table 13-4 compares and contrasts domestic abuse with elder abuse.

Table 13-4. Domestic and Elder Abuse

Domestic Abuse	Elder Abuse
85% female victims Risks include 16–25 years of age, recent separation, children < 12 years, homelessness, pregnancy Signs include • Evasiveness, hesitancy • Inconsistent explanations • Frequent ED visits • Injury to trunk, extremities	Includes physical, emotional, sexual, financial, abandonment, violation of personal rights Signs include • Soft-tissue injuries • Untreated medical problems • Withdrawal • Lack of personal hygiene

Nursing Interventions for the Abused Patient

- Interview patient privately
- Utilize therapeutic communication
  - Involves exploring how the person actually feels while interpreting spoken words, gestures, and facial expressions. Do they match?
  - In a case where the patient's words do not match the gestures or facial expressions, further explore how the person actually feels.
  - For therapeutic communication to be effective, the nurse needs to be aware of how he/she appears to the patient as well as be able to assess the overall message communicated by the patient, such as fear, pain, sadness, anxiety, or apathy.
- Provide support
- Do not judge
- Document assessment, referrals
- Refer to social service
- Elder abuse is expected to be reported to adult protective services by law

SUBSTANCE DEPENDENCE

- Patients admitted to critical care for acute physiologic problems may have treatment complicated by chronic dependence on opiates, benzodiazepines, nicotine, alcohol, and other substances.
- The chronic dependence will need to be identified, withdrawal symptoms differentiated from acute physiologic problems, and withdrawal symptoms controlled as part of the overall plan of care.

Signs of Alcohol Withdrawal

- Minor, initial signs (first 6–36 hours without alcohol) include tremulousness, mild anxiety, headache, diaphoresis, palpitations, anorexia, GI upset; mental status is normal
- Seizures may occur during the first 48 hours
- "Alcoholic hallucinosis" after 12–48 hours without alcohol may occur, with visual, auditory, and/or tactile hallucinations; normal orientation and normal vital signs
- Delirium tremens (DTs) may occur 48–96 hours without alcohol with delirium, agitation, tachycardia, hypertension, fever, diaphoresis
  - Mortality rate of ~5%

RISKS OF DTs

- The presence of a concurrent illness
- A history of sustained drinking
- A history of previous DTs
- Age greater than 30
- The presence of significant alcohol withdrawal in the presence of an elevated alcohol level
- Present with acute illness already in withdrawal, last alcohol consumption greater than 2 previous days

☆ Treatment of Alcohol Withdrawal

- Preventative therapy for patients with known heavy alcohol intake or previous history of DTs with oral benzodiazepines such as lorazepam (Ativan), diazepam (Valium), or chlordiazepoxide (Librium)
  - Benzodiazepines enhance the effect of the neurotransmitter gamma-aminobutyric acid (GABA) at the $GABA_A$ receptor, resulting in sedative, hypnotic (sleep-inducing), anxiolytic (antianxiety), anticonvulsant, and muscle relaxant properties.
- Symptom-triggered treatment with benzodiazepines using a valid tool
  - Clinical Institute Withdrawal Assessment for Alcohol—Revised (CIWAS-Ar), is a valid tool to measure alcohol withdrawal severity. The tool relies on the patient being capable of answering. The tool is **not** valid if the patient cannot answer questions, e.g., receiving mechanical ventilation and disoriented.
  - Richmond Agitation-Sedation Scale (RASS) appropriate for the critical care setting, with a goal score of 0 to –2.
- Phenobarbital for refractory DTs
- Restore volume deficits due to diaphoresis, lack of oral intake, insensitive loss
- ☆ Glucose and thiamine to prevent Wernicke's encephalopathy (gait disturbances, nystagmus, eye muscle paralysis) and Korsakoff syndrome (decreased spontaneity, amnesia, denial of memory loss by making up facts)
- Multivitamins with folate
- Correct potassium, magnesium, phosphate deficiencies
- Provide as quiet an environment as possible
- Evaluate need for restraints for patient safety, especially until agitation is controlled
- Remove restraints once sedation is achieved as resistance against restraints may lead to temperature increase or rhabdomyolysis and may cause physical injury
- Following acute treatment, follow-up treatment should be planned
  - Encourage and support abstinence
  - Involve family, social services

Benzodiazepine Withdrawal

- Identify a history of chronic benzodiazepine use, by patient or family report
- Signs and symptoms onset may occur 2 days up to 21 days after last dose of benzodiazepine depending on the half-life and amount of the benzodiazepine that was taken chronically
- Signs and symptoms include tremors, anxiety, perceptual disturbances, psychosis, and seizures

MANAGEMENT OF BENZODIAZEPINE WITHDRAWAL

- The goal is to prevent or eliminate symptoms without causing respiratory depression or moderate to deep sedation.
- Administer a benzodiazepine, the same agent the patient was taking chronically, or a long-acting one such as chlordiazepoxide (Librium) as patient condition warrants.

Signs of Opiate Withdrawal

- Approximately the first 24 hours—fear of withdrawal, anxiety, drug craving
- Insomnia, restlessness, yawning, lacrimation, rhinorrhea, diaphoresis may follow
- Severe signs include vomiting, diarrhea, fever, chills, muscle spasm, tremor, tachycardia, hypertension

PREVENTION/MANAGEMENT OF OPIATE WITHDRAWAL

- Administer opiates, preferably long-acting such as methadone, in doses needed to control patient symptoms; may then gradually taper

Now that you have reviewed key behavioral concepts, go to the Behavioral Practice Questions. Answer the questions, and then check your answers. Continue to review the information until you get at least 80% on the practice questions.

BEHAVIORAL PRACTICE QUESTIONS

1. A 79-year-old female is admitted from home with acute prerenal failure secondary to severe dehydration. The patient has a history of dementia and is cared for at home by family members. During the admission assessment, the nurse notices pressure ulcers and bruising on wrists bilaterally. The nurse suspects elder abuse. Which of the following is the most appropriate intervention?

   (A) Contact the physician to report the possibility of abuse.
   (B) Provide emotional support to the patient.
   (C) Discuss your findings with the family.
   (D) Contact social services to call adult protective services.

2. Development of delirium has been shown to have a negative effect on patient outcome. Therefore, it is important to PREVENT delirium. Which of the following is an effective strategy to prevent delirium?

   (A) Restrain wrists loosely to provide safety.
   (B) Maintain a target of deep sedation for most patients.
   (C) Encourage communication and reorient repetitively.
   (D) Maintain bedrest until weaned off ventilator and pressors.

3. A 69-year-old female is admitted with suicide attempt after being found at home unresponsive by her husband with an open bottle of zolpidem (Ambien). On entering the room, the patient greets the nurse cheerfully and claims it was all a "big mistake," stating that she would never want to end her life. Which of the following should be included in the patient's plan of care?

   (A) Stay with the patient until she swallows her scheduled medications.
   (B) Update the patient's husband that the patient is not depressed.
   (C) Advise the patient that she will need to be honest in order to improve.
   (D) Provide privacy in order to increase the patient's self-esteem.

4. A 45-year-old male patient is admitted with acute respiratory failure secondary to pneumonia. He has demonstrated signs of mild delirium thought to be due to alcohol withdrawal, and haloperidol has been added to the plan of care. The nurse knows that which of the following is important to this patient's plan of care?

   (A) The benzodiazepines will need to be discontinued.
   (B) The patient will need to be monitored more closely for stroke.
   (C) The QT interval will need to be measured regularly.
   (D) The amoxicillin will need to be switched to erythromycin.

5. A patient with a long history of alcohol abuse may develop gait disturbances due to deficiency of thiamine that, in turn, affects glucose metabolism. Gait disturbance is a sign of which of the following problems?

   (A) Grey Turner's sign
   (B) Wernicke's encephalopathy
   (C) alcohol poisoning
   (D) Korsakoff syndrome

6. A patient has suddenly become verbally aggressive and loud. Which of the following is the best strategy the nurse may use at this time?

(A) Speak loudly to the patient.
(B) Restrain the patient.
(C) Stand directly in front of the patient.
(D) Provide direct care with a colleague.

ANSWER KEY

1. **D**   2. **C**   3. **A**   4. **C**   5. **B**   6. **D**

ANSWERS EXPLAINED

1. **(D)** The RN is obligated to report elder abuse, either directly to state adult protective services or through social services. This should be done without consulting the family or the physician. Although the patient requires emotional support, this alone will not address the cause of the problem.

2. **(C)** Studies have shown that engaging patients in communication and frequent reorientation will help prevent delirium. Restraining patients, deep sedation, and lack of mobility will all increase the incidence of delirium.

3. **(A)** Patients who have attempted suicide have been known either to hoard medications to use in a future suicide attempt or be suspicious of medication ordered by health-care providers. The patient is most likely depressed as evidenced by actions. Her statement otherwise is not to be entirely believed. Confrontation is most likely not therapeutic. Patients who have attempted suicide should not be left alone.

4. **(C)** Haloperidol (Haldol) has the potential to prolong the QT interval and result in a life-threatening arrhythmia, torsades de pointes ventricular tachycardia. Benzodiazepines are needed in acute alcohol withdrawal syndromes in order to prevent complications such as seizures. The patient's diagnosis and addition of haloperidol does not lead to increased risk of stroke. Erythromycin is not recommended during treatment with haloperidol as it may also prolong the QT interval.

5. **(B)** Gait disturbance is one of several signs of Wernicke's encephalopathy, which is due to severe lack of thiamine. The remaining 3 choices do not result in gait changes and/or are not due to alcohol abuse.

6. **(D)** When more than one caregiver is in the room, the patient is less likely to be aggressive. The remaining 3 choices may provoke aggression or put the nurse into an unsafe position.

Professional Caring and Ethical Practices

14

Don't worry about failures, worry about the chances you miss when you don't even try.

—Jack Canfield

PROFESSIONAL CARING AND ETHICAL PRACTICES TEST BLUEPRINT

Professional Caring and Ethical Practices 20% of total test   **30 Questions**

→ Advocacy/moral agency (3%)
→ Caring practices (4%)
→ Collaboration (4%)
→ Systems thinking (2%)
→ Response to diversity (2%)
→ Clinical inquiry (2%)
→ Facilitation of learning (3%)

OVERVIEW

The AACN places a great deal of importance on the nurses' ability to provide care to critically ill patients and their families beyond the physiological realm. The nurses' ability to assess the entire patient situation is expected. Novice critical care nurses tend to focus on learning the many clinical issues and management of symptoms. As nurses progress from novice to competent to expert level of nursing practice, they increase their ability to see the whole patient and consider patient characteristics beyond the physiologic. The competencies are described in the AACN Synergy Model for Patient Care, which can be found at *www.aacn.org*. The test questions will expect you to include all of the patient's characteristics, not just the physiological, when planning care.

TEST PREPARATION

- Read the Synergy Model, but do not attempt to memorize it. Simply understand the AACN's philosophy on professional caring and ethical practices.
- Review the concepts presented in this section.
- Answer the practice questions, and review the answers to identify areas you may need to review.

- Although there are as many professional caring and practices questions as there are cardiovascular questions, you will not need to study this section as many hours as the cardiovascular section, probably one-half the time.
- Familiarize yourself with the AACN Practice Alerts that are related to professional caring and ethical practices. The Practice Alerts are available at *www.aacn.org* and can be saved as PDFs for your files.
  - "Family Presence During Resuscitation and Invasive Procedures"
  - "Family Visitation in the Adult ICU"

NURSE CHARACTERISTICS NECESSARY TO PROVIDE PROFESSIONAL CARING AND ETHICAL PRACTICES

Clinical Judgment

The ability to synthesize and interpret multiple pieces of data, critical thinking

- At the expert level of practice, the nurse interprets multiple, sometimes conflicting, data and makes decisions based on a grasp of the whole picture; can anticipate problems based on previous experience
- Helps the patient and family see the "big picture"
- Takes time to develop
- For example, when caring for a patient with multisystem organ dysfunction with comorbidities, the less-experienced nurse will focus solely on the immediate physiologic instability of the patient. This will be reflected in patient/family communication. The expert nurse will address the physiologic instability but also realize the impact of the comorbidities and include this when communicating with the patient and family.

Advocacy and Moral Agency

Works on behalf of others; represents concerns of others, including patient/family and other nurses; able to identify and help resolve ethical issues

- At the expert level of practice, the nurse advocates from the patient/family perspective, even when different from personal values
- May work to suspend rules to work for the benefit of the patient/family
- The integrity of the family system is crucial to the long-term patient outcome, i.e., the patient support system is always considered in the plan of care
- Empowers the patient/family to speak for themselves
- For example, if the wife of an unresponsive ventilator patient requests to use an herbal remedy ointment known to be a cure in their culture, the less-experienced nurse might tactfully explain it is not allowed and support the rules. The expert nurse would understand the importance to the wife and explain that she/he would consult a pharmacist to see if the ointment is safe. If it is safe to use, the expert nurse will allow the wife to apply it under supervision.

Caring Practices

Creates a compassionate, supportive, and therapeutic environment for patients/family; prevents unnecessary suffering

- Able to engage the patient/family and aware of patient/family needs, able to anticipate needs
- Coordinates care to provide comfort for patient/family, even at time of death
- Ensures that **all** patients and families understand that palliative options exist to relieve suffering at the end of life
- For example, if a young adult athlete has an acute traumatic injury that may impact his/her future ability to play sports and exhibits "difficult" behavior, the less-experienced nurse may sympathize and do what is necessary and attempt to meet demands. The expert nurse will understand the behavior may be a symptom of grief and loss and will encourage the patient to express feelings related to loss. The nurse may also seek expert consultation and engage the rehab team early in the patient's treatment.

Collaboration

Works with others in a manner that promotes/encourages each person's contributions toward achieving optimal, realistic goals

- Initiates collaboration, does not wait for others to reach out
- Seeks opportunities to teach, coach, and mentor
- Seeks opportunities to be taught, coached, and mentored
- Values consistent communication
- For example, if the nephrologist explains to the wife of an 89-year-old unresponsive patient with metastatic cancer that hemodialysis is required and will provide a chance for improvement and the wife expresses doubt after the physician leaves the room, the nurse with less experience may either comfort the wife or perhaps contradict what the physician has explained. The expert nurse will seek to collaborate with the physician. The expert nurse will discuss the prognosis, the wife's hesitancy to continue with dialysis, and work for a better solution.

Systems Thinking

Manages environmental and system resources to meet patient/family needs; considers factors outside the unit; considers the hospital as a whole, the community

- Able to navigate through the system on behalf of the patient/family
- Considers factors outside the immediate unit
- Sees the patient/family in the "big picture," not only in terms of the immediate unit environment
- Understands the impact on processes and system influence on human error and efficiency
- In a culture of patient safety:
  - When errors are made, the response is to analyze the system processes that led to the error (not punitive).
  - The number of incident reports or patient safety event reports generally increases in a culture of safety since reports are made to assess and identify how processes can be improved to prevent future errors, not to target individuals.

- For example, a patient received 2 stents during a PCI procedure for acute coronary syndrome and will need to take clopidogrel. The patient does not have health insurance. The nurse with less experience may not realize the cost of the drug and not be aware of resources that can be recommended to the patient. The expert nurse may be aware of a special program sponsored by a pharmaceutical company. The expert nurse may consult with the social services or discharge planner to attempt to get financial assistance for the patient.

Response to Diversity

Recognize, appreciate, and incorporate differences into the plan of care. Differences include age, gender, race, cultural differences, ethnicity, lifestyle, educational level, socioeconomic status, values, and beliefs

- Does not expect patients/family to be the same as healthcare providers, able to explore and identify differences
- Accepts the patient/family individualized response to acute illness and modifies the plan of care to accommodate the patient/family
- For example, a patient's family may have what seems to be an unrealistic expectation for recovery, which is frustrating to healthcare providers. The nurse with less experience may experience frustration and provide explanations in the same manner as for all other patients. The experienced nurse may attempt to identify where the family is "coming from," get background information, and then revise explanations to them accordingly.

Facilitation of Learning

Promotes learning of patients, family, nursing staff, and members of healthcare team, both formally and informally

- Creatively finds opportunities for providing accurate information
- Adapts educational programs to the patient/family need/situation
- Obtains input from patient/family when setting educational goals
- Collaborates with all members of the healthcare team and incorporates healthcare goals into the patients' educational plan
- For instance, the patient may have 3 major risk factors for coronary artery disease status post PCI with stent deployment. The inexperienced nurse might provide all of the available written resources on risk factor modification and advise the patient to attend cardiac rehab after discharge. The expert nurse will ask the patient which of the risk factors he/she wants to target the most and advise based on patient motivation as well as seriousness of risk factor, e.g., smoking more serious than sedentary lifestyle. The advantages of the cardiac rehab program will be discussed and arrangements made for the rehab staff to visit the patient prior to discharge.

Clinical Inquiry

Questions and evaluates practice, maintains familiarity with professional literature, shares best practices

- Identifies circumstances when standards and guidelines may be improved upon or deviated from to address individualized patient situations or populations
- Stays current with new, updated, or revised evidence-based practice and incorporates into practice
- According to the Synergy Model, the domains of clinical judgment and clinical inquiry converge at the expert level and cannot be separated
- For example, the inexperienced nurse may continue to determine correct placement of an enteral feeding tube by auscultation of air. If aware that it is no longer evidence based, the inexperienced nurse may continue to perform air insufflation since all other nurses use the technique. An expert nurse will be aware that studies show this is not an accurate method for determining feeding tube placement, bring in the literature, share the information with staff, and engage in the process to update hospital procedures.

Patient Characteristics

In addition to nurse characteristics that affect professional caring and ethical practice, AACN has identified patient characteristics (other than physiological) that the nurse needs to consider when planning care. If only physiological problems are identified without consideration of nonclinical individual differences, the outcome will be negatively affected. The characteristics include:

- Resiliency: the patient's ability to "bounce back"
- Vulnerability: susceptibility to actual or potential stressors
- Stability: ability to maintain equilibrium (not only physiological)
- Complexity: family interactions, environment
- Resource availability: of patient **and** family (personal, fiscal, technical, social)
- Participation in care: extent that patient and family are engaged in care
- Participation in decision making: extent that patient and family are engaged in making decisions
- Predictability: the degree to which the outcome is expected, events expected

> Now that you have reviewed key professional caring and ethical practices, go to the Professional Caring and Ethical Practices Practice Questions. Answer the questions, and then check your answers. Continue to review the information until you get at least 80% on the practice questions.

PROFESSIONAL CARING AND ETHICAL PRACTICES
PRACTICE QUESTIONS

1. A nurse colleague is having difficulty with a patient's family and requests assistance from the more experienced nurse. The best approach for the experienced nurse would be:

   (A) offer to speak with the family.
   (B) advise she/he ignore the family's behavior.
   (C) suggest use of active-listening techniques.
   (D) suggest the patient assignment be changed.

2. The healthcare team believes that the patient with multisystem organ dysfunction will not survive and is dying. Which of the following is the most appropriate at this time?

   (A) Avoid discussion of death as it is upsetting to the wife.
   (B) Ensure the wife understands the availability of palliative care at the end of life.
   (C) Refer family questions to the attending physician.
   (D) Portray the hopelessness of the situation so the wife accepts the reality of the situation.

3. Upon entering the room of a patient receiving mechanical ventilation, the nurse notes that the nursing assistant allowed the patient to remain supine and did not elevate the head of the bed to at least 30 degrees after leaving. The best response would be to elevate the head of the bed and:

   (A) mention the omission by the nursing assistant to the charge nurse.
   (B) point out the omission to the nursing assistant later in the shift.
   (C) advocate for a policy change related to nursing assistant responsibility.
   (D) explain to the nursing assistant the rationale for elevation of the head of the bed for ventilator patients.

4. The nurse is approached by the family during active resuscitation for full cardio-pulmonary arrest and requests to be present. The nurse's best response would be:

   (A) call security.
   (B) allow them to stay as long as they do not interfere.
   (C) follow the current hospital policy.
   (D) explain that the physician in charge does not permit family presence during CPR.

5. The 25-year-old male patient is recovering from septic shock. His mother has a homeopathic ointment and is applying it to the patient's hands and feet "for the swelling." The nurse should:

   (A) take the ointment from the mother and explain it is not allowed.
   (B) instruct the mother to withhold ointment use until the pharmacist is consulted.
   (C) allow the mother to continue to use the ointment since it is comforting her.
   (D) explain that the ointment will not be of any help to the patient's edema.

6. The nurse reads a meta-analysis of a clinical intervention that supports its adoption in a nursing procedure. The most effective action to be taken by the nurse is:

    (A) bring a copy of the study with a request to nursing and physician leadership to consider revision of the current nursing procedure.
    (B) incorporate the clinical intervention into practice.
    (C) discuss the clinical intervention with the charge nurse.
    (D) assume the nursing leadership will be adopting the new practice in the near future.

7. While receiving a report from the nurse working the previous shift, the nurse notes that her colleague provided a sedative drug but no analgesic to the post-op patient. The best response would be to:

    (A) point out to the nurse that omission of analgesia post-op is negligent.
    (B) consider the previous shift was busier than usual and provide the analgesic as soon as possible.
    (C) point out to the nurse that it appears as if an analgesic was not given, inquire why, and then explain the importance of post-op analgesia.
    (D) report the omission to the charge nurse.

8. Which of the following statements related to patient characteristics is TRUE?

    (A) The quadriplegic patient admitted with septic shock has low resiliency.
    (B) The patient with multiple comorbidities has low complexity.
    (C) The patient admitted with multiple fractures and no other problems has low predictability.
    (D) Restricted family visitation improves patient resource availability.

9. The family of a patient in critical, unstable condition is critical of the hospital and nursing staff and is highly distraught. What is the most appropriate response?

    (A) Explain all interventions in detail.
    (B) Listen to the family's concerns, and provide reassurance.
    (C) Provide information on the hospital's clinical excellence.
    (D) Call the nursing supervisor to meet with the family.

10. The wife of a 29-year-old critically ill trauma patient requests that she be able to bring in their 9-month-old daughter for the patient to see. The patient, who is lightly sedated, nods "yes" when asked if he wants to see his daughter. Which of the following would be the nurse's best response?

    (A) Explain that children under the age of 12 cannot visit.
    (B) Ignore the policy, and allow the wife to bring in their daughter.
    (C) Explain to the wife that the patient will not remember the visit.
    (D) Tell the wife the physician and charge nurse will be consulted to request permission.

11. The nurse receives information from her colleague at 0700 that during the previous shift, the 21-year-old female patient admitted with acute complications related to sickle cell crisis has not reported a pain score of less than 8 (on a 0–10 scale). The attending physician was contacted at 0500 for additional analgesia but stated, "The order is adequate; the patient is drug-seeking." On the initial shift assessment, the patient rates pain as a "9." The best response by the day shift nurse would be:

(A) explain to the patient that the physician has been notified but no further orders were received.

(B) reassure the patient that the next dose of analgesia is due in an hour.

(C) call the physician, report the current assessment, and recommend the analgesia order felt to be most appropriate for the patient's pain.

(D) contact the nurse manager and explain the situation.

12. The patient reported to the nurse that the physician told him he would be transferred to the step-down unit later in the evening, but the wife was told the patient would be transferred the next day. The nurse should:

(A) explain to them both that physicians often change their minds after getting more information.

(B) contact the physician to clarify the plan of care.

(C) tell the patient and wife to wait and see what is decided.

(D) contact the charge nurse to discuss the matter.

13. A nurse has found out about an innovative IV tubing label system from a nurse colleague friend who works at another hospital. The nurse feels strongly that the innovative system would promote patient safety and would like to be able to use the system in his/her unit. The best approach to use to get the new system would be:

(A) obtain written information and samples of the system and present to nursing leadership.

(B) advise the unit manager that the current IV labeling system is not safe, citing examples.

(C) complete an incident report each time a nurse colleague forgets to label IV tubing.

(D) point out to colleagues the multiple problems with the unit's current IV labeling system.

14. The nursing staff are reacting negatively when assigned a patient with a large family who have been labeled "demanding." The best resolution would be:

(A) hold a team conference to discuss the issue.

(B) rotate the patient assignment from day to day.

(C) meet with the family and explain that the demands need to cease.

(D) request a psychiatric consult from the attending physician.

15. The nurse does not understand the physician's plan of care and treatments ordered for the patient. It is the nurse's responsibility to:

(A) plan to look up the patient diagnosis and treatment after work.

(B) complete the orders as written.

(C) tell the charge nurse to reassign the patient to another nurse.

(D) approach the physician and seek to understand the plan of care.

16. One of the newer nurses continues to struggle when setting up the IV infusion pump despite several explanations and provision of written material. The optimal strategy for the more experienced nurse would be:

(A) provide coaching while he/she sets up a pump.

(B) obtain a video.

(C) report to the manager.

(D) demonstrate how it is done.

17. Which of the following statements is TRUE?

(A) Speaking up when safety lapses are identified increases error.

(B) It is easier to assess system problems as the source of medication errors than take a punitive approach.

(C) Family presence benefits the family, not the patient.

(D) The AACN expects nurses to consider non-physiological patient characteristics as well as physiological data.

18. The nurse discovers that a medication error was made as the infusion pump was programmed incorrectly 30 minutes ago. The patient has not experienced any adverse reaction and is stable. The nurse should:

(A) continue to monitor the patient for adverse effects and notify the physician if adverse effects occur.

(B) report the error to the physician but do not mention it to the patient.

(C) contact the pharmacist to determine the next steps.

(D) notify the physician, tell the patient of the error, and complete a safety event report.

19. A patient arrives on the critical care unit from the post-anesthesia recovery unit (PACU) with a chest tube drainage system never seen before by the nurse receiving the patient. The nurse's best response would be:

(A) request the nurse from the PACU explain the system operation and answer questions as the system is reviewed.

(B) call the charge nurse into the room and explain the situation.

(C) call the surgeon and explain how disruptive and unsafe the use of the new system has been.

(D) assume the new drainage system is similar to those you have used in the past.

20. Several nurse colleagues of a nurse who has attained certification have asked what the value of certification is. The certified nurse's best response would be that certification:

(A) validates clinical skills.
(B) is a process that leads to higher levels of professionalism.
(C) provides fiscal awards.
(D) contributes to the professional reputation of the hospital.

21. The nurse is caring for a 71-year-old male with respiratory failure secondary to pneumonia and requires mechanical ventilation. The patient is married with 9 children and 20 grandchildren. Many of them are either coming to see the patient or calling to inquire about the patient. Which of the following is the best response to this situation?

(A) Ask security to intervene.
(B) Ask the family to leave the hospital, limiting the visits to 2 to 3 family members in the hospital at the same time.
(C) Answer questions succinctly as they arise, and take calls if not busy providing patient care.
(D) Ask the family to decide on one spokesperson and communicate in the plan of care who the spokesperson is.

22. The critical care unit upgraded the patient beds, and the beds have many new features. All nurses received education on the new beds. On the first day at work with the new beds, the nurse realizes that most of the education was forgotten. The nurse should:

(A) complain to colleagues that the education took place too far in advance of actual use.
(B) make a point to review the new bed at some point during the shift.
(C) request that the unit educator or another nurse colleague who worked with the beds during the previous shift review essential operations.
(D) look up the bed vendor on the Internet as soon as possible.

23. The unit education committee is developing written resources for patients with heart failure. An effective approach would include:

(A) shrinking the information so it fits on one page.
(B) using more pictures than words.
(C) developing an online program.
(D) ensuring the material is written at a fourth-grade reading level.

24. The nurse and her ICU colleagues have seen what they feel is an increase in lapses in care by the Emergency Department nurses. The most effective course of action would be:

(A) document all of the problems and send to Risk Management.
(B) ask the unit manager to set up a meeting between the leadership and staff representatives from each unit to plan a course of action.
(C) request that the ED receive more education.
(D) arrange to have all ICU nurses ask more detailed questions of the ED when getting a report on patient status prior to receiving the patient.

25. The nurse has reason to believe one of her nurse colleagues is diverting controlled substances. The nurse should:

(A) report her suspicions to the nurse manager.
(B) approach the colleague to discuss her suspicions.
(C) call security.
(D) not take any action until more information is obtained.

26. Nurse staffing and patient assignments are best based on:

(A) nurse/patient ratio.
(B) patient acuity.
(C) nurse seniority.
(D) patient characteristics.

27. The physician orders a medication that is not considered compatible with another medication the patient is already receiving. The nurse should:

(A) call the pharmacist to get information.
(B) ask the physician to explain the order.
(C) ask a nurse colleague what she/he thinks of the order.
(D) administer the medication as ordered.

28. A 25-year-old female patient sustained a double amputation due to a traumatic injury. She seems withdrawn and with poor self-esteem related to body image although she has a strong family support system, good health insurance, and no previous health problems. An effective strategy for this patient would be:

(A) ask for an order for an antidepressant.
(B) point out to the patient what she has in her life for which she can be grateful.
(C) encourage the patient to participate in care and provide options.
(D) ask for a psychiatric consult.

29. A 25-year-old Mexican-American trauma patient is unable to make decisions for himself. His wife seems to understand English and nods "yes" that she understands. However, she speaks in only short sentences and does not ask questions. The best course of action would be to:

(A) request an interpreter.
(B) attempt to contact an English-speaking family member.
(C) call a phlebotomist who speaks Spanish.
(D) continue to speak English with the wife as long as she does not object.

30. The attending physician of a patient with multisystem problems continues to express hope of a positive outcome to the patient's husband. However, the consultants have portrayed a more bleak outcome to the husband. The patient's husband has expressed his frustration to the nurse. The nurse's best response would be:

(A) support the attending's opinions when speaking with the husband.
(B) support the consultants' opinions when speaking to the husband.
(C) contact the attending physician and express concern regarding conflicting information provided to the husband by physicians.
(D) empathize with the husband and explain this often happens when multiple physicians are providing care.

ANSWER KEY

1. **C**	6. **A**	11. **C**	16. **A**	21. **D**	26. **D**
2. **B**	7. **C**	12. **B**	17. **D**	22. **C**	27. **B**
3. **D**	8. **A**	13. **A**	18. **D**	23. **D**	28. **C**
4. **C**	9. **B**	14. **A**	19. **A**	24. **B**	29. **A**
5. **B**	10. **D**	15. **D**	20. **B**	25. **A**	30. **C**

ANSWERS EXPLAINED

1. **(C)** Most difficult situations are related to communication gaps, and listening is a major part of communication. This response demonstrates the nursing characteristic of facilitating learning. Choices (A) and (D) do not provide an opportunity for the nurse colleague to develop professionally. Choice (B) is avoidance behavior.

2. **(B)** All critically ill patients and families, even those in situations where the outcome is unsure and may not be the "end of life," are entitled to palliative care, which provides a plan for the family. The choice illustrates advocacy and caring nurse characteristics. Choice (A) is not a solution for the family and is not helpful. Choice (C) is not a strategy of a proactive professional nurse. Choice (D), although it may be honest, is not helpful for the family.

3. **(D)** The nursing assistant must understand the importance of elevating the head of the bed for this patient population in order to prevent ventilator-associated complications. The correct choice also demonstrates the nurse's ability to teach. Choice (A) is passive. Choice (B) is not optimal as the ward may get too busy or the nurse may forget, plus coaching should be done as close to the situation as possible. Choice (C) is not

a solution. Elevation of the head of the bed is a responsibility able to be delegated to unlicensed assistants.

4. **(C)** Although choice (B) may be considered, this is not the time to allow the family's presence since systems are not in place that would ensure a good experience. Choice (A) is an overreaction. Choice (D) is not a valid reason to prevent the family's presence.

5. **(B)** As long as homeopathic remedies are not harmful to the patient, allowing the family to practice within its culture is acceptable. Choices (A) and (D) do not acknowledge cultural diversity. Choice (C) is not correct as some homeopathic remedies may harm the patient, especially when used in conjunction with some medical therapies already in use.

6. **(A)** Choices (C) and (D) are not effective strategies. Choice (B) may contradict current policy that, despite being outdated, cannot be ignored without special physician approval.

7. **(C)** Choice (C) gives the nurse the chance to teach plus provides an opportunity to hear the colleague's point of view. Choices (A) and (D) are not effective strategies. Choice (B) is passive behavior and ignores the opportunity for coaching.

8. **(A)** This patient has 2 major problems that will decrease his ability to "bounce back" and have a positive outcome. The plan of care should optimally take this into consideration. The remaining 3 choices are not accurate.

9. **(B)** This strategy allows the family to be heard and also allows the nurse to show a degree of empathy. The remaining 3 choices do not acknowledge the family's stress or provide support.

10. **(D)** Choices (A) and (C) do not attempt to provide patient-centered care. Choice (B), although acknowledging the patient's and wife's needs, may send the wrong message regarding hospital policies in general. Plus choice (B) shows a lack of ability to collaborate on the part of the nurse.

11. **(C)** This strategy, unlike the other choices, puts the patient's needs first. It has the potential to get a more appropriate order for the patient going forward.

12. **(B)** This choice is the most collaborative and direct approach.

13. **(A)** Although this choice requires the most effort, it is the one most likely to result in an improvement over the current process.

14. **(A)** The team needs to discuss strategies for handling this type of situation because the solution that all can support might be used in the future for similar situations. Choice (B) prevents continuity of care. Choice (C) does not consider the family's needs. Choice (D) implies the issue is all the "fault" of the family. A social worker or psychiatric specialist may be consulted, but that alone would not be the solution.

15. **(D)** The professional nurse needs to collaborate actively to ensure understanding and facilitate her/his own learning. The other choices are not effective strategies for ensuring the nurse understands the plan of care.

16. **(A)** This allows visual, auditory, and sensory learning. It also provides immediate feedback to the learner. All of these factors are principles of effective adult learning. The other choices do not provide multiple learning modalities.

17. **(D)** Choice (A) is not correct because speaking up decreases error. Choice (B) is not correct because system assessments are more difficult. Choice (C) is incorrect because family presence benefits both the patient and the family.

18. **(D)** Transparency (notification of both the physician and the patient) is the appropriate response to committing a patient error, even if the patient does not experience adverse effects.

19. **(A)** The best immediate solution for the patient is for the nurse to get information on the new collection system and get questions answered from a more knowledgeable source. Introducing new equipment without preparation will need to be addressed by unit leadership in order to prevent a repeat incident in the future.

20. **(B)** Certification does **not** validate clinical skills and does **not** guarantee fiscal rewards, although it may. Certification is not directly associated with the hospital's reputation. The "journey" of attaining certification results in the professional growth of the nurse.

21. **(D)** This will help control the volume of family the nurse will need to communicate with, allowing the nurse to care for the patient yet provide a means to include the family. The other 3 choices do not provide an organized approach for the nursing staff plus meet the family's needs.

22. **(C)** This is the best strategy. It will allow the nurse to care for the patients safely during the present shift. The remaining choices are not effective, safe strategies.

23. **(D)** In order for educational materials to meet requirements for the majority of the population, information needs to be written at a fourth-grade reading level. The other 3 choices do not provide an effective strategy for patient/family comprehension by the majority of the adult population.

24. **(B)** Collaboration between the 2 units will provide the most effective solution.

25. **(A)** Diversion of controlled substances is not an issue that is dealt with collaboratively between the 2 nurses. Suspicions need to be pursued for the safety of the patients and the nurse who may be diverting the drugs. Human resources has the knowledge and expertise for handling these situations.

26. **(D)** Basing resources on the individual needs of the patient is most likely to provide quality care.

27. **(B)** The nurse is responsible for understanding the plan of care. The best strategy is to collaborate actively with the physician. If, after doing this, the nurse still has doubts, they need to be taken up the chain of command.

28. **(C)** Active participation and providing choices may allow some patient control and decrease passivity, which may improve self-esteem.

29. **(A)** It is the nurse's responsibility to ensure the family (or patient) understands the information and that the nurse's communication is delivered accurately and objectively. The remaining 3 choices do not ensure accuracy and objectively.

30. **(C)** The goal is to provide realistic, consistent information to the patient's husband. The best strategy for the nurse to achieve this is to express concerns directly to the physician and contribute feedback as well as possible recommendations about the situation.

Practice Tests

ANSWER SHEET
Practice Test 1

1. Ⓐ Ⓑ Ⓒ Ⓓ
2. Ⓐ Ⓑ Ⓒ Ⓓ
3. Ⓐ Ⓑ Ⓒ Ⓓ
4. Ⓐ Ⓑ Ⓒ Ⓓ
5. Ⓐ Ⓑ Ⓒ Ⓓ
6. Ⓐ Ⓑ Ⓒ Ⓓ
7. Ⓐ Ⓑ Ⓒ Ⓓ
8. Ⓐ Ⓑ Ⓒ Ⓓ
9. Ⓐ Ⓑ Ⓒ Ⓓ
10. Ⓐ Ⓑ Ⓒ Ⓓ
11. Ⓐ Ⓑ Ⓒ Ⓓ
12. Ⓐ Ⓑ Ⓒ Ⓓ
13. Ⓐ Ⓑ Ⓒ Ⓓ
14. Ⓐ Ⓑ Ⓒ Ⓓ
15. Ⓐ Ⓑ Ⓒ Ⓓ
16. Ⓐ Ⓑ Ⓒ Ⓓ
17. Ⓐ Ⓑ Ⓒ Ⓓ
18. Ⓐ Ⓑ Ⓒ Ⓓ
19. Ⓐ Ⓑ Ⓒ Ⓓ
20. Ⓐ Ⓑ Ⓒ Ⓓ
21. Ⓐ Ⓑ Ⓒ Ⓓ
22. Ⓐ Ⓑ Ⓒ Ⓓ
23. Ⓐ Ⓑ Ⓒ Ⓓ
24. Ⓐ Ⓑ Ⓒ Ⓓ
25. Ⓐ Ⓑ Ⓒ Ⓓ
26. Ⓐ Ⓑ Ⓒ Ⓓ
27. Ⓐ Ⓑ Ⓒ Ⓓ
28. Ⓐ Ⓑ Ⓒ Ⓓ
29. Ⓐ Ⓑ Ⓒ Ⓓ
30. Ⓐ Ⓑ Ⓒ Ⓓ
31. Ⓐ Ⓑ Ⓒ Ⓓ
32. Ⓐ Ⓑ Ⓒ Ⓓ
33. Ⓐ Ⓑ Ⓒ Ⓓ
34. Ⓐ Ⓑ Ⓒ Ⓓ
35. Ⓐ Ⓑ Ⓒ Ⓓ
36. Ⓐ Ⓑ Ⓒ Ⓓ
37. Ⓐ Ⓑ Ⓒ Ⓓ
38. Ⓐ Ⓑ Ⓒ Ⓓ

39. Ⓐ Ⓑ Ⓒ Ⓓ
40. Ⓐ Ⓑ Ⓒ Ⓓ
41. Ⓐ Ⓑ Ⓒ Ⓓ
42. Ⓐ Ⓑ Ⓒ Ⓓ
43. Ⓐ Ⓑ Ⓒ Ⓓ
44. Ⓐ Ⓑ Ⓒ Ⓓ
45. Ⓐ Ⓑ Ⓒ Ⓓ
46. Ⓐ Ⓑ Ⓒ Ⓓ
47. Ⓐ Ⓑ Ⓒ Ⓓ
48. Ⓐ Ⓑ Ⓒ Ⓓ
49. Ⓐ Ⓑ Ⓒ Ⓓ
50. Ⓐ Ⓑ Ⓒ Ⓓ
51. Ⓐ Ⓑ Ⓒ Ⓓ
52. Ⓐ Ⓑ Ⓒ Ⓓ
53. Ⓐ Ⓑ Ⓒ Ⓓ
54. Ⓐ Ⓑ Ⓒ Ⓓ
55. Ⓐ Ⓑ Ⓒ Ⓓ
56. Ⓐ Ⓑ Ⓒ Ⓓ
57. Ⓐ Ⓑ Ⓒ Ⓓ
58. Ⓐ Ⓑ Ⓒ Ⓓ
59. Ⓐ Ⓑ Ⓒ Ⓓ
60. Ⓐ Ⓑ Ⓒ Ⓓ
61. Ⓐ Ⓑ Ⓒ Ⓓ
62. Ⓐ Ⓑ Ⓒ Ⓓ
63. Ⓐ Ⓑ Ⓒ Ⓓ
64. Ⓐ Ⓑ Ⓒ Ⓓ
65. Ⓐ Ⓑ Ⓒ Ⓓ
66. Ⓐ Ⓑ Ⓒ Ⓓ
67. Ⓐ Ⓑ Ⓒ Ⓓ
68. Ⓐ Ⓑ Ⓒ Ⓓ
69. Ⓐ Ⓑ Ⓒ Ⓓ
70. Ⓐ Ⓑ Ⓒ Ⓓ
71. Ⓐ Ⓑ Ⓒ Ⓓ
72. Ⓐ Ⓑ Ⓒ Ⓓ
73. Ⓐ Ⓑ Ⓒ Ⓓ
74. Ⓐ Ⓑ Ⓒ Ⓓ
75. Ⓐ Ⓑ Ⓒ Ⓓ
76. Ⓐ Ⓑ Ⓒ Ⓓ

77. Ⓐ Ⓑ Ⓒ Ⓓ
78. Ⓐ Ⓑ Ⓒ Ⓓ
79. Ⓐ Ⓑ Ⓒ Ⓓ
80. Ⓐ Ⓑ Ⓒ Ⓓ
81. Ⓐ Ⓑ Ⓒ Ⓓ
82. Ⓐ Ⓑ Ⓒ Ⓓ
83. Ⓐ Ⓑ Ⓒ Ⓓ
84. Ⓐ Ⓑ Ⓒ Ⓓ
85. Ⓐ Ⓑ Ⓒ Ⓓ
86. Ⓐ Ⓑ Ⓒ Ⓓ
87. Ⓐ Ⓑ Ⓒ Ⓓ
88. Ⓐ Ⓑ Ⓒ Ⓓ
89. Ⓐ Ⓑ Ⓒ Ⓓ
90. Ⓐ Ⓑ Ⓒ Ⓓ
91. Ⓐ Ⓑ Ⓒ Ⓓ
92. Ⓐ Ⓑ Ⓒ Ⓓ
93. Ⓐ Ⓑ Ⓒ Ⓓ
94. Ⓐ Ⓑ Ⓒ Ⓓ
95. Ⓐ Ⓑ Ⓒ Ⓓ
96. Ⓐ Ⓑ Ⓒ Ⓓ
97. Ⓐ Ⓑ Ⓒ Ⓓ
98. Ⓐ Ⓑ Ⓒ Ⓓ
99. Ⓐ Ⓑ Ⓒ Ⓓ
100. Ⓐ Ⓑ Ⓒ Ⓓ
101. Ⓐ Ⓑ Ⓒ Ⓓ
102. Ⓐ Ⓑ Ⓒ Ⓓ
103. Ⓐ Ⓑ Ⓒ Ⓓ
104. Ⓐ Ⓑ Ⓒ Ⓓ
105. Ⓐ Ⓑ Ⓒ Ⓓ
106. Ⓐ Ⓑ Ⓒ Ⓓ
107. Ⓐ Ⓑ Ⓒ Ⓓ
108. Ⓐ Ⓑ Ⓒ Ⓓ
109. Ⓐ Ⓑ Ⓒ Ⓓ
110. Ⓐ Ⓑ Ⓒ Ⓓ
111. Ⓐ Ⓑ Ⓒ Ⓓ
112. Ⓐ Ⓑ Ⓒ Ⓓ
113. Ⓐ Ⓑ Ⓒ Ⓓ
114. Ⓐ Ⓑ Ⓒ Ⓓ

115. Ⓐ Ⓑ Ⓒ Ⓓ
116. Ⓐ Ⓑ Ⓒ Ⓓ
117. Ⓐ Ⓑ Ⓒ Ⓓ
118. Ⓐ Ⓑ Ⓒ Ⓓ
119. Ⓐ Ⓑ Ⓒ Ⓓ
120. Ⓐ Ⓑ Ⓒ Ⓓ
121. Ⓐ Ⓑ Ⓒ Ⓓ
122. Ⓐ Ⓑ Ⓒ Ⓓ
123. Ⓐ Ⓑ Ⓒ Ⓓ
124. Ⓐ Ⓑ Ⓒ Ⓓ
125. Ⓐ Ⓑ Ⓒ Ⓓ
126. Ⓐ Ⓑ Ⓒ Ⓓ
127. Ⓐ Ⓑ Ⓒ Ⓓ
128. Ⓐ Ⓑ Ⓒ Ⓓ
129. Ⓐ Ⓑ Ⓒ Ⓓ
130. Ⓐ Ⓑ Ⓒ Ⓓ
131. Ⓐ Ⓑ Ⓒ Ⓓ
132. Ⓐ Ⓑ Ⓒ Ⓓ
133. Ⓐ Ⓑ Ⓒ Ⓓ
134. Ⓐ Ⓑ Ⓒ Ⓓ
135. Ⓐ Ⓑ Ⓒ Ⓓ
136. Ⓐ Ⓑ Ⓒ Ⓓ
137. Ⓐ Ⓑ Ⓒ Ⓓ
138. Ⓐ Ⓑ Ⓒ Ⓓ
139. Ⓐ Ⓑ Ⓒ Ⓓ
140. Ⓐ Ⓑ Ⓒ Ⓓ
141. Ⓐ Ⓑ Ⓒ Ⓓ
142. Ⓐ Ⓑ Ⓒ Ⓓ
143. Ⓐ Ⓑ Ⓒ Ⓓ
144. Ⓐ Ⓑ Ⓒ Ⓓ
145. Ⓐ Ⓑ Ⓒ Ⓓ
146. Ⓐ Ⓑ Ⓒ Ⓓ
147. Ⓐ Ⓑ Ⓒ Ⓓ
148. Ⓐ Ⓑ Ⓒ Ⓓ
149. Ⓐ Ⓑ Ⓒ Ⓓ
150. Ⓐ Ⓑ Ⓒ Ⓓ

Practice CCRN Test 1

15

PRACTICE TEST 1

Directions: This is the first of two, 150-question comprehensive practice tests. Do not attempt to complete these tests until you have reviewed each section of the book and have completed the tests related to each section. The pretest questions and the questions that follow each section focus more on "facts." Questions found in each final comprehensive test require application, evaluation, and analysis of knowledge. Master the book contents until you can achieve a score of at least 80% on the comprehensive tests prior to taking the CCRN® exam.

1. After attending an educational session that reviewed drug dosing and provided a review of the literature, the nurse would like to start using the admission weight to calculate drug dosing during titration of vasoactive drugs rather than the current practice of using daily weights. What would be the most effective next step for the nurse to take to implement this change?

(A) Begin adaptation of the concept by using the admission weight for patients.
(B) Identify key stakeholders related to the proposed change of practice.
(C) Ask the attending physician on rounds his/her thoughts about the practice.
(D) Discuss the educational session with nurse colleagues.

2. Which of the following is indicated during the embolization of an AV malformation procedure?

(A) phenytoin
(B) fibrinolytic
(C) fluids
(D) heparin

3. The patient with a urinary tract infection presented with a temp of 39°C, heart rate 132/minute, respiratory rate of 24, and B/P of 78/49. The patient received 2 L of 0.9 NS within 1 hour. The B/P is now 100/52, heart rate 118/minute, and respiratory rate of 20/minute. It seems this patient has:

(A) bacteremia.
(B) severe sepsis.
(C) sepsis.
(D) septic shock.

4. A patient was 48-hours post aortic valve replacement. Which of the following would be a major goal for this patient?

(A) diuretic therapy
(B) stabilize blood pressure
(C) prophylactic antibiotics
(D) prevent thrombus

PRACTICE CCRN TEST 1 267

5. A patient with hypoxic encephalopathy has been opening eyes to touch for the past 24 hours. The patient now withdraws to painful stimulus, has developed unequal pupils, and has positive Babinski. Which of the following interventions should the nurse anticipate?

(A) ventriculostomy, oxygen, steroids
(B) thiazide diuretic, sedation, pitressin (Vasopressin)
(C) osmotic diuretic, intubation, and monitor pCO_2
(D) lumbar puncture and increase FiO_2

6. A 19 year old, admitted with sickle cell crisis and acute kidney injury, requests to use a phone to update her friends on her condition. The best response of the nurse would be to:

(A) explain to the patient that calls can be made when transferred from the critical care unit.
(B) allow the patient to make the calls to meet the patient's need for social support.
(C) explain to the patient that she needs to rest in order for the analgesic medication to take effect.
(D) allow the patient to make the calls to meet the patient's need to reduce anxiety.

7. The patient is administered tensilon 2 mg IV as part of a "tensilon test." The patient develops increased muscle weakness, drooling, and lacrimation and has an emesis. The patient has signs of which of the following?

(A) myasthenia crisis
(B) anaphylactic reaction
(C) cholinergic crisis
(D) Trousseau sign

8. The patient has cardiogenic shock and cardiogenic pulmonary edema. Which of the following therapies would be most effective for this patient?

(A) ventricular assist device to increase coronary artery perfusion
(B) beta blocker to increase cardiac contractility
(C) alpha-adrenergic drug to increase coronary artery perfusion
(D) angiotensin-converting enzyme inhibitors to decrease afterload

9. The patient has a diagnosis of pulmonary aspiration. Which of the following is correctly related to pulmonary aspiration?

(A) It will not occur with an endotracheal tube or nasogastric tube in place.
(B) Aspiration is most commonly seen in the left lung.
(C) It may be chronic in certain patient populations.
(D) Aspiration, by definition, involves infection.

10. The patient has a history of chronic respiratory failure secondary to COPD and now has acute respiratory failure secondary to pneumonia. On arrival to the critical care unit, his ABGs were pH 7.29, $PaCO_2$ 77, PaO_2 51, HCO_3 31. He is receiving noninvasive ventilation with settings of FiO_2 0.40, IPAP of 12 cm, and EPAP of 5 cm. After 1 hour of therapy, the patient's ABG results are 7.20, $PaCO_2$ 89, PaO_2 48, and HCO_3 32.

What is the correct evaluation of this data?

(A) Alveolar hyperventilation is getting worse; BiPAP settings need adjustment.
(B) Metabolic acidosis is worse; the FiO_2 needs to be increased.
(C) Alveolar hypoventilation is getting worse; the patient needs to be intubated.
(D) The pH is acceptable for a patient with COPD; continue current therapy.

11. Which of the following is true related to plateau pressure?

(A) It is a pressure used to calculate static compliance and reflects pressure in the lungs.
(B) It is a pressure used to calculate vital capacity and reflects pressure in the lungs.
(C) It is a pressure used to calculate dynamic compliance and reflects pressure in the airways.
(D) It is a pressure used to measure tidal volume and reflects pressure in the airways.

12. The patient is admitted with salicylate overdose. Which of the following treatments are most effective for this patient?

(A) *N*-acetylcysteine, support airway, fluids
(B) gastric lavage, antidote, fluids
(C) activated charcoal, urine alkalinization, dialysis
(D) support airway, gastric lavage, ethanol

13. Which of the following patients who have sustained multiple trauma is most likely to have a poor outcome based on patient characteristics?

(A) the college graduate
(B) the owner of a successful business
(C) the married man
(D) the homeless man

14. A 68-year-old male is admitted with acute ST elevation myocardial infarction. The patient had a successful PCI with stent deployment and today has demonstrated anger and withdrawal. The patient has a history of depression and was taking an SSRI medication prior to admission. The nurse knows that a successful strategy for dealing with this patient would be to:

(A) provide environmental stimulation.
(B) encourage decision making.
(C) encourage expressing his feelings.
(D) provide solitude.

15. The patient has acute right ventricular infarct and RV failure. Which of the following is an indication that this patient's condition has improved?

(A) The PAOP has decreased.
(B) The RA pressure has decreased.
(C) The RV pressure has increased.
(D) The PA diastolic has decreased.

16. At 1-day status post AAA repair with a Dacron graft, the patient's serum BUN and creatinine increase and urine output decreases. Which of the following is the most likely etiology?

(A) acute renal failure
(B) graft rejection
(C) septic shock
(D) acute hemorrhage

17. The patient complains of chest pain with deep inspiration, worse when lying supine. There is a friction rub on auscultation and sinus tachycardia. Which of the following would you expect to find on the stat 12-lead ECG?

(A) ST depression in V1–V4
(B) ST elevation in II, III, aVF, and V2–V5
(C) ST depression rV2, rV3
(D) ST elevation in II, III, aVF

18. The trauma patient's morning labs return with the following values:

Hemoglobin 8.2 g/dL; hematocrit 30%; platelets 50,000/mcL; PTT 50 sec; INR 3.0 sec; fibrinogen 150 mg/dL; fibrin split products 45 mcg/dL

What is most likely the cause of the patient's lab profile?

(A) autoimmune reaction
(B) consumption of clotting factors
(C) occult blood loss
(D) drug reaction

19. The patient has a temporary transvenous VVI pacemaker with a set rate of 72/minute and an mA of 5. The monitor shows 1:1 pacing at the set rate. The physician asks the nurse to determine the capture threshold. Which of the following should the nurse do?

(A) Slowly increase the sensitivity until the heart rate increases.

(B) Slowly decrease the sensitivity until the capture is lost.

(C) Slowly increase the mA output until the native beats are seen.

(D) Slowly decrease the mA output until the capture is lost.

20. A 24-year-old female patient is in the ICU status post ruptured spleen. Radiographic studies done in the ED demonstrated old, healed rib and arm fractures. The patient has had frequent ED visits, and there is suspicion of domestic abuse. The patient reported tripping down the stairs as the cause of her current injuries. The husband is constantly at the patient's bedside. Which of the following is the most effective strategy for the nurse caring for the patient?

(A) Arrange for social services to interview the patient privately.

(B) Explain to the patient and husband the healthcare provider's suspicion of abuse.

(C) Inform the patient and husband that the local authorities have been called.

(D) Restrict the husband from visiting the patient.

21. A 70 kg patient with ARDS is mechanically ventilated on the following settings: FiO_2 70%, tidal volume 450 mL, assist control 10/min, PEEP 20. On these settings, the patient's PaO_2 mmHg is 76 and $PaCO_2$ is 58 mmHg. The patient's core temp is 37°C, heart rate 116, and BP 78/58. Which of the following interventions should the nurse now anticipate?

(A) Decrease PEEP to decrease intrathoracic pressure.

(B) Administer 500 mL fluid bolus of normal saline.

(C) Initiate a norepinephrine drip to maintain SBP of 80 mmHg.

(D) Increase tidal volume to 750 mL.

22. Which of the following is accurate regarding nursing responsibilities related to brain death?

(A) Report loss of brain-stem reflexes (gag, corneal) to the physician.

(B) Obtain the order from the physician to call the organ procurement agency.

(C) Request permission from the family to remove the ventilator.

(D) Ensure the patient receives an EEG, transcranial Doppler, and cerebral angiogram.

23. A 70 kg patient with ARDS is intubated and mechanically ventilated. The patient is on continuous infusions of opiate, sedative, and neuromuscular blocking drugs. Plateau pressure is 45 cm H_2O. The PaO_2 is 60. The physician orders the following ventilator settings: SIMV mode, tidal volume 700 mL, rate 12/minute, FiO_2 1.00, PEEP 15. Which of the following needs to be discussed with the physician?

(A) the ventilator mode

(B) the tidal volume

(C) the PEEP

(D) the FiO_2

24. Which of the following is an appropriate strategy when providing mechanical ventilation for the patient with status asthmaticus?

(A) provide long inspiratory time and short expiratory time
(B) utilize PEEP of 10–15 cm
(C) use low respiratory rates
(D) set tidal volume 10–12 mL/kg

25. A large (32 mm) V-wave appears on the pulmonary arterial occlusive pressure (PAOP) tracing of an unstable patient after an extensive inferior wall myocardial infarction. This finding is consistent with:

(A) cardiogenic shock.
(B) congestive heart failure.
(C) pericarditis.
(D) mitral regurgitation.

26. A patient is admitted with serum calcium of 15.1 mEq/L. Which of the following interventions should the nurse anticipate?

(A) rule out hypermagnesemia, administer vitamin D
(B) treat hypoalbuminemia
(C) emergent hemodialysis, rule out hyperphosphatemia
(D) rule out hypokalemia, then administer diuretics

27. Which of the following patients is most likely to experience a heart block?

(A) cardiac transplant
(B) CABG
(C) mitral valve repair
(D) ventricular septal defect repair

28. A patient with a head injury was admitted last night. This morning she is increasingly less responsive, and her right pupil has become unresponsive to light. Now her systolic pressure has increased, heart rate has slowed, and respirations have slowed. These vital sign changes are referred to as:

(A) Battle's sign.
(B) Cushing's triad.
(C) halo sign.
(D) Chvostek sign.

29. A 68-year-old patient is admitted with syndrome of inappropriate antidiuretic hormone (SIADH). Which of the following lab findings and interventions would the nurse anticipate for this patient?

(A) serum sodium low, serum osmolality low, urine output low, order for phenytoin (Dilantin)
(B) serum sodium elevated, serum osmolality elevated, urine output low, order for pitressin
(C) serum sodium low, urine specific gravity low, urine output elevated, order for 3% saline
(D) serum sodium elevated, urine output elevated, hypokalemia, arterial pH low

30. The patient with chronic alcohol abuse is admitted with a serum phosphorous of 1.8 mEq/L. The nurse will need to observe the patient closely for:

(A) massive diarrhea.
(B) hypoventilation.
(C) tetany.
(D) ventricular arrhythmias.

31. Which of the following nursing behaviors is usually most helpful to patients and families regarding end-of-life decisions?

    (A) avoiding the use of words such as death, dying, and suffering
    (B) consulting clergy for support
    (C) acting as an arbitrator between family members
    (D) requesting that only one person be the spokesperson

32. A patient is receiving patient controlled analgesia, morphine 1 mg per hour IV infusion, and 2 mg every 15 minutes as PRN bolus doses. The patient is having episodes of sleep apnea and is arousable only by touch. Priority interventions include:

    (A) stop the continuous infusion and give naloxone slow IV until patient awakens.
    (B) decrease the morphine continuous infusion rate to 0.5 mg per hour and continue to monitor.
    (C) discontinue the PRN bolus doses and give naloxone 2 mg IV bolus.
    (D) discontinue PCA, check SpO_2, and give naloxone

33. Which of the following is contraindicated when providing enteral feeding?

    (A) Check for gastric residuals every 4 hours.
    (B) Use a small-bore duodenal feeding tube.
    (C) Keep the head of the bed flat.
    (D) Ensure free water is provided.

34. Massive atelectasis occurs in adult respiratory distress syndrome. What are the two major causes of this alveolar collapse?

    (A) increased pulmonary vascular resistance and increased pulmonary compliance
    (B) increased pulmonary compliance and pulmonary edema
    (C) surfactant deficiency and pulmonary edema
    (D) mucous plugs and bronchospasm

35. A patient admitted status post gunshot wound to the chest 2 days ago is now exhibiting signs of restlessness, hypertension, tachycardia, yawning, lacrimation, and rhinorrhea. Which of the following should be included in the nurse's plan of care?

    (A) assess further for history of opiate abuse
    (B) provide scheduled pain medication
    (C) ensure there is an order for sedation and administer sedative
    (D) discuss the need for an antihypertensive agent with the physician

36. A 74-year-old female reports explosive diarrhea for several days. She is lethargic, mucous membranes dry and sticky, dark amber urine with 40 mL output in the past hour, specific gravity 1.035, BUN 65, creatinine 2.9. Vital signs are temp 38°C, HR 130, RR 24, B/P 90/40. Which of the following should the nurse anticipate administering?

    (A) antibiotics
    (B) nutrition
    (C) isotonic fluids
    (D) furosemide

37. Which of the following pathophysiological conditions will cause refractory hypoxemia not treatable with oxygen alone?

(A) shunt
(B) hyperventilation
(C) diffusion defects
(D) V/Q mismatch

38. Review the following parameters of patients with acute pancreatitis on admission. Which patient has the poorest prognosis according to Ranson's criteria?

(A) WBC 15,000; glucose 280; LDH 400; age 45
(B) WBC 22,000; glucose 190; LDH 250; age 50
(C) WBC 32,000; glucose 220; LDH 400; age 60
(D) WBC 19,000; glucose 250; LDH 250; age 65

39. A patient with a history of heart failure and MI presents following an episode of syncope. The assessment 2 hours later demonstrates:

BP 134/64 (supine); 110/70 (sitting)
HR 115 with weak, thready pulse (supine); 130 (sitting)
RR 32 and shallow
U/O 30 mL over the past 2 hours
Breath sounds: clear

The patient most likely requires:

(A) vasodilators.
(B) loop diuretics.
(C) IV fluids.
(D) vasopressors.

40. Which of the following is a priority assessment for the patient with myasthenia gravis?

(A) pulse oximetry
(B) vital capacity
(C) respiratory rate
(D) lung sounds

41. The patient is status post stroke and has been advanced to oral feedings after successfully completing a swallow study. The nurse knows that the patient needs to be closely monitored for signs of pulmonary aspiration. Which of the following is the earliest indication that the patient may be aspirating oral feedings?

(A) tachypnea and tachycardia
(B) coughing and positive sputum cultures
(C) oxygen desaturation
(D) right middle lobe infiltrate on chest radiograph

42. While getting a 71-year-old male patient's history, the patient tells the nurse that he has mitral stenosis. The nurse would anticipate which of the following findings?

(A) systolic murmur, sinus bradycardia
(B) systolic murmur, atrial fibrillation
(C) diastolic murmur, atrial fibrillation
(D) diastolic murmur, sinus bradycardia

43. Which of the following patients will require 0.9 NS at 1 mL/kg before and after a CT scan with infusion?

(A) elderly patient taking NSAIDs for arthritis every 6 hours
(B) patient with hypertension
(C) male patient taking beta-adrenergic blocker
(D) patient with acute coronary syndrome

44. The patient was admitted status post motor vehicle crash. The patient sustained an intracranial bleed, is hypotensive, and is tachycardic. The patient's clinical status is most likely due to which of the following?

(A) intracranial hemorrhage
(B) neurogenic shock
(C) shock from multiple trauma
(D) brain herniation

45. The 19-year-old male patient was admitted with DKA for the third time in the past 4 months. The patient told you that he is considering dropping out of college, cannot concentrate on his studies, has had insomnia, and is just "sick of it all." Which of the following would be the best response by the nurse?

   (A) Consult with the physician regarding initiation of an antidepressant.
   (B) Consult with the endocrinologist regarding the patient's symptoms.
   (C) Consult with the physician regarding a psychiatric consult.
   (D) Provide emotional support, and encourage the patient to be positive.

46. Twelve hours after admission for traumatic injury, the patient's arterial blood gas showed the following results:

   pH   7.48
   PCO₂   28
   pO₂   68
   HCO₃   25

   Which of the following interventions are most appropriate at this time?

   (A) consider intubation, assess blood pressure
   (B) increase FiO₂, assess electrolytes
   (C) consider sedation, assess blood sugar
   (D) increase FiO₂, assess for pain

47. The patient is admitted postoperatively after surgery for a crush injury of the lower left leg sustained in a motor vehicle crash. Which of the following is indicated for prevention of a deep-vein thrombosis?

   (A) compression stockings
   (B) pneumatic compression device to the right extremity
   (C) daily low molecular weight heparin
   (D) daily warfarin

48. Abdominal auscultation of a patient with early mechanical obstruction would likely reveal which of the following?

   (A) normal bowel sounds
   (B) hyperactive bowel sounds
   (C) hypoactive bowel sounds
   (D) absent bowel sounds

49. The patient was admitted with an acute anterior wall myocardial infarction and suddenly develops a loud holosystolic murmur, loudest at the left sternal border, 5th intercostal space, tachypnea, and bibasilar crackles. Which of the following would provide the most definitive diagnosis of this problem?

   (A) decreased cardiac output
   (B) increased oxygen saturation in the pulmonary artery and the right ventricle
   (C) central venous pressure less the pulmonary artery diastolic pressure
   (D) decreased arterial saturation

50. The patient receiving mechanical ventilation is receiving a propofol drip at 50 mcg/kg/min in order to maintain a RASS score of –1 to –2. The patient becomes agitated with a RASS score of +3 and behavioral pain scale (BPS) of 10 (range 3–13). The SpO₂ and breath sounds are unchanged. The blood pressure and heart rate are somewhat higher. Which of the following interventions would be appropriate?

   (A) increase the propofol infusion to 60 mcg/kg/min
   (B) give lorazepam 2 mg IV
   (C) give morphine 2 mg IV
   (D) order an arterial blood gas STAT

51. Which of the following statements related to care of the patient with a chest tube is TRUE?

(A) Clamp the tube during patient transport.
(B) Position tubing in a dependent loop.
(C) Avoid high airway pressures.
(D) Place the collection chamber onto the cart during transport.

52. Which of the following may be the result of pulmonary hypertension?

(A) pulmonic stenosis
(B) left ventricular failure
(C) tricuspid regurgitation
(D) increased lung compliance

53. Which of the following interventions would the nurse anticipate for the patient with intracerebral hemorrhage?

(A) STAT MRI of the brain
(B) correction of coagulopathy
(C) surgical evacuation of the hematoma
(D) nitroprusside (Nipride) for immediate correction of hypertension

54. The patient with a history of alcohol abuse sustained a traumatic injury and was admitted to the ICU. Which of the following is most likely to prevent development of delirium tremens (DTs)?

(A) thiamine
(B) phenobarbital
(C) fluids
(D) benzodiazepines

55. The patient is receiving a heparin infusion status post pulmonary embolism. The latest lab results reveal a sudden drop in platelet count to 80,000/mcL from 280,000/mcL the previous day. The nurse would anticipate receiving which of the following physician orders?

(A) begin an argatroban infusion
(B) hold all anticoagulant
(C) infuse platelets
(D) continue heparin, order labs for heparin antibodies

56. The 49-year-old male patient was admitted in a stuporous state with a blood alcohol level of 250 mg/dL. Which of the following is most likely to be a part of his treatment plan?

(A) naloxone activated charcoal, sodium bicarb
(B) romazicon, lactulose, calcium gluconate
(C) dialysis, cooling, potassium
(D) fluids, thiamine, phosphate

57. The nurse is preparing to suction the patient receiving mechanical ventilation with history of increased ICP due to head injury. Which of the following interventions is contraindicated for this patient?

(A) increase the FiO_2 to 100% during suctioning
(B) provide sedation
(C) limit the procedure to 1 to 2 quick passes
(D) stimulate coughing

58. What lab value would differentiate diabetic ketoacidosis from hyperosmolar hyperglycemic state (HHS)?

(A) serum glucose of 600 mg/dl
(B) serum K^+ of 4.0 mEq/L
(C) positive serum ketones
(D) serum osmolality of 320 mOsm/L

59. The 70-year-old patient is admitted with a serum glucose of 850 mg/dL, history of Type II diabetes, and obtunded mental status. Which of the following laboratory findings would be expected?

    (A) pH 7.35, sodium 150 mEq/L, BUN 10 mEq/L
    (B) pH 7.25, potassium 3.2 mEq/L, serum osmolality 160 mOsm/kg
    (C) pH 7.35, potassium 5.9 mEq/L, sodium 128 mEq/L
    (D) pH 7.25, potassium 6.2 mEq/L, serum osmolality 310 mOsm/kg

60. A 28-year-old woman is in the ICU with a gunshot wound to the head. One week after admission, the physician has declared the patient brain dead. The nurse is present when the diagnosis is shared with the patient's mother. Which is one of the first issues the nurse needs to anticipate?

    (A) the need to document this physician-family discussion
    (B) the need to initiate discussion related to organ donation
    (C) that the family may request a second opinion
    (D) that the hospital ethics committee should be contacted

61. Which of the following is most likely to result in airflow obstruction?

    (A) tracheostomy tube and secretions
    (B) endotracheal tube and bronchospasm
    (C) bronchospasm and opiate overdose
    (D) pulmonary embolus and hypoxemia

62. The patient develops PSVT, and synchronized cardioversion is being considered. Which of the following would be a contraindication to the cardioversion?

    (A) digoxin level of 4.0 mg/dL
    (B) potassium level of 5.1 mEq/L
    (C) magnesium level of 2.6 mg/dL
    (D) creatinine level of 3.1 mg/dL

63. The orientee asks the preceptor how IABP therapy will benefit the patient who was just admitted from the cardiac catheterization suite. The preceptor's best response would be:

    (A) it will increase the patient's myocardial oxygen supply.
    (B) it will increase coronary artery perfusion during systole.
    (C) it will increase the patient's left ventricular filling volume.
    (D) it will increase the left ventricular diastolic pressure.

64. A shift of the oxyhemoglobin dissociation curve to the right will result in:

    (A) improved SaO_2.
    (B) worsening SaO_2.
    (C) decreased release of oxygen from hemoglobin.
    (D) decreased release of 2, 3-DPG in the serum.

65. The patient in septic shock received a pulmonary artery catheter. Which of the hemodynamic profiles would the patient most likely exhibit?

    (A) SVR 1400 dynes/s/cm^{-5}, cardiac output 5 L/min, SvO_2 58%
    (B) SVR 1800 dynes/s/cm^{-5}, cardiac output 6 L/min, SvO_2 60%
    (C) SVR 500 dynes/s/cm^{-5}, cardiac output 7 L/min, SvO_2 78%
    (D) SVR 700 dynes/s/cm^{-5}, cardiac output 2 L/min, SvO_2 68%

66. The patient was admitted with a serum glucose of 498 mg/dL. After 2 hours of therapy with 5 units/hour of regular insulin, the patient's glucose is 478 mg/dL. Which of the following interventions is appropriate at this time?

(A) Add subcutaneous sliding scale coverage, and continue to monitor.
(B) Continue the insulin infusion at the current dose, and continue to monitor.
(C) Increase the insulin infusion to 7 units/hour, and continue to monitor.
(D) Increase the insulin infusion to 10 units/hour, and continue to monitor.

67. A patient is admitted with a right cerebral hemisphere stroke. Assessment would reveal:

(A) dilated left pupil and left-sided paresis or plegia.
(B) dilated left pupil and right-sided paresis or plegia.
(C) dilated right pupil and left-sided paresis or plegia.
(D) dilated right pupil and right-sided paresis or plegia.

68. When there is a drop in cardiac output, which of the following is a normal compensatory response?

(A) increased oxygen extraction
(B) decreased oxygen consumption
(C) decreased heart rate
(D) increased oxygen delivery

69. A 19-year-old female is admitted with Type I diabetes to the critical care unit. The family reported she was home with a "chest cold" today and became very lethargic after dinner. Blood glucose is 490 mEq/dL and serum positive for ketones. What is the most likely cause of the patient's current symptoms?

(A) dietary noncompliance
(B) insulin omission
(C) infection
(D) dehydration

70. On arrival to the ICU from the cardiac catheterization lab where the patient had a diagnostic right heart catheterization and a percutaneous coronary intervention, the cardiologist informed the nurse that the patient had an elevated left ventricular filling pressure and a low cardiac output. Which of the following therapies would be beneficial for this patient?

(A) left ventricular afterload reduction
(B) heart rate reduction
(C) left ventricular preload elevation
(D) negative inotropic therapy

71. Which of the following assessment findings would indicate the presence of a massive hemothorax?

(A) absent breath sounds on affected side; hyperresonance to percussion; tracheal deviation toward affected side
(B) decreased excursion on affected side; dullness to percussion; tracheal deviation toward affected side
(C) absent breath sounds on affected side; dullness to percussion; tracheal deviation toward unaffected side
(D) decreased excursion on unaffected side; hyperresonance to percussion; tracheal deviation toward unaffected side

72. The patient has acute renal failure secondary to septic shock, had prolonged hypotension, and now requires hemodialysis with a BUN of 90 mg/dL and a creatinine of 9.2 mg/dL. Which of the following would you expect this patient to have?

(A) low urine osmolality, high urine sodium concentration
(B) high urine osmolality, high urine sodium concentration
(C) low urine osmolality, low urine sodium concentration
(D) high urine osmolality, low urine sodium concentration

73. The patient had an episode of chest pain at rest with ST elevation on the ECG. The chest pain was relieved, and the ST segments normalized after administration of nitroglycerin sublingual. The patient most likely had:

   (A) stable angina.
   (B) ST-elevation myocardial infarction.
   (C) Prinzmetal's or variant angina.
   (D) Wellen's syndrome.

74. The patient develops abdominal pain, shortness of breath, and fever during administration of a blood transfusion. What is the priority nursing intervention?

   (A) Administer oxygen.
   (B) Contact the physician.
   (C) Administer acetaminophen.
   (D) Stop the transfusion.

75. Which of the following acid-base abnormalities is most often seen in the patient with chronic alcoholism?

   (A) pH 7.28; pCO_2 35; HCO_3 19
   (B) pH 7.50; pCO_2 30; HCO_3 29
   (C) pH 7.31; pCO_2 51; HCO_3 25
   (D) pH 7.46; pCO_2 49; HCO_3 31

76. The patient has an esophageal-balloon tube (Sengstaken-Blakemore) for treatment of bleeding esophageal varices. What nursing assessment/intervention is specific to the care of the patient with this type of tube?

   (A) Ensure suction is maintained.
   (B) Monitor for recurrent bleeding.
   (C) Initiate fluid resuscitation as needed.
   (D) Keep scissors at the bedside.

77. The 28-year-old male patient with muscular dystrophy is admitted with acute respiratory failure secondary to heart failure. He tells you that he is tired of frequent hospitalizations related to his disease and does not want invasive or noninvasive ventilation as he is tired of living. Which of the following would be the best response of the nurse?

   (A) "You will need to sign a 'No CPR' form as soon as possible."
   (B) "You are very uncomfortable right now and will feel differently when you are feeling better."
   (C) "This is an acute problem that can be resolved with treatment and allow you to return home to your family."
   (D) "Have you discussed this decision with your family and physician?"

78. Which of the following patients has delirium?

   (A) The patient has become lethargic and is inattentive.
   (B) The patient is unresponsive.
   (C) The patient is acutely agitated and attentive.
   (D) The patient's baseline mental status has not changed.

79. The patient received 10 units of packed red blood cells for traumatic injury. Which of the following therapies should the nurse anticipate?

   (A) platelets and fresh frozen plasma
   (B) protamine zinc
   (C) albumin
   (D) calcium and hetastarch

80. Desirable blood pressure ranges vary depending on the neurological problem and need to be clarified with the physician. Which of the following blood pressure (B/P) ranges is CORRECT?

    (A) treat B/P for an acute ischemic stroke patient, not a candidate for thrombolytic therapy, if greater than 200–220 mmHg systolic or 100 mmHg diastolic
    (B) keep systolic B/P greater than 180 mmHg for an acute ischemic stroke patient who is a candidate for thrombolytic therapy
    (C) keep systolic B/P for a patient with acute subarachnoid hemorrhage, pre-op, 160–180 mmHg
    (D) keep systolic B/P less than 120 mmHg to prevent vasospasm after subarachnoid hemorrhage

81. Positive pressure ventilation (PPV) was initiated for the patient. Which of the following would be expected?

    (A) decreased carbon monoxide
    (B) decreased carbon dioxide
    (C) decreased plateau pressure
    (D) decreased airway secretions

82. Which of the following is treated with surgery?

    (A) basilar skull fracture
    (B) linear skull fracture
    (C) vasospasm
    (D) A-V malformation

83. A 59-year-old male is admitted with ST elevation in V2, V3, and V4. IV thrombolytic therapy was started in the ED. Indications of successful reperfusion would include all of the following EXCEPT:

    (A) pain cessation.
    (B) absence of troponin elevation.
    (C) reversal of ST segment elevation with return to baseline.
    (D) short runs of ventricular tachycardia.

84. The patient with lung cancer is status post right thoracotomy with removal of the middle and lower right lung lobes. What is the purpose of the patient's 2 chest tubes?

    (A) provide normal ventilation
    (B) restore negative pleural pressure
    (C) improve lung compliance
    (D) drain pleural fluid

85. The critical care leadership of a medical center with several ICUs has assembled a committee to decide on how to implement the use of a new patient transfer device to the critical care units. Which of the following would be an important initial action of the committee?

    (A) Benchmark with area hospitals that have already implemented use of the new device.
    (B) Consult with the manufacturer regarding available printed user guides and sample procedures that are available.
    (C) Check for any national safety warnings related to the new piece of equipment.
    (D) Include nurses from all units that will use the new transfer device on the committee.

86. PEEP is beneficial for the treatment of the patient with pneumonia, ALI, or ARDS because of which of the following effects?

    (A) decrease in pulmonary shunt
    (B) increase in dead space ventilation
    (C) increase in alveolar recruitment
    (D) decrease in capillary leak

87. A 79-year-old male comes to the critical care unit with left-sided paralysis and paresthesia, eye deviation to the right, and a dilated right pupil. He cannot remember falling and has no signs of physical trauma. His family states he has been "acting differently" for approximately 1 month. Patient denies headache. Based on this information, he probably has which of the following?

    (A) a left-hemispheric epidural hematoma
    (B) a right-hemispheric subdural hematoma
    (C) a basilar skull fracture
    (D) central herniation

88. A patient is suspected of having appendicitis with intestinal perforation. Which description of abdominal pain is most specific to peritoneal irritation?

    (A) lessened while lying still with knees flexed
    (B) generalized of the abdominal area
    (C) of greater than 6 hours' duration
    (D) becoming increasingly severe

89. Which of the following best characterizes acute lung injury (ALI)?

    (A) tachypnea, unilateral pulmonary edema on chest X-ray
    (B) decreased compliance, hypercapnea, infection
    (C) elevated PAOP, bilateral infiltrates on chest X-ray, pO_2 less than 60 mmHg
    (D) refractory hypoxemia, decreased FRC, acute physiologic problem

90. The 23-year-old patient with head trauma begins to have polyuria with 900 mL of urine output in 1 hour, urine specific gravity 1.001, and serum osmolality elevated. Which of the following interventions would be expected for this patient?

    (A) administer 3% saline
    (B) administer phenytoin
    (C) administer pitressin
    (D) administer dextrose 5% in water

91. The patient complains of chest tightness, shortness of breath, and difficulty breathing shortly after the IV antibiotic is initiated. Hives have appeared across the face and chest. Vital signs include a B/P of 84/34, heart rate 130/min, sinus tachycardia, respiratory rate 28/min with wheezing, SpO_2 94% on room air. Which of the following interventions are most appropriate for the patient?

    (A) stat ECG, aspirin, oxygen, pressor
    (B) albuterol, steroids, oxygen, fluids
    (C) fluids, oxygen, CT of the chest, oxygen, heparin
    (D) epinephrine IM, steroids IV, antihistamine, fluids

92. The patient presents with mental status change and history of headache, the carboxyhemoglobin level is 45%, and the pulse oximeter is reading 98%. What is the priority treatment for this patient?

    (A) provide 100% FiO_2
    (B) provide mechanical ventilation
    (C) provide 40% FiO_2
    (D) administer naloxone (Narcan)

93. A patient is admitted with chest pain and ST elevation in II, III, aVF. He is receiving dobutamine at 10 mcg/kg/min and nitroglycerin at 20 mcg/min. His blood pressure is 90/60, sinus tachycardia at 110/minute. A pulmonary artery catheter is inserted and the following are obtained:

RAP = 16 mmHg, PAOP = 5 mmHg, PAP = 26/10 mmHg, cardiac index = 1.9 L/min/m²

The patient has jugular venous distention in a semi-Fowler's position; tall, peaked P-waves are seen in lead II. Which of the following therapies is indicated for this patient?

(A) Increase the dobutamine infusion to 20 mcg/kg/minute, and infuse 50 mL saline.
(B) Begin a milrinone infusion at 0.5 mcg/kg/minute after a loading dose of 50 mcg/kg.
(C) Discontinue the nitroglycerin, and infuse 500 mL normal saline.
(D) Discontinue dobutamine, and start a dopamine infusion at 10 mcg/kg/minute.

94. Which of the following is true of epidural hematoma?

(A) The patient's level of consciousness will change before pupillary changes.
(B) It may occur up to a month after the injury.
(C) There is risk of uncal herniation of the brain.
(D) Muscle weakness will occur on the side of the injury.

95. An 81-year-old male patient was admitted with sinus arrest. The cardiologist has recommended to the patient that he receive a permanent pacemaker. The patient, with a history of hypertension and Type II diabetes, told the physician he does not want a pacemaker, that he would rather "let Mother Nature take its course." What would the best approach be for the nurse to take regarding the patient's decision?

(A) Explain to the patient that he might die without the pacemaker.
(B) Explain the consequences of the patient's decision to the family, and advise them to persuade the patient to agree to the procedure.
(C) Explore the reason for the patient's decision, and provide information on what is involved during the procedure and the usual recovery.
(D) Advise the patient that a "no CPR" order will be needed in order to limit treatment that will prevent his heart from stopping.

96. The nurse caring for the patient after coronary artery bypass graft (CABG) surgery should:

(A) anticipate possible drop in blood pressure during rewarming.
(B) strip chest tubes hourly to maintain patency.
(C) maintain blood sugar 150–200 mg/dL with insulin infusion.
(D) maintain serum potassium 3.0–4.0 mEq/dL to prevent arrhythmias.

97. Unlike the patient with systolic dysfunction, the patient with diastolic heart failure may benefit from:

(A) digoxin.
(B) calcium-channel blocker.
(C) ACE inhibitor.
(D) dobutamine.

98. The patient is admitted with bleeding esophageal varices. Which of the following is a sign of compensation for hypovolemic shock?

(A) decrease in renin secretion
(B) increase in reabsorption of sodium and water
(C) vasodilation
(D) capillary fluid shift to interstitial space

99. The patient with status asthmaticus requires mechanical ventilation. Which of the following needs to be utilized?

(A) increased inspiratory phase
(B) increased PEEP
(C) increased expiratory phase
(D) increased rate

100. The patient has a right middle and lower-lobe bacterial pneumonia and is expectorating rust-colored sputum. Which intervention is most appropriate for this patient?

(A) Provide antibiotic therapy to cover MRSA.
(B) Turn the patient to the left to prevent hypoxemia.
(C) Hold enoxaparin prescribed for DVT prophylaxis.
(D) Maintain the head of the bed less than 30 degrees.

101. The patient had a pulmonary artery catheter and the following values were obtained on the initial shift assessment:

Blood pressure 82/48, heart rate 126/minute, pulmonary artery pressure 22/10, right atrial pressure 1 mmHg, pulmonary artery occlusive pressure 4 mmHg, cardiac output 3 L/minute, and systemic vascular resistance 1,600 dynes/s/cm^{-5}

The patient requires administration of:

(A) a fluid bolus of 500 ml 0.9 normal saline.
(B) dopamine at 5 mcg/kg/min.
(C) dobutamine (Dobutrex) at 10 mcg/kg/min.
(D) nitroprusside (Nipride) at 1 mcg/kg/min.

102. A patient has been admitted to the ICU with a diagnosis of esophageal varices and upper GI bleeding, the third such admission in the previous year. She is hemodynamically stable, and there is no evidence of active bleeding at this time. Which question will provide the nurse with information to ensure that her patient understands her diagnosis?

(A) Why do you think you are sick?
(B) When did you experience your first symptoms?
(C) Does anyone else in your family have this bleeding problem?
(D) Do you consume alcohol on a regular basis?

103. Asthma is best characterized by which of the following?

(A) alveolar thickening and destruction
(B) bronchial swelling and spasm
(C) alveoli filled with fluid or exudate
(D) loss of supporting fibers for the bronchiolar walls

104. The patient has an oxygen saturation of 85%. Which of the following problems will require treatment other than an increase in the FiO_2 in order to correct the hypoxemia?

(A) V/Q imbalance
(B) right to left shunting
(C) alveolar hypoventilation
(D) impaired diffusion

105. Which of the following statements are accurate related to delirium?

(A) Hypoactive delirium is easier to identify than hyperactive or mixed delirium.
(B) Haloperidol is an effective treatment for delirium.
(C) Deep sedation will prevent delirium.
(D) Severity of illness on admission is a more significant risk for delirium than age.

106. A patient's abdominal assessment reveals complaint of dull abdominal pain, abdominal distention, low-pitched bowel sounds, and report of change in bowel habits. The patient most likely has which of the following problems?

(A) large bowel obstruction
(B) acute pancreatitis
(C) small bowel obstruction
(D) acute appendicitis

107. The patient admitted with traumatic injury and multiple fractures has become increasingly tachypneic with a decrease in SpO_2 requiring an increase in FiO_2 to 5 L/nasal cannula. ABGs are obtained with the following results: pH 7.52, pCO_2 29, pO_2 48, HCO_3 25. Lungs, previously clear, have bibasilar crackles, and the chest X-ray demonstrates a ground-glass appearance. The patient most likely has developed which of the following?

(A) pneumothorax
(B) acute lung injury
(C) pulmonary embolus
(D) pneumonia

108. Which of the following may prevent vasospasm following subarachnoid hemorrhage secondary to ruptured aneurysm?

(A) nimodipine (Nimotop)
(B) loop diuretic, e.g., furosemide (Lasix)
(C) aminocaproic acid (Amicar)
(D) osmotic diuretic, e.g., mannitol

109. The patient is admitted with the diagnosis of acute tubular necrosis (ATN). Which of the following findings would this patient be expected to manifest?

(A) hypermagnesemia, acidosis, hyperkalemia
(B) azotemia, hypocalcemia, alkalosis
(C) hypokalemia, acidosis, hypertension
(D) hyperkalemia, hypomagnesemia, acidosis

110. The preceptor for a new nurse notices that the orientee is using the printed waveform strip of the CVP to determine the reading rather than using the digital readout on the monitor. When questioned about this practice, the orientee states that he had heard that assessing the printed waveform is more accurate than using the digital display on the monitor. The preceptor has never heard of this practice. What should the preceptor do?

(A) Instruct the new nurse on the usual unit practice of using the digital display of the pressure on the monitor.
(B) Use the waveform strip to get the pressure and look at the digital readout on the monitor and then compare readings.
(C) Design a research study to compare the relationship between obtaining CVP measurements using the printed waveform vs. the digital display.
(D) Review the current literature to identify evidence and recommendations related to this practice.

111. The patient with a history of schizophrenia is admitted with hyperglycemic hyperosmolar state (HHS), blood glucose of 800. Which of the following is a priority nursing intervention?

    (A) Contact the patient's psychiatrist.
    (B) Assess all home medications.
    (C) Hold psychiatric medications.
    (D) Apply a vest restraint.

112. The patient is admitted with a serum sodium of 118 mEq/L and serum osmolality of 249 mOsm/kg. Which of the following intravenous fluids is contraindicated?

    (A) normal saline solution (0.9% NaCl)
    (B) 3% saline solution
    (C) lactated Ringer's solution
    (D) dextrose in water (D_5W)

113. The patient is admitted status post motor vehicle crash with a left linear temporal skull fracture, stable mental status on admission. One hour after admission, he developed a right arm motor drift, dilated left pupil, and decreased level of consciousness. Which of the following interventions would the nurse anticipate?

    (A) cerebral arteriography and arterial stenting
    (B) emergent burr hole and clot evacuation
    (C) lower head of the bed and osmotic diuretic administration
    (D) intubation and ventriculostomy

114. The nurse is initiating a vasopressin drip for the patient with GI bleeding. What is a priority assessment specific to the patient receiving this medication?

    (A) monitor for hypotension
    (B) monitor ECG for ST changes
    (C) monitor for cardiac arrhythmia
    (D) monitor for bowel obstruction

115. The patient is describing an episode of chest pain. Which of the following would most likely indicate coronary artery disease as the etiology?

    (A) The pain is associated with nausea, extreme fatigue, and radiates to the right arm.
    (B) The pain is burning, started after eating, and was relieved by an antacid.
    (C) The pain is squeezing, going to the back, and associated with shortness of breath.
    (D) The pain is sharp, worse with deep inspiration, and relieved by turning to the side.

116. Preload and afterload are affected by various interventions. Which of the following statements is accurate?

    (A) Afterload is increased by nitroglycerin (Tridil).
    (B) Afterload is decreased by enalaprilat (Vasotec).
    (C) Preload is increased by furosemide (Lasix).
    (D) Preload is decreased with fluid administration.

117. Which of the following patients (all of whom are receiving mechanical ventilation for pneumonia) described below has the greatest complexity?

    (A) the woman with 3 school-age children, whose husband died 6 months ago, and who just lost her job
    (B) the man who just retired, is married, has a company pension, and owns his home
    (C) the woman with 2 school-age children who is going through a contentious divorce and who works for a law firm
    (D) the man who is the caregiver for his wife with dementia, and whose eldest daughter is caring for his wife while he is hospitalized

118. A patient is admitted with COPD exacerbation and worsening dyspnea. Admitting vital signs are temp 38.1°C, heart rate 120/minute, B/P 180/80, SpO_2 90% on 2L/min per nasal cannula, respiratory rate 35/minute and slightly labored. Initial ABGs are pH 7.33, $PaCO_2$ 49, PaO_2 61, SaO_2 87%, HCO_3 35. Which intervention should the nurse anticipate based on this information?

(A) intubation related to the hypercarbia
(B) aggressive diuresis
(C) provide sedation
(D) increase O_2 to 4L per nasal cannula

119. The patient admitted with pneumonia and subsequent alcohol withdrawal is receiving a lorazepam (Ativan) drip at 4 mg/hour in order to maintain a RASS score of –1 to –2. The patient suddenly becomes agitated, RASS score +2, all physiological and environmental causes have been ruled out as the cause of the agitation. The most appropriate lorazepam (Ativan) adjustment would be to:

(A) increase infusion to 5 mg/hour.
(B) give 2 mg IV, increase the infusion to 5 mg/hour.
(C) give 5 mg IV, increase the infusion to 5 mg/hour.
(D) increase the infusion to 6 mg/hour.

120. The patient was admitted with diabetic ketoacidosis, serum glucose 450 mg/dL, and pH 7.12. The latest serum glucose is 160 mg/dL (was 275 mg/dL 1 hour previous), the anion gap is 22 mEq/dL, and the venous CO_2 is 14 mmol/kg. Which of the following interventions is most appropriate at this time?

(A) Discontinue the insulin infusion.
(B) Lower the insulin infusion dose.
(C) Administer sodium bicarbonate.
(D) Increase the insulin infusion dose.

121. A patient is admitted to the ICU after a motor vehicle crash related to excessive consumption of alcohol. The patient has had several previous traffic violations related to alcohol consumption, and the driver of another car in the crash had critical injuries. During the nurse's initial assessment, the patient is awake, oriented, and lying quietly. What would be the optimal approach for the nurse to use at this time?

(A) Enter the room, but avoid talking about the most recent incident.
(B) Discuss nonthreatening topics such as the weather to engage in conversation.
(C) Provide nonjudgmental encouragement aimed at reducing or ceasing alcohol consumption.
(D) Ask the patient if he would like to talk about what happened.

122. The nurse evaluates results of the patient's lumbar puncture and anticipates the physician will order antibiotics. Which of the following results explains the nurse's evaluation of the CSF report?

(A) protein elevated
(B) clear in color
(C) glucose 30 mg/dL
(D) WBC elevated

123. The cardiac monitor shows a pacer spike before the P-wave, a spike before the QRS, and the heart rate increases with activity. The patient has which type of pacemaker?

(A) abnormally functioning AAI pacemaker
(B) abnormally functioning VVD pacemaker
(C) normally functioning VVI pacemaker
(D) normally functioning DDD pacemaker

124. The patient is admitted with ripping upper-back pain, blood pressure 198/106, heart rate 102, respiratory rate 22. A 7 cm thoracic aneurysm is identified on CT. Which of the following is contraindicated?

    (A) morphine for pain
    (B) labetalol infusion
    (C) immediate surgery
    (D) surgery in the morning

125. The patient has intracranial pressure monitoring in progress. The nurse knows that the pCO_2 should be maintained at which of the following?

    (A) greater than 35 mmHg
    (B) between 25 mmHg and 30 mmHg
    (C) less than 25 mmHg
    (D) between 30 mmHg and 35 mmHg

126. The patient was admitted 2 days ago with ST elevation in II, III, and aVF. Two days later, the patient developed hypotension, tachypnea, hypoxemia, and a new loud holosystolic murmur at the apex. The definitive treatment for the patient will be:

    (A) percutaneous coronary intervention.
    (B) intra-aortic balloon pump therapy.
    (C) surgery.
    (D) intubation and mechanical ventilation.

127. Which of the following patients has the least resiliency?

    (A) the 80-year-old male with STEMI, no comorbidities
    (B) the 48-year-old female with multiple fractures and hypertension
    (C) the 78-year-old female with lung cancer and severe sepsis
    (D) the 59-year-old male with DKA and drug abuse

128. The patient with chronic renal failure is admitted to the critical care unit with an acute MI. Which of the following is known to result in the highest incidence of death for the patient with chronic renal failure?

    (A) infection
    (B) azotemia
    (C) fluid overload
    (D) electrolyte imbalance

129. Despite emergent PCI and dobutamine infusion, the patient with acute anterior wall myocardial infarction remained hypotensive. An intra-aortic balloon (IAB) is inserted via left femoral artery. The immediate effect of IABP therapy is:

    (A) decreased preload and myocardial oxygen consumption.
    (B) decreased preload and afterload.
    (C) decreased afterload and improved coronary artery perfusion.
    (D) decreased afterload and increased myocardial contractility.

130. The patient is receiving amiodarone. Which of the following assessments are important?

    (A) PR interval, renal function, blood pressure
    (B) QRS interval, liver function, lung sounds
    (C) QT interval, thyroid function, heart rate
    (D) ST segment, pulmonary function, urine output

131. A patient is 1 day post open heart surgery. The patient's spouse inquires if she might bring in the patient's favorite CD of classical music to help control the pain. Which of the following is the nurse's best response?

(A) "Use of music may reduce pain and tension."

(B) "We will give your spouse as much pain medication as needed. Music will not be necessary."

(C) "There are no studies to suggest that it will help manage postoperative pain."

(D) "We can try it, but the portable radio or CD player will require approval by the biomedical department before it can be used."

132. Which of the following is an abnormal reflexive response in the adult?

(A) The toes flare up toward the patient's head in response to plantar stimulation.

(B) The eyes turn toward the right when cold water is injected into the right ear.

(C) The eye blinks when the cornea is touched.

(D) Gagging occurs when the endotracheal tube is suctioned.

133. The patient has an ankle/brachial index of 0.8. Which of the following is important in the care of this patient?

(A) Place the bed in reverse Trendelenburg.

(B) Provide an antihypertensive.

(C) Elevate the lower extremities.

(D) Elevate the affected arm.

134. A 24-year-old man was admitted after a fight. He sustained multiple rib fractures on the left and multiple abrasions on his face and body. He is complaining of sharp left shoulder pain, present at rest or with movement. Which of the following should you suspect?

(A) fractured scapula

(B) ruptured spleen

(C) rotator cuff injury

(D) pulmonary contusion

135. The preceptor overhears the orientee give an update on the patient status post full cardiac arrest to the patient's family when they arrived. Although there was return of circulation, the patient was not responsive, receiving mechanical ventilation, and the clinical hypothermia protocol was ordered. The preceptor felt the orientee's update was more positive than it should have been. What would be the best approach for the preceptor to take at this time?

(A) While the orientee is still in the room, tell the family it will be best to wait for the attending physician to come in and provide an update to the family.

(B) While the orientee is still in the room, introduce herself to the family, explaining the preceptor/orientee relationship, and provide a more accurate update.

(C) Ask the orientee to go get something from the storeroom. After the orientee leaves the room, introduce herself to the family, explain the preceptor/ orientee relationship, and provide a more accurate update.

(D) Ask the orientee to go get something from the storeroom, tell the family the attending physician is on the way to provide them with an update, and coach the orientee after leaving the room.

136. The patient presents with an overdose of an unknown substance. The patient is hypertensive, tachycardic, temperature normal. Skin is warm, flushed, pupils equal and reactive with eyes flickering up and down. Patient experienced a seizure shortly after arrival. Which of the following agents has the patient most likely taken?

   (A) PCP
   (B) heroin
   (C) LSD
   (D) amphetamines

137. The patient with dilated cardiomyopathy is most likely to have which of the following?

   (A) diastolic murmur, loudest at the right sternal border, left ventricular hypertrophy on the ECG
   (B) systolic murmur, loudest at the apex, enlarged cardiac silhouette on chest radiograph
   (C) diastolic murmur, loudest at the apex, normal ejection fraction
   (D) systolic murmur, loudest at the left sternal border, S4

138. Which of the following would warrant an immediate call to the neurosurgeon postoperatively?

   (A) ICP 15 mmHg, cerebral perfusion pressure 100 mmHg
   (B) temperature increase to 39.8°C from 37.2°C.
   (C) urine output of 100 mL in past hour and urine specific gravity of 1.010
   (D) patient arouses with voice, previously aroused with shaking

139. The patient with abdominal trauma is experiencing acute left shoulder pain. Which of the following might cause this symptom?

   (A) diaphragmatic irritation
   (B) ruptured bladder
   (C) liver contusion
   (D) ruptured kidney

140. Nursing measures to optimize cerebral perfusion pressure (CPP) include:

   (A) turn the patient every hour.
   (B) prevent MAP greater than 65 mmHg.
   (C) maintain $PaCO_2$ less than 30 mmHg.
   (D) maintain neutral head position.

141. The physician advises intubation and mechanical ventilation for the patient with asthma. The patient's respiratory rate is 28/minute and is currently receiving 3L/nasal cannula oxygen. Which of the following arterial blood gases best supports the decision to place an endotracheal tube?

   (A) pH, 7.41; $PaCO_2$, 39 mmHg; PaO_2, 83 mmHg
   (B) pH, 7.50; $PaCO_2$, 29 mmHg; PaO_2, 72 mmHg
   (C) pH, 7.46; $PaCO_2$, 33 mmHg; PaO_2, 62 mmHg
   (D) pH, 7.36; $PaCO_2$, 41 mmHg; PaO_2, 62 mmHg

142. The nurse assessing a patient with acute coronary syndrome needs to know that:

   (A) there are always acute ECG changes, chest pain, and positive troponin.
   (B) the standard of care for a NSTEMI is emergent reperfusion within 90 minutes.
   (C) the most common cause is plaque rupture and most common complication is arrhythmias.
   (D) it includes stable angina, unstable angina, NSTEMI, and STEMI.

143. Which of the following patients will most likely need hemodialysis?

    (A) the patient with BUN of 88 mg/dL, creatinine of 3.8 mg/dL

    (B) the patient with metabolic alkalosis and hypokalemia

    (C) the patient with aspirin overdose, BUN 15 mg/dL, creatinine 1.5 mg/dL

    (D) the patient with serum potassium 5.8 mEq/L and normal ECG

144. The Type II diabetic patient presents with serum glucose of 1,050 mg/dL, negative ketones. Which of the following is the priority intervention for this patient?

    (A) insulin

    (B) bicarbonate

    (C) potassium

    (D) fluid replacement

145. The patient with acute pancreatitis has the following assessment:

Vital signs: Temp 37°C, B/P 98/65, heart rate 110/minute, respiratory rate 28/minute, SpO_2 89%, FiO_2 of 2 L/nasal cannula

Labs: WBC 19,000, hemoglobin 9.0 g/dL, hematocrit 40%; Na^+ 145 mEq/L, K^+ 3.0 mEq/L, Ca^{++} 7.8 mEq/L, glucose 220 mg/dL

Assessment: Lungs with left lower lobe crackles, abdomen with Cullen's sign

In addition to pancreatitis, the patient most likely has which of the following?

    (A) hemorrhagic shock, stress hyperglycemia, hypoxemia, the patient needs blood

    (B) hypovolemic shock, diabetes, severe sepsis, the patient needs antibiotics

    (C) SIRS, hemorrhagic pancreatitis, MODS, the patient needs fluids

    (D) dehydration, ARDS, stress hyperglycemia, the patient needs intubation

146. The patient receiving intracranial pressure monitoring has sustained A-waves on the intracranial pressure (ICP) monitor. Which of the following interventions is contraindicated?

    (A) Discontinue opiate and sedating drugs.

    (B) Administer mannitol.

    (C) Infuse isotonic solutions.

    (D) Drain CSF from the ventricular catheter.

147. The patient arrives in the critical care unit 4 hours postpartum with bleeding thought to be secondary to severe uterine atony. Blood pressure is 78/40, heart rate 140/min, respiratory rate 30/min. The hemoglobin is 11.2 g/dL. Which of the following interventions is appropriate?

    (A) The patient has lost 1,500–2,000 mL of blood and is at high risk for DIC. Initiate fluid resuscitation, transfuse blood, and check coagulation profile.

    (B) The patient has lost 500–1,000 mL of blood and is at high risk for septic shock. Initiate fluid resuscitation, give pressors, and obtain blood cultures.

    (C) The patient has lost 250–500 mL of blood and is at high risk for pulmonary embolism. Initiate fluid resuscitation, get a chest CT, and obtain D-dimer.

    (D) The patient has lost over 2,000 mL of blood and is at high risk for uterine rupture. Initiate fluid resuscitation, transfuse blood, and obtain ultrasound of abdomen.

148. The decision has been made to wean a patient from the ventilator. Which of the following would be an indication to stop the weaning trial?

(A) development of paradoxical breathing pattern with accessory muscle use

(B) the patient remains disoriented with demonstration of mild anxiety and agitation

(C) a productive cough with activation of the ventilator alarm within the first 5 minutes of the weaning trial

(D) increase in heart rate from 82 per minute to 96 per minute within the first 5 minutes of the weaning trial

149. The patient presents with blood pressure 232/129 and acute chest pain. Which of the following would be the agent of choice to use for this patient?

(A) nicardipine (Cardene)

(B) labetalol (Normadyne)

(C) nitroprusside (Nipride)

(D) diltiazem (Cardizem)

150. Which of the following findings would be expected on chest auscultation of the patient with systolic heart failure?

(A) an S4 at the apex of the heart

(B) a systolic murmur at the apex of the heart

(C) a diastolic murmur at the left sternal border

(D) an S3 at the apex of the heart

1.	B	39.	C	77.	D	115.	C
2.	D	40.	B	78.	A	116.	B
3.	B	41.	A	79.	A	117.	A
4.	D	42.	C	80.	A	118.	D
5.	C	43.	A	81.	B	119.	B
6.	B	44.	C	82.	D	120.	B
7.	C	45.	C	83.	B	121.	D
8.	A	46.	D	84.	B	122.	C
9.	C	47.	C	85.	D	123.	D
10.	C	48.	B	86.	C	124.	D
11.	A	49.	B	87.	B	125.	D
12.	C	50.	C	88.	A	126.	C
13.	D	51.	C	89.	D	127.	C
14.	C	52.	C	90.	C	128.	A
15.	B	53.	B	91.	D	129.	C
16.	A	54.	D	92.	A	130.	C
17.	B	55.	A	93.	C	131.	A
18.	B	56.	D	94.	C	132.	A
19.	D	57.	D	95.	C	133.	A
20.	A	58.	C	96.	A	134.	B
21.	B	59.	C	97.	B	135.	B
22.	A	60.	C	98.	B	136.	A
23.	B	61.	B	99.	C	137.	B
24.	C	62.	A	100.	B	138.	B
25.	D	63.	A	101.	A	139.	A
26.	D	64.	B	102.	A	140.	D
27.	C	65.	C	103.	B	141.	D
28.	B	66.	D	104.	B	142.	C
29.	A	67.	C	105.	D	143.	C
30.	B	68.	A	106.	A	144.	D
31.	C	69.	C	107.	B	145.	C
32.	A	70.	A	108.	A	146.	A
33.	C	71.	C	109.	A	147.	A
34.	C	72.	A	110.	D	148.	A
35.	A	73.	C	111.	B	149.	B
36.	C	74.	D	112.	D	150.	D
37.	A	75.	A	113.	B		
38.	C	76.	D	114.	B		

1. **(B)** The experienced nurse realizes that an organizational change, to be effective, will require input from the key stakeholders and their acceptance of the proposed change. Changing one's own practice, although admirable, will not affect broad-based change and may even cause confusion. Although getting a physician's thoughts is interesting, the response alone will not affect organizational change. Discussing the idea with nurse colleagues provides information on possible resistance, but it is not the optimal broad-based approach required to be effective.

2. **(D)** Anticoagulation will prevent clot formation. The remaining 3 choices are not indicated during embolization of an AV malformation.

3. **(B)** The patient meets criteria for SIRS, has a source of infection, and has signs of organ dysfunction (hypotension). The blood pressure responded to fluid administration. Bacteremia is bacteria cultured from the blood, which this patient has not yet evidenced. Sepsis would not include signs of organ dysfunction. The patient does not have septic shock at this time since pressors are not yet indicated.

4. **(D)** Clot formation on the valve is a major complication of valvular replacement, especially a mechanical valve. Therefore, anticoagulation will be needed. Fluid overload, labile B/P, and infection are all possible complications. However, they are not as likely as thrombus formation and resultant stroke (if related to the aortic valve).

5. **(C)** The patient exhibits signs of increased ICP, and each intervention in choice (C) will decrease ICP. Steroids, vasopressin, thiazide diuretics, and lumbar puncture are not interventions for increased ICP.

6. **(B)** Social support is very important for the young adult to cope. A request to call friends is evidence of this need. Choices (A) and (C) do not provide the patient the opportunity to utilize social support. The scenario does not indicate that the patient is anxious as shown in choice (D).

7. **(C)** The tensilon test is done to differentiate which type of crisis the patient is having, one of undertreatment or one of overtreatment. If the patient develops the signs described (worsening of signs), it is a cholinergic crisis. If the patient improves, it would be a sign of a myasthenic crisis. An anaphylactic reaction would be manifested by airway constriction and hypotension. Trousseau sign is manifested by carpal spasm when a blood pressure cuff is inflated in the presence of hypocalcemia.

8. **(A)** Mechanical devices such as a VAD or IABP will increase coronary artery perfusion, a positive hemodynamic effect in the setting of cardiogenic shock. Alpha-adrenergic drugs such as phenylephrine or norepinephrine constrict arteries, decrease perfusion, and increase the work of the heart. Beta blockers decrease myocardial contractility. Afterload reduction will decrease the work of the heart; this effect alone will decrease blood pressure and coronary perfusion.

9. **(C)** Aspiration may be chronic in patients with history of stroke, Parkinson's, or end-stage dementia. Presence of an ETT or NG tube increases the risk of aspiration, especially when the ETT cuff is not adequately inflated or large-diameter NG tubes are used. Aspiration is most common in the right lung, not the left lung. Aspiration often results

in infection, although initially it is a chemical insult to the lung tissue that may cause clinical signs and symptoms.

10. **(C)** The patient did not respond to noninvasive ventilation as the $PaCO_2$ increased, respiratory acidosis is worse, and severe hypoxemia was not corrected. BiPAP should not be continued. It is not a metabolic acidosis. The pH is not acceptable.

11. **(A)** The plateau pressure reflects lung pressure and is needed to calculate static (lung) compliance. It is not used to calculate vital capacity, dynamic compliance, or tidal volume. Peak inspiratory pressure is used to calculate dynamic compliance.

12. **(C)** Salicylate overdose will cause renal failure. Activated charcoal will help neutralize salicylates. Alkalinization of urine by administration of sodium bicarbonate in the intravenous fluids will protect the kidneys. Emergent dialysis will ensure clearance of salicylates. The remaining choices will not protect the kidneys from the effects of salicylic acid.

13. **(D)** The homeless man has the least resources available of those listed. The lack of resiliency needs to be assessed when planning care.

14. **(C)** Just the verbalization of feeling will often decrease the patient's depressed state. Additionally, the medication will need to be restarted. The remaining strategies would not be effective in dealing with depression.

15. **(B)** The RA pressures are elevated in RV failure secondary to RV infarct, and a decrease is evidence that treatment is effective. The PAOP is a left heart pressure. It is often already low in the setting of RV infarct/failure since the preload to the left heart drops. A further decrease is not warranted. An increase in RV pressure is a sign of worsening RV failure. The PAD is already low with RV infarct, and a further decrease is not desirable.

16. **(A)** During a AAA repair, there may be prolonged decreased perfusion to the renal artery and resulting damage to renal tubules. This population is at high risk of acute renal failure. The remaining 3 choices are less common than renal failure.

17. **(B)** The patient has pericarditis, and the expected ECG change is global ST elevation. Choice (A) is seen in anterior wall ischemia or NSTEMI. Choice (C) is associated with RV ischemia/infarct. Choice (D) is seen with acute inferior wall STEMI.

18. **(B)** The patient has DIC, a problem that causes excessive clotting resulting in consumption of clotting factors, the eventual inability to clot, and bleeding. The lab profile reveals a coagulopathy. However, the key parameter is the elevated fibrin split products (also known as fibrin degradation products) of 45 mcg/dL (normal is less than 10 mcg/dL), which is evidence of excessive clot breakdown. The remaining 3 choices would not elevate the fibrin split products.

19. **(D)** Capture threshold is assessed by decreasing (not increasing) the mA until pacer spikes are seen without a QRS. This is the point at which the capture is lost. The output is then set at about double the capture threshold. This may prevent loss of capture even if fibrinous crust overgrows on the surface of the electrode. The pacing (or sensing) threshold is assessed by adjusting the sensitivity.

20. **(A)** The problem will be best addressed if the wife feels safe enough to discuss her situation openly with a professional able to help her and takes steps to prevent future

occurrences. The social worker knows available resources and can conduct a private interview. The remaining 3 choices use confrontation of one type or another and provide less of a chance for a long-term solution.

21. **(B)** The primary problem is hypotension, and it should be treated with fluids. Although reduction of PEEP would most likely increase the B/P, it would result in de-recruitment of alveoli and hypoxemia. A norepinephrine drip should be initiated only if fluids alone do not correct the hypotension. An increase in tidal volume would not increase the B/P and would cause volutrauma in the patient with ARDS.

22. **(A)** The absence of gag and corneal reflexes in a patient who recently had the reflexes needs to be further investigated. The RN should not need a physician order to call the organ procurement agency. If brain death has been diagnosed, the family should be prepared for the clinical diagnosis of brain death. However, requesting permission to remove the ventilator is not a family decision. Confirmatory tests such as described in choice (D) may be hospital policy. However, they are not needed to make the diagnosis of brain death.

23. **(B)** The patient with ARDS needs to receive 4–5 mL/kg tidal volume in order to prevent volutrauma. This patient is receiving 10 mL/kg tidal volume, and this level needs to be reduced. The mode of ventilation and both PEEP and FiO$_2$ settings are acceptable.

24. **(C)** The patient with asthma requires longer expiratory time in order to decrease air trapping. A lower respiratory rate will help provide this. Short expiratory time, PEEP, and larger tidal volumes will all promote air-trapping or auto-PEEP. This will increase intrathoracic pressure, decrease venous return, and reduce cardiac output.

25. **(D)** Large V-waves are produced by regurgitant flow backward into the left atrium during left ventricular systole. The other 3 choices do not cause this backflow of blood and the resultant large V-waves.

26. **(D)** Hypercalcemia may be associated with hypokalemia. Therefore, hypokalemia must be ruled out prior to initiating diuretic therapy (a treatment for hypercalcemia) in order to prevent life-threatening arrhythmias.

27. **(C)** The aortic, tricuspid, and mitral valves are anatomically located near conduction pathways. Therefore, the patient who has undergone mitral valve repair may develop heart block post-procedure, which is thought to be due to a local effect on conduction pathways.

28. **(B)** The systolic pressure increases in order to try to perfuse the brain better as pressure in the cranial vault increases. This widens the pulse pressure. Heart rate slowing and respiratory depression are the other 2 signs of the triad. Battle's sign is a sign of a basilar skull fracture. Halo sign is seen when CSF is put on sterile white gauze and results in a red center color surrounded by yellow. Chvostek sign is a cheek/facial spasm caused by low serum calcium.

29. **(A)** SIADH causes excessive production of antidiuretic hormone, which results in fluid retention, dilutional hyponatremia, low serum osmolality, and elevated urine specific gravity. Dilantin will decrease production of ADH. The serum sodium would NOT be elevated, the urine output would not be elevated, nor would urine specific gravity be low. SIADH does not cause hypokalemia or acidosis.

30. **(B)** Hypophosphatemia results in muscle weakness that may affect the diaphragm and result in hypoventilation. Low serum phosphorous causes constipation, not diarrhea. It results in depressed deep tendon reflexes, not tetany. Low serum phosphorous does not cause ventricular arrhythmias.

31. **(C)** When end-of-life decisions are required, a certain amount of family conflict usually occurs. The experienced nurse knows how to arbitrate in these matters. Choice (A) is not an effective strategy. Clergy may be consulted but only if this is the family's wishes. A request that only one person be the spokesperson is an effective strategy for routine communication with a large family. However, when end-of-life decisions are necessary, all stakeholders need to have a voice.

32. **(A)** The patient has signs of sedation that precede hypoventilation, plus signs of sleep apnea that increase the risk of hypoventilation. The continuous infusion needs to be discontinued, not reduced. Sedation needs to be gradually (not suddenly) reversed. The patient will still need analgesia with PRN doses. A drop in SpO_2 is a late sign of hypoventilation. Although it is not a choice in this scenario, ideally the patient should have continuous waveform capnography.

33. **(C)** The head of the bed should be kept at least > 30 degrees elevation when providing enteral feeding in order to prevent aspiration. Choices (A), (B), and (D) are correct interventions for the patient receiving enteral nutrition.

34. **(C)** ARDS destroys Type II alveolar cells, which results in decreased surfactant production and atelectasis. Additionally, capillary "leak" occurs at normal left heart pressures, resulting in noncardiogenic pulmonary edema. The pulmonary vascular resistance does increase. ARDS results in decreased pulmonary compliance, not increased pulmonary compliance, Mucous plugs are not associated with ARDS, although bronchospasm may be present, secondary to the pulmonary edema.

35. **(A)** Although restlessness, hypertension, and tachycardia may be signs of other problems, including delirium, the additional signs of lacrimation, yawning, and rhinorrhea are classic signs of opiate withdrawal. The patient will need higher doses of opiate to manage the pain due to the injury and surgical procedure. Then the opiate dose will need to be gradually tapered. The remaining 3 choices will not address the withdrawal from opiates.

36. **(C)** The patient is dehydrated and shows signs of acute prerenal failure. Administration of isotonic fluids will restore vascular volume, increase urine output, and correct the tachycardia, hypotension, BUN, and creatinine. The etiology of the diarrhea needs to be addressed as this is the primary problem. The remaining 3 choices will not correct the immediate acute symptoms.

37. **(A)** A shunt requires more than oxygen to correct hypoxemia, for example, PEEP therapy. Hyperventilation reduces the pCO_2, not the pO_2. Diffusion defects may produce hypoxemia but respond to oxygen therapy. A V/Q mismatch that results in hypoxemia will respond to oxygen administration.

38. **(C)** Ranson's criteria are used to evaluate the patient with acute pancreatitis upon admission and during the next 48 hours. Upon admission, the greater the number of the following parameters that are positive at admission, the higher the morbidity:

WBC > 16,000/mm^3, glucose > 200 mg/dL, LDH > 350, and age > 60 years. Choice (C) is positive for all 4 parameters.

39. **(C)** The decrease in blood pressure and increase in heart rate with position change (orthostatic hypotension), clear lungs, and low urine output are signs of hypovolemia. Vasodilators or diuretics will exacerbate the problem. Vasopressors will only further elevate the SVR, increasing the work of the heart.

40. **(B)** Muscle weakness may develop with myasthenia gravis. Routine vital capacity monitoring will identify diaphragmatic weakness earlier than will pulse oximetry, respiratory rate, or lung sounds.

41. **(A)** The lung injury sustained will first manifest itself with an increase in heart rate and respiratory rate. Coughing is also an early sign, although positive sputum cultures take time. Oxygen desaturation and infiltrates on the chest radiograph occur hours to days later.

42. **(C)** Murmurs of stenosis occur when the valve is open, and the mitral valve is open during the filling phase of the heart cycle. Chronic resistance produced by stenosis of the mitral valve will result in an enlarged left atrium, which in turn may lead to atrial fibrillation, not sinus bradycardia. During systole, the mitral valve is closed. Therefore, mitral regurgitation would cause a systolic murmur.

43. **(A)** Age and use of NSAIDs are risks for contrast-induced nephropathy. The remaining choices are not risks for this problem.

44. **(C)** Tachycardia and hypotension are signs of hypovolemia, not intracranial hemorrhage in which the amount of blood loss is small; neurogenic shock and brain herniation result in bradycardia. Brain herniation also results in widening pulse pressure.

45. **(C)** The patient is exhibiting signs of depression and perhaps suicidal tendencies and needs to be evaluated by a psychiatric expert in order to determine the treatment options. Beginning antidepressants without an expert evaluation would not be the best strategy. The endocrinologist, although able to manage the DKA, is not the best person to assess the patient's signs of depression. Emotional support, although helpful, will not get at the cause of the patient's depression.

46. **(D)** The ABG demonstrates an uncompensated respiratory alkalosis. Common causes of this problem include hypoxemia (which the patient has) and pain (which the patient is at risk for considering the diagnosis). The patient does not require intubation as there is hyperventilation, not hypoventilation. Blood pressure abnormalities will not cause uncompensated respiratory alkalosis. Electrolyte abnormalities and blood sugar abnormalities do not cause respiratory alkalosis.

47. **(C)** Pharmacological prophylaxis is superior to mechanical prophylaxis for DVT. Low molecular weight heparin daily or unfractionated heparin every 8 or 12 hours are the agents of choice. Compression stockings alone are effective for only select, lower-risk patients. Pneumatic compression devices need to be used bilaterally on lower extremities at all times except when walking, not on only one extremity. Warfarin is used for the treatment of DVT and PE, not for prophylaxis.

48. **(B)** Early in the obstruction, bowel sounds are increased. Later the bowel sounds become diminished. A small bowel obstruction generally causes high-pitched sounds. A large bowel obstruction typically has low-pitched sounds.

49. **(B)** The clinical picture is one of ventricular septal defect (based on location of the murmur and the patient's chief presenting problem). The O_2 saturation on the right side of the heart would be expected to be higher than normal if arterial blood from the left ventricle is shunting into the right ventricle.

50. **(C)** The patient is demonstrating agitation (RASS score +3), and it is due to pain (BPS of 10). Therefore, an analgesic is indicated for the patient's agitation. An increase in the propofol dose or lorazepam administration would not address the pain. There is no indication that the agitation is due to a gas exchange problem. Therefore, a stat ABG is not indicated.

51. **(C)** High airway pressures may lead to an air leak. Choices (A), (B), and (D) are all contraindicated in the care of the patient with a chest tube.

52. **(C)** The pulmonary pressures get increasingly high with pulmonary hypertension, which causes right ventricular strain and dilation, which in turn may result in an inability of the tricuspid valve to close fully. Pulmonary hypertension does not cause pulmonic stenosis, left ventricular failure, or increased lung compliance. Right ventricular failure and decreased lung compliance are more likely.

53. **(B)** Any sign of coagulopathy needs to be rapidly corrected in order to prevent a larger hematoma. Brain MRI is not indicated. CT is done. Surgical evacuation of hematoma may be done in select cases if thought to decrease neurological injury. Nitroprusside is not the agent of choice to decrease B/P for cerebral hematoma. Labetalol is the drug of choice.

54. **(D)** The "adrenergic storm" of DTs is best addressed by benzodiazepines. They enhance the effect of the neurotransmitter gamma-aminobutyric acid (GABA) at the GABA receptors, resulting in sedative, hypnotic (sleep-inducing), anxiolytic (antianxiety), anticonvulsant, and muscle relaxant properties. Thiamine will be needed to prevent Wernicke's encephalopathy. Fluids will be needed to prevent dehydration. Phenobarbital has been used for extreme cases. However, benzodiazepines are the treatment of choice for prevention and treatment of DTs.

55. **(A)** The patient has most likely developed heparin-induced thrombocytopenia. A direct thrombin inhibitor (DTI) needs to be started, and heparin must be immediately discontinued. The patient will still require an anticoagulant but not heparin. Platelets are not indicated for HIT unless the patient has life-threatening bleeding or may be considered if the platelets drop to less than 10,000/mcL.

56. **(D)** The patient has signs of acute alcohol poisoning and may have a history of chronic alcohol abuse. He needs fluids to prevent hypovolemia, thiamine to prevent Wernicke's encephalopathy in the event the patient has chronic alcohol abuse and thiamine deficiency, and phosphate as chronic alcohol abuse often results in hypophosphatemia. The remaining 3 choices do not include effective interventions.

57. **(D)** Stimulation of the cough reflex will increase the ICP. Occasionally, lidocaine is ordered to be given prior to suctioning this patient population. The remaining choices are appropriate for the patient with increased ICP.

58. **(C)** Positive serum ketones are not seen in HHS, but ketones are always positive in DKA. The other 3 choices may be seen in either DKA **or** HHS and are not differentiation signs.

59. **(C)** The patient most likely has HHS. Although the patient may still produce some insulin, the problem develops less rapidly than DKA and the serum glucose is greater than that of DKA. Additionally, acidosis is not present, serum osmolality is high due to fluid loss, serum potassium may be elevated due to insufficient insulin production (not due to acidosis as in DKA), and sodium is often low due to loss in urine.

60. **(C)** The nurse who has experience in these situations will realize that many families, when faced with the diagnosis of brain death, may request another opinion. Documentation of the discussion is done in all circumstances. Discussion of organ donation will need to be addressed after the family has processed the information or prior to making the diagnosis. Not every brain death diagnosis requires an ethics consult.

61. **(B)** The endotracheal tube (ETT) has a narrow diameter and is longer than the normal airway, resulting in increased dead space. Bronchospasm narrows airways. Both decrease airflow. A tracheostomy tube is shorter than an ETT and therefore results in less dead space and does not obstruct airflow. Opiate overdose does not affect airflow; it decreases ventilation. A pulmonary embolus does not affect airflow; it increases dead space due to obstruction of a pulmonary vessel and pulmonary perfusion. Hypoxemia results in pulmonary vasculature constriction but does not affect air flow.

62. **(A)** If synchronized cardioversion is attempted in the presence of digoxin toxicity, ventricular tachycardia or fibrillation may result. The remaining 3 options would not be contraindications to synchronized cardioversion.

63. **(A)** When the balloon inflates during diastole, coronary artery perfusion is increased, which increases the myocardial oxygen supply. This occurs during diastole, not systole. It does not increase the LV filling volume. It will not increase the LV diastolic pressure. IAB therapy will actually help to decrease LV diastolic pressure after several hours of therapy.

64. **(B)** A right shift of the oxyhemoglobin dissociation curve allows hemoglobin to more easily release oxygen to the tissues, which can decrease the SaO_2 of hemoglobin. A right shift of the oxyhemoglobin dissociation curve does **not** improve the SaO_2. It does **not** decrease the release of oxygen from hemoglobin. It increases oxygen release. A right shift does **not** decrease the release of 2,3-DPG. It increases 2,3-DPG release, which results in hemoglobin more readily releasing oxygen from hemoglobin.

65. **(C)** The endotoxins present in sepsis may cause massive vasodilation and loss of vascular tone, which will decrease the SVR. The decreased SVR results in an increase in cardiac output (although there is shunting of blood at the capillary level that can result in uneven tissue perfusion at the capillary level). The SvO_2 is elevated due to poor oxygen consumption and utilization at the cellular level. The other 3 profiles are not representative of septic shock.

66. **(D)** The dose should be doubled in order to achieve a decrease in serum glucose of 50–75 mg/dL per hour. This patient has decreased serum glucose by only 20 mg/dL in 2 hours. The remaining choices would not achieve the desired goal.

67. **(C)** If the injury is on the right, pupil changes—if present—are ipsilateral and motor changes are contralateral. The remaining 3 choices do not meet these criteria.

68. **(A)** Oxygen utilization is about 300 mL/min, whereas oxygen delivery is ~ 1,000 mL/min. If the CO decreases, myocardial extraction will increase. (The heart rate will also increase.) A drop in oxygen consumption and a decrease in heart rate do **not** occur with a drop in CO. If the CO drops, oxygen delivery will decrease, not increase.

69. **(C)** Infection is the most common cause of DKA. In this case, the patient had evidence of an infection. Even when symptoms of an infection are not reported in the history, all patients with DKA need to be assessed for infection. Although the other choices may cause DKA, there is no evidence of these causes in the scenario.

70. **(A)** An elevated LV filling pressure (PAOP) and a decrease in cardiac output would benefit from decreased SVR (LV afterload). A vasodilating drug such as an ACE inhibitor (or mechanically with intra-aortic balloon therapy) would provide this effect. Heart rate reduction might benefit diastolic filling but not necessarily help an elevated LV filling pressure. Elevation of the LV preload or negative inotropic therapy would make the problem worse.

71. **(C)** A massive hemothorax will push the mediastinum toward the unaffected side, which will push the trachea to the unaffected side. A simple pneumothorax without massive pleural fluid collection or tension due to air that cannot escape will pull the trachea toward the affected side.

72. **(A)** The patient has intrarenal failure as evidenced by the 10:1 BUN to creatinine ratio. In intrarenal failure, the tubular basement membrane is damaged and the tubules are no longer able to concentrate urine or hold onto sodium. The remaining choices do not meet both of these criteria.

73. **(C)** ST segment elevation that normalizes and chest pain is relieved after administration of nitroglycerin are indicative of Prinzmetal's angina. Stable angina occurs with activity; it is predictable. STEMI does not respond to NTG with normalization of ST segments and complete pain relief. Wellen's syndrome does not present with ST elevation but rather a biphasic T-wave specific to leads V1, V2.

74. **(D)** The patient has signs and symptoms of a blood transfusion reaction. No further blood should be infused when a reaction is suspected. The remaining interventions will be required. However, the priority intervention is to address the source of the problem, the blood transfusion, which may be life threatening.

75. **(A)** The chronic alcohol abuser is likely to have chronic liver disease that may result in elevated lactate and cause a metabolic acidosis. Choice (A) demonstrates uncompensated metabolic acidosis. The remaining choices do not demonstrate metabolic acidosis. Choice (B) is combined metabolic and respiratory alkalosis. Choice (C) is uncompensated respiratory acidosis. Choice (D) is partially compensated metabolic alkalosis.

76. **(D)** In the event the tube becomes displaced and moves up, the esophageal balloon may obstruct the airway and result in an acute airway emergency. The scissors would be needed to cut the esophageal balloon immediately. The remaining interventions may be needed, but they are not specific to the esophageal balloon tube.

77. **(D)** Gathering information is more important at this point than giving information. Telling the patient how he/she will feel is not advisable.

78. **(A)** There is an acute change in level of consciousness (altered mental status) and inattention, both of which are required in order to make the diagnosis of delirium. Unresponsiveness alone does not meet criteria for delirium. If the patient is attentive, delirium cannot be present. If the baseline mental status is unchanged, delirium is not present.

79. **(A)** Packed RBCs have had platelets and plasma removed. Therefore, these components will need to be replaced following transfusion of multiple units of packed RBCs. Because of the citrate present in banked blood that binds with calcium and magnesium, the patient will also need to be closely monitored for hypocalcemia and hypomagnesemia. Protamine zinc is used to reverse heparin. Albumin is not needed following multiple transfusions of PRBCs. Hetastarch is not needed.

80. **(A)** Abrupt lowering of the B/P to normal in the presence of an acute ischemic stroke may decrease perfusion to the area of injury and result in greater brain injury. Elevated B/P is contraindicated for the patient who is a candidate for thrombolytic therapy. The patient with acute SAH requires treatment of elevated B/P pre-op in order to prevent further bleeding. The B/P needs to be somewhat elevated after repair of acute SAH rather than < 120 mmHg systolic as normal to low B/P is thought to contribute to cerebral vasospasm.

81. **(B)** Positive pressure ventilation will assist in "blowing off" CO_2. The remaining choices would not be expected with the initiation of positive pressure ventilation (PPV).

82. **(D)** A-V malformation is treated surgically. Basilar skull fracture is not treated surgically unless there is sign of infection or persistent CSF leakage. Linear skull fracture is not surgically treated unless cranial depression is 5 mm or greater. Vasospasm is not treated surgically, although interventional radiologic treatment may be attempted to relieve spasm in select cases.

83. **(B)** The patient is having an anterior wall myocardial infarction. Even with reperfusion achieved in a timely manner, the cardiac biomarkers (troponin) will be elevated. When the artery opens, choices (A), (C), and (D) **will** occur.

84. **(B)** Chest tubes do not affect ventilation or lung compliance. Although there may be a small amount of pleural drainage S/P thoracotomy, pleural drainage is not the main purpose of the chest tubes.

85. **(D)** Inclusion of all key stakeholders is effective for successful implementation of a change. Choices (A), (B), and (C) should have been done prior to making the decision to purchase and implement the device.

86. **(C)** Although PEEP is the therapy used for ALI/ARDS that results in a shunt, PEEP does not necessarily decrease the shunt itself. Rather, PEEP improves the severe hypoxemia

by its ability to increase alveolar recruitment. PEEP does not increase dead space ventilation or decrease capillary leak.

87. **(B)** The problem seems to be right hemispheric in that the paralysis is on the left (contralateral), eyes look to the right (the problem side), and pupil changes are ipsilateral (right pupil). Additionally, a subdural hematoma develops slower and may even be chronic. Epidural hematoma usually develops with trauma and acutely, plus signs do not support a left-sided problem. Basilar skull fracture would present with raccoon eyes, Battle's sign, and perhaps otorrhea or rhinorrhea. Central herniation would present with bilateral pupil changes, bilateral Babinski, and Cushing's triad.

88. **(A)** The abdominal pain of peritonitis is exacerbated by movement of the peritoneum. Therefore lying still with knees flexed would lessen the pain. Coughing, flexing hips up, and positive rebound maneuver will increase the pain. Peritonitis may be generalized or localized, is not related to time duration, and does not necessarily become increasingly severe.

89. **(D)** Pulmonary edema is not unilateral but is always bilateral. It is not always associated with infection. By definition, the PAOP in ALI/ARDS is normal or low, not elevated. Elevated PAOP with pulmonary edema is due to left ventricular failure.

90. **(C)** The patient is exhibiting signs of diabetes insipidus (DI) in which there is insufficient production of antidiuretic hormone (ADH), most likely due to the head trauma. Pitressin is a form of ADH and is the treatment of choice. The massive diuresis will result in elevated serum sodium, therefore 3% saline is not appropriate. Phenytoin may cause DI and is **not** a treatment. The main complication of DI is hypovolemic shock. Therefore, a hypotonic solution such as D_5W would not be indicated for DI.

91. **(D)** The clinical signs and symptoms indicate an allergic reaction and anaphylactic shock. The epinephrine, steroids, and antihistamine will counteract the effects of the massive histamine release. Fluids will address the hypotension and relative hypovolemia caused by the massive dilatation. The remaining responses include options not indicated or helpful for anaphylaxis.

92. **(A)** Delivery of the highest FiO_2 possible will help replace the carbon monoxide binding to the hemoglobin. If a hyperbaric oxygen chamber is accessible within approximately 30 minutes, the patient should be transferred for treatment. Mechanical ventilation will provide 100% FiO_2; however, the patient does not need assistance with ventilation. In addition, 40% FiO_2 is not enough; naloxone is indicated for opiate overdose.

93. **(C)** The patient is having an acute inferior myocardial infarction. The elevated RAP, JVD, and tall peaked P-waves are clinical indications of RV failure, most likely secondary to RV infarct. Preload reduction (nitroglycerin) will further decrease LV filling and cardiac output. Therefore, it should be discontinued, and fluid boluses will help to increase the LV preload. Dobutamine has a mild dilating effect and may further decrease the blood pressure. Therefore, an increase in dose would not be advisable. Starting milrinone would provide no benefits at this time. Dopamine 20 mcg/kg/min is a high dose. If dopamine (a pressor) is needed, it would be started at 5 mcg/kg/min, not at 10 mcg/kg/min.

94. **(C)** Epidural hematoma is due to meningeal artery injury. The meningeal artery runs along the temporal lobe, the uncal area of the brain. Epidural hematoma is one brain injury in which pupillary change on the side of the injury will change **before** sustained change in LOC, which makes choice (A) incorrect. Choice (B) is not correct as epidural hematoma is an acute arterial bleed, not chronic. Muscle weakness caused by an epidural hematoma will cause contralateral weakness, therefore choice (D) is not correct.

95. **(C)** An assessment of why the patient made his decision will help the nurse better intervene, and providing information will better help the patient to make an informed decision. Attempting to motivate the patient with fear or using family influence may cause problems in the future even if the patient agrees to the procedure.

96. **(A)** As the patient temperature rises, vasoconstriction that was present at lower temperatures decreases with a possible drop in blood pressure. Chest tubes should not be stripped. A blood sugar of 150–200 mg/dL is too high for a post-op CABG surgery patient. Serum potassium needs to be close to 4.0 mEq/dL, and 3.0–4.0 mEq/dL is too low.

97. **(B)** Calcium-channel blockers help to decrease pressure/stiffness and help LV filling in the presence of diastolic heart failure. Calcium-channel blockers are not helpful for systolic dysfunction. Digoxin and dobutamine are positive inotropic drugs. They will increase LV wall tension and may exacerbate symptoms. ACE inhibitors are not harmful to the patient with diastolic heart failure, but they are not a first-line agent for diastolic failure.

98. **(B)** Volume depletion will activate the renin-angiotensin-aldosterone system (RAAS). This results in aldosterone release, causing sodium and water retention in an effort to increase vascular volume. Renin is increased, not decreased. The vasculature constricts. It does not dilate. Capillary fluid shift to the interstitial space would worsen the hypovolemia.

99. **(C)** Air trapping and auto-PEEP are the most lethal results of status asthmaticus, and a longer exhalation time will address this problem. The remaining 3 choices may increase air trapping and auto-PEEP.

100. **(B)** Gravity affects pulmonary perfusion, and it is best to have the "good lung down." For this patient, that would be the left side. There is not enough information available to indicate MRSA coverage is needed. No contraindications are indicated in the scenario that would lead to the decision to withhold DVT prophylaxis. The rust-colored sputum may be due to *Streptococcus pneumoniae* bacterial pneumonia. The head of the bed should be kept at least 30 degrees, not less.

101. **(A)** The hemodynamic profile is one of hypovolemia. Fluid boluses should be given until the blood pressure, CVP, and PAOP increase and heart rate and SVR decrease. A vasopressor (dopamine) will constrict an already constricted vasculature and decrease tissue perfusion. Administration of a positive inotrope (dobutamine) will not correct the main problem of hypovolemia and will further increase the heart rate. Administration of a potent dilator (nitroprusside) will further decrease perfusion.

102. **(A)** The question relates to assessing the patient's knowledge of the diagnosis of esophageal varices. Therefore, asking why she thinks she is sick is the most open-ended

approach. Inquiring about symptoms or family history will not provide the information the nurse needs. Inquiry related to alcohol consumption, although related to the diagnosis, does not assess the patient's understanding of the diagnosis.

103. **(B)** Asthma results in bronchospasm, bronchial swelling, and mucous plugging. Asthma does not result in alveolar thickening and destruction, alveoli filled with exudate, or loss of supporting fibers for bronchiolar walls.

104. **(B)** A shunt requires PEEP therapy, not oxygen alone, to correct the hypoxemia. V/Q imbalance will respond to an increase in FiO_2. Alveolar hypoventilation requires a definitive treatment to address ventilation, but the resultant hypoxemia will improve with oxygen administration. Impaired diffusion will respond to oxygen administration.

105. **(D)** Although age is a risk for developing delirium, studies have found that severity of illness upon admission to be an even greater risk for developing delirium. The remaining 3 choices are not accurate statements related to delirium.

106. **(A)** Pain is boring with acute pancreatitis and bowel habits are not remarkable. Bowel sounds are more likely to be high pitched with small bowel obstruction, and projectile vomiting is more common than change in bowel habits. Abdominal distention is not generally seen with appendicitis.

107. **(B)** The development of bibasilar crackles, the "ground glass" appearance on the chest X-ray, and refractory hypoxemia are not typical of the other 3 choices.

108. **(A)** Nimodipine (Nimotop) is a calcium-channel blocker that targets cerebral vessels and prevents constriction. Loop diuretics and osmotic diuretics may result in hypovolemia and increase the vessel spasm. Amicar prevents bleeding.

109. **(A)** The patient with ATN is unable to eliminate magnesium and potassium. Bicarbonate regulation is lost, resulting in a metabolic acidosis. These factors eliminate one or more elements of choices (B), (C), and (D).

110. **(D)** The preceptor, with an open mind, will need to review the literature on the topic before forming an opinion on the practices unfamiliar to her. Choice (A) refuses to acknowledge that perhaps there is a better way to obtain the CVP value. Choice (B) may sound reasonable, but the literature on the topic needs to be consulted. Choice (C) may be decided upon but only **after** the preceptor becomes more familiar with the present research on the topic.

111. **(B)** Although admitted with the acute problem of HHS, the patient's comorbidity (schizophrenia) needs to be treated during the acute care hospital stay. Continuation of home meds (as long as they will not exacerbate the acute problem) will prevent the need of a psychiatric consult. Holding psychiatric meds is not necessarily indicated; the patient is not demonstrating a need for a restraint.

112. **(D)** D_5W is contraindicated because it is a hypotonic solution that would exacerbate the low serum osmolality of this patient. The remaining 3 types of fluid may be chosen depending on other factors and would not harm the patient.

113. **(B)** The nature of the injury and subsequent clinical signs indicate epidural hematoma. Arteriogram would not be needed. A CT of the head would be less invasive and confirm the diagnosis. The head of the bed should be kept at least 30 degrees, not low-

ered in order to facilitate venous drainage from the head. Although the patient is exhibiting signs of increased ICP, emergent surgery would be the definitive treatment rather than intubation/ventriculostomy.

114. **(B)** Vasopressin may cause myocardial ischemia that would result in chest pain and/or ST changes on the ECG. The doses used do not generally cause hypertension. Although coronary artery ischemia might result in cardiac arrhythmia, the signs of ischemia would occur first and more reliably. Vasopressin does not result in bowel obstruction.

115. **(C)** Choice (A) is incorrect because pain due to CAD does not radiate to the right arm. Choice (B) is incorrect because it describes the pain of indigestion or acid reflux. Choice (D) is not correct because it describes the pain typical of pericarditis.

116. **(B)** Enalaprilat (Vasotec) is an angiotensin-converting enzyme inhibitor drug that prevents the conversion of angiotensin I to angiotensin II (a potent vasoconstrictor) and thereby causes vasodilation and a decrease in SVR. The other 3 choices are incorrect because afterload is **decreased** by nitroglycerin (high dose NTG). Preload is **decreased** by furosemide and is **increased** with fluids.

117. **(A)** This patient has additional life stressors that add to the complexity of her care. This complexity needs to be considered when planning her care.

118. **(D)** The ABG demonstrates partially compensated respiratory acidosis and hypoxemia. The FiO_2 should be increased and patient response assessed. Intubation is not indicated as the hypercapnea is mild. The clinical picture does not support cardiogenic pulmonary edema as the source of the patient's problem. Therefore, diuresis is not indicated. Sedation will worsen the hypoventilation.

119. **(B)** The patient requires a higher dose of lorazepam. An increase in the infusion rate needs to be preceded by a 2 mg bolus dose. An increase of the infusion drip rate alone will not be effective since it will take an hour for the increased dose to get infused. A bolus dose of 5 mg is not indicated. An increase in the rate to 6 mg/hr alone will not be effective.

120. **(B)** The serum glucose should be decreased by about 50–75 mg/dL per hour for the patient with DKA. Therefore, in this situation, the insulin infusion needs to be decreased. Insulin infusion should be continued, not stopped, until the acidosis is resolved. In this case, acidosis is still present as evidenced by the anion gap and venous CO_2. Bicarbonate administration is not indicated in this situation. nor should the insulin infusion be increased.

121. **(D)** Choices (A) and (B) are passive strategies and do not provide the patient the opportunity to share feelings. At this point, encouragement is not an effective strategy. Being nonjudgmental is important, but the patient requires more than encouragement at this point.

122. **(C)** CSF with glucose less than 60% of the serum glucose is an indication of bacterial meningitis rather than viral meningitis. Elevated protein is present in both viral and bacterial meningitis. Clear CSF is a sign of viral meningitis. Elevated WBC is present in both viral and bacterial meningitis.

123. **(D)** The spike before the P-wave is evidence of atrial pacing. The spike before the QRS is evidence of ventricular pacing. An increase in heart rate with activity demonstrates

the ability to respond to a need for a higher heart rate. Choices (A), (B), and (C) do not illustrate the pacer spikes and increase in heart rate as described.

124. **(D)** The clinical picture is one of a dissection of the aneurysm, which is a surgical emergency. The patient requires immediate surgery in order to have the best outcome. Therefore, waiting until the next day is contraindicated. The other 3 choices **are** indicated.

125. **(D)** Hypoventilation should be avoided in order to prevent an increase in ICP secondary to resulting vasodilation. Hyperventilation beyond pCO_2 30 may decrease O_2 delivery to the brain due to vasoconstriction caused by alkalosis.

126. **(C)** The patient had an acute inferior wall MI. The sudden change in condition is most likely due to acute mitral valve regurgitation secondary to papillary muscle dysfunction. With hypotension, the MV regurgitation is massive and is most likely a surgical emergency. A PCI is not indicated as there is not recurrence of ST elevation. Although IABP therapy and mechanical ventilation might help, they are not definitive treatments for this life-threatening problem.

127. **(C)** All factors, including age, acute illness, chronic illnesses, and support system need to be assessed when looking at patient resiliency.

128. **(A)** Infection is the leading cause of death for the patient with chronic renal failure, which is what this question is asking. The remaining choices are complications of renal failure but do not cause the greatest number of deaths.

129. **(C)** When the intra-aortic balloon closes right before systole begins, the LV afterload is decreased. When the balloon inflates during diastole, coronary artery perfusion is increased. Preload may eventually decrease as coronary artery perfusion increases and afterload has decreased. However, this is an indirect effect of IAB therapy. The balloon does not directly increase myocardial contractility.

130. **(C)** Amiodarone may prolong the QT interval, and a 200 mg tablet is estimated to contain about 75 mg of organic iodide. This may result in amiodarone-induced thyrotoxicosis (AIT) or amiodarone-induced hypothyroidism (AIH), both of which can develop in apparently normal thyroid glands or in glands with preexisting abnormalities. Amiodarone does not affect PR interval or renal function. It does not affect the QRS interval, liver function, or lung sounds. It also does not affect the ST segment or urine output. Amiodarone might decrease B/P if a large dose (300 mg) is given in a rapid IV to a patient with a pulse and could affect pulmonary function (fibrosis) when used orally for long periods of time.

131. **(A)** The experienced nurse will know that there have been studies done on the effects of music on critically ill patients and would advise the spouse that this is a good idea. Choices (B) and (C) are not evidence based. The nurse should ensure that processes are in place to provide non-pharmacological therapy that is evidence based and know how to make that therapy happen without going into details with the spouse.

132. **(A)** Flaring of toes up toward the patient's head is a Babinski reflex, which is not normal in the adult. The remaining choices describe normal reflexive responses. Choice (B) is a normal oculovestibular reflex in the unconscious patient. Choice (C) is a normal corneal reflex. Choice (D) describes a normal gag reflex.

133. **(A)** An ankle/brachial index (ABI) < 1 is a sign of peripheral arterial disease (PAD). The patient with PAD needs to have the feet kept lower than the heart level in order to allow gravity to increase perfusion to the lower extremities. An ABI < 1 is not an indication of hypertension. Elevation of the lower extremities may worsen perfusion. The ABI has nothing to do with arm perfusion.

134. **(B)** The sharp pain to the left shoulder (Kehr's sign) is one sign of a ruptured spleen. The other sign is a distended abdomen with absent bowel sounds. The remaining choices would not cause the same symptoms at rest.

135. **(B)** This strategy is the most transparent approach to use with the family and is also a role-modeling opportunity for the orientee. Choice (A) abdicates nursing involvement in the plan of care. Choice (C) may spare the orientee some embarrassment but may send the wrong message to the family and decrease trust. Choice (D) again abdicates nursing engagement with the family.

136. **(A)** Eye flickering and seizure are most typical of PCP overdose.

137. **(B)** As the left ventricle dilates, complete closure of the mitral valve is impeded, which prevents normal closing of the mitral valve leaflets and causes mitral regurgitation. This resultant murmur is a systolic murmur heard loudest at the apex of the heart and the LV is enlarged.

138. **(B)** Temperature elevation increases the cerebral oxygen requirements and may increase mortality of patients with neuro problems. The pressures described in choice (A) are normal. Urine assessments described in choice (C) are normal. A patient now arousable with voice who had previously required shaking, choice (D), is a sign of improvement in arousability.

139. **(A)** Injury that results in diaphragmatic irritation, e.g., splenic rupture, will result in referred pain to the left shoulder, also known as Kehr's sign. The remaining 3 choices do not cause left shoulder pain.

140. **(D)** CPP (MAP minus ICP) would be lowered due to an increase of ICP that might result if the head is bent or flexed. A neutral head position facilitates venous drainage from the brain and prevents elevated ICP. Although the patient still needs to be repositioned, it does not necessarily need to be hourly. The MAP needs to be kept > 65 mmHg, not lower. A $PaCO_2$ < 30 mmHg will lower ICP by causing vasoconstriction of brain vessels. However, this will decrease blood flow to the brain and cause hypoxemia.

141. **(D)** Normalization of the $PaCO_2$ and hypoxemia for the tachypneic patient with an asthma exacerbation is a sign that the patient is tiring and may need mechanical support. Choice A shows $PaCO_2$ normalization; however, the PaO_2 is acceptable; choice B shows a respiratory alkalosis, an early finding in an asthma exacerbation; choice C shows hypoxemia, which is a worrisome sign, but hyperventilation is still present, a sign the patient is still able to maintain ventilation.

142. **(C)** Chest pain may not always be present. Emergent reperfusion is **not** indicated for a NSTEMI. Stable angina is **not** considered ACS since it is not usually due to plaque rupture.

143. **(C)** The patient with confirmed aspirin overdose will require immediate dialysis in order to prevent renal tubular damage. The patient in choice (A) has a 20:1 BUN to cre-

atinine ratio and most likely needs fluids, not dialysis. The patient in choice (B) needs potassium replacement. The patient in choice (D) has hyperkalemia but does not have ECG changes. Therefore, strategies other than dialysis are indicated.

144. **(D)** The patient most likely has HHS, and the most serious complication is hypovolemic shock. Therefore, fluid replacement is paramount. Insulin administration is needed but is secondary to fluid administration. Bicarbonate is not needed as serious acidosis is not present. Potassium replacement will most likely not be needed.

145. **(C)** The patient has SIRS as evidenced by the increased heart rate, respiratory rate, and WBCs. There is evidence of hemorrhagic pancreatitis as evidenced by Cullen's sign (discoloration around the umbilicus). There is evidence of multisystem organ dysfunction as evidenced by low SpO_2 and hypotension. Fluids are indicated as there are massive fluid shifts with acute pancreatitis with resultant hypovolemia. The patient does not have hemorrhagic shock, does not have diabetes, and does not need antibiotics. The patient is at high risk for ARDS but does not yet have refractory hypoxemia and bilateral infiltrates.

146. **(A)** Sustained A-waves on the ICP tracing are "awful," a sign of very elevated ICP B-waves are "bad." C-waves are OK. Discontinuation of opiate and sedating drugs would **not** be indicated in the presence of A-waves/elevated ICP. The remaining 3 choices **would** be indicated in the presence of A-waves/increased ICP.

147. **(A)** The patient has hypovolemic shock secondary to hemorrhage. A blood loss of 1,500 mL is generally required in order for compensatory responses to fail and for the patient to be hypotensive. Aggressive fluid administration is needed, and blood needs to be given. Since the sudden massive blood loss will use up coagulation factors, the patient needs to be monitored closely for development of DIC. Choices (B) and (C) are not correct since the estimated blood loss is not accurate and there are no signs of septic shock or of pulmonary embolism. Uterine rupture, choice (D), is not suspected.

148. **(A)** Paradoxical breathing pattern is evidence that the main muscle of ventilation, the diaphragm, is tiring. The remaining 3 choices are not criteria that support discontinuation of the spontaneous breathing trial.

149. **(B)** The patient has hypertensive crisis as evidenced by high blood pressure and signs of end-organ damage (chest pain). The labetalol (which is a beta blocker) will help lower the blood pressure plus provide some anti-ischemic effect, which the patient most likely needs in the presence of chest pain. Although nicardipine is an antihypertensive and can prevent chest pain, it is not recommended for hypertensive crisis and active chest pain. Nitroprusside is indicated for hypertensive crisis but is not recommended for cardiac ischemia. Diltiazem may be used for hypertension but not for hypertensive crisis.

150. **(D)** An S3 heart sound at the apex is thought to be due to high pressure within the LV present in heart failure. S4 is usually due to hypertension or acute MI. A systolic murmur at the apex is usually due to mitral valve regurgitation. A diastolic murmur at the left sternal border is usually due to tricuspid valve disease.

1. Ⓐ Ⓑ Ⓒ Ⓓ	39. Ⓐ Ⓑ Ⓒ Ⓓ	77. Ⓐ Ⓑ Ⓒ Ⓓ	115. Ⓐ Ⓑ Ⓒ Ⓓ
2. Ⓐ Ⓑ Ⓒ Ⓓ	40. Ⓐ Ⓑ Ⓒ Ⓓ	78. Ⓐ Ⓑ Ⓒ Ⓓ	116. Ⓐ Ⓑ Ⓒ Ⓓ
3. Ⓐ Ⓑ Ⓒ Ⓓ	41. Ⓐ Ⓑ Ⓒ Ⓓ	79. Ⓐ Ⓑ Ⓒ Ⓓ	117. Ⓐ Ⓑ Ⓒ Ⓓ
4. Ⓐ Ⓑ Ⓒ Ⓓ	42. Ⓐ Ⓑ Ⓒ Ⓓ	80. Ⓐ Ⓑ Ⓒ Ⓓ	118. Ⓐ Ⓑ Ⓒ Ⓓ
5. Ⓐ Ⓑ Ⓒ Ⓓ	43. Ⓐ Ⓑ Ⓒ Ⓓ	81. Ⓐ Ⓑ Ⓒ Ⓓ	119. Ⓐ Ⓑ Ⓒ Ⓓ
6. Ⓐ Ⓑ Ⓒ Ⓓ	44. Ⓐ Ⓑ Ⓒ Ⓓ	82. Ⓐ Ⓑ Ⓒ Ⓓ	120. Ⓐ Ⓑ Ⓒ Ⓓ
7. Ⓐ Ⓑ Ⓒ Ⓓ	45. Ⓐ Ⓑ Ⓒ Ⓓ	83. Ⓐ Ⓑ Ⓒ Ⓓ	121. Ⓐ Ⓑ Ⓒ Ⓓ
8. Ⓐ Ⓑ Ⓒ Ⓓ	46. Ⓐ Ⓑ Ⓒ Ⓓ	84. Ⓐ Ⓑ Ⓒ Ⓓ	122. Ⓐ Ⓑ Ⓒ Ⓓ
9. Ⓐ Ⓑ Ⓒ Ⓓ	47. Ⓐ Ⓑ Ⓒ Ⓓ	85. Ⓐ Ⓑ Ⓒ Ⓓ	123. Ⓐ Ⓑ Ⓒ Ⓓ
10. Ⓐ Ⓑ Ⓒ Ⓓ	48. Ⓐ Ⓑ Ⓒ Ⓓ	86. Ⓐ Ⓑ Ⓒ Ⓓ	124. Ⓐ Ⓑ Ⓒ Ⓓ
11. Ⓐ Ⓑ Ⓒ Ⓓ	49. Ⓐ Ⓑ Ⓒ Ⓓ	87. Ⓐ Ⓑ Ⓒ Ⓓ	125. Ⓐ Ⓑ Ⓒ Ⓓ
12. Ⓐ Ⓑ Ⓒ Ⓓ	50. Ⓐ Ⓑ Ⓒ Ⓓ	88. Ⓐ Ⓑ Ⓒ Ⓓ	126. Ⓐ Ⓑ Ⓒ Ⓓ
13. Ⓐ Ⓑ Ⓒ Ⓓ	51. Ⓐ Ⓑ Ⓒ Ⓓ	89. Ⓐ Ⓑ Ⓒ Ⓓ	127. Ⓐ Ⓑ Ⓒ Ⓓ
14. Ⓐ Ⓑ Ⓒ Ⓓ	52. Ⓐ Ⓑ Ⓒ Ⓓ	90. Ⓐ Ⓑ Ⓒ Ⓓ	128. Ⓐ Ⓑ Ⓒ Ⓓ
15. Ⓐ Ⓑ Ⓒ Ⓓ	53. Ⓐ Ⓑ Ⓒ Ⓓ	91. Ⓐ Ⓑ Ⓒ Ⓓ	129. Ⓐ Ⓑ Ⓒ Ⓓ
16. Ⓐ Ⓑ Ⓒ Ⓓ	54. Ⓐ Ⓑ Ⓒ Ⓓ	92. Ⓐ Ⓑ Ⓒ Ⓓ	130. Ⓐ Ⓑ Ⓒ Ⓓ
17. Ⓐ Ⓑ Ⓒ Ⓓ	55. Ⓐ Ⓑ Ⓒ Ⓓ	93. Ⓐ Ⓑ Ⓒ Ⓓ	131. Ⓐ Ⓑ Ⓒ Ⓓ
18. Ⓐ Ⓑ Ⓒ Ⓓ	56. Ⓐ Ⓑ Ⓒ Ⓓ	94. Ⓐ Ⓑ Ⓒ Ⓓ	132. Ⓐ Ⓑ Ⓒ Ⓓ
19. Ⓐ Ⓑ Ⓒ Ⓓ	57. Ⓐ Ⓑ Ⓒ Ⓓ	95. Ⓐ Ⓑ Ⓒ Ⓓ	133. Ⓐ Ⓑ Ⓒ Ⓓ
20. Ⓐ Ⓑ Ⓒ Ⓓ	58. Ⓐ Ⓑ Ⓒ Ⓓ	96. Ⓐ Ⓑ Ⓒ Ⓓ	134. Ⓐ Ⓑ Ⓒ Ⓓ
21. Ⓐ Ⓑ Ⓒ Ⓓ	59. Ⓐ Ⓑ Ⓒ Ⓓ	97. Ⓐ Ⓑ Ⓒ Ⓓ	135. Ⓐ Ⓑ Ⓒ Ⓓ
22. Ⓐ Ⓑ Ⓒ Ⓓ	60. Ⓐ Ⓑ Ⓒ Ⓓ	98. Ⓐ Ⓑ Ⓒ Ⓓ	136. Ⓐ Ⓑ Ⓒ Ⓓ
23. Ⓐ Ⓑ Ⓒ Ⓓ	61. Ⓐ Ⓑ Ⓒ Ⓓ	99. Ⓐ Ⓑ Ⓒ Ⓓ	137. Ⓐ Ⓑ Ⓒ Ⓓ
24. Ⓐ Ⓑ Ⓒ Ⓓ	62. Ⓐ Ⓑ Ⓒ Ⓓ	100. Ⓐ Ⓑ Ⓒ Ⓓ	138. Ⓐ Ⓑ Ⓒ Ⓓ
25. Ⓐ Ⓑ Ⓒ Ⓓ	63. Ⓐ Ⓑ Ⓒ Ⓓ	101. Ⓐ Ⓑ Ⓒ Ⓓ	139. Ⓐ Ⓑ Ⓒ Ⓓ
26. Ⓐ Ⓑ Ⓒ Ⓓ	64. Ⓐ Ⓑ Ⓒ Ⓓ	102. Ⓐ Ⓑ Ⓒ Ⓓ	140. Ⓐ Ⓑ Ⓒ Ⓓ
27. Ⓐ Ⓑ Ⓒ Ⓓ	65. Ⓐ Ⓑ Ⓒ Ⓓ	103. Ⓐ Ⓑ Ⓒ Ⓓ	141. Ⓐ Ⓑ Ⓒ Ⓓ
28. Ⓐ Ⓑ Ⓒ Ⓓ	66. Ⓐ Ⓑ Ⓒ Ⓓ	104. Ⓐ Ⓑ Ⓒ Ⓓ	142. Ⓐ Ⓑ Ⓒ Ⓓ
29. Ⓐ Ⓑ Ⓒ Ⓓ	67. Ⓐ Ⓑ Ⓒ Ⓓ	105. Ⓐ Ⓑ Ⓒ Ⓓ	143. Ⓐ Ⓑ Ⓒ Ⓓ
30. Ⓐ Ⓑ Ⓒ Ⓓ	68. Ⓐ Ⓑ Ⓒ Ⓓ	106. Ⓐ Ⓑ Ⓒ Ⓓ	144. Ⓐ Ⓑ Ⓒ Ⓓ
31. Ⓐ Ⓑ Ⓒ Ⓓ	69. Ⓐ Ⓑ Ⓒ Ⓓ	107. Ⓐ Ⓑ Ⓒ Ⓓ	145. Ⓐ Ⓑ Ⓒ Ⓓ
32. Ⓐ Ⓑ Ⓒ Ⓓ	70. Ⓐ Ⓑ Ⓒ Ⓓ	108. Ⓐ Ⓑ Ⓒ Ⓓ	146. Ⓐ Ⓑ Ⓒ Ⓓ
33. Ⓐ Ⓑ Ⓒ Ⓓ	71. Ⓐ Ⓑ Ⓒ Ⓓ	109. Ⓐ Ⓑ Ⓒ Ⓓ	147. Ⓐ Ⓑ Ⓒ Ⓓ
34. Ⓐ Ⓑ Ⓒ Ⓓ	72. Ⓐ Ⓑ Ⓒ Ⓓ	110. Ⓐ Ⓑ Ⓒ Ⓓ	148. Ⓐ Ⓑ Ⓒ Ⓓ
35. Ⓐ Ⓑ Ⓒ Ⓓ	73. Ⓐ Ⓑ Ⓒ Ⓓ	111. Ⓐ Ⓑ Ⓒ Ⓓ	149. Ⓐ Ⓑ Ⓒ Ⓓ
36. Ⓐ Ⓑ Ⓒ Ⓓ	74. Ⓐ Ⓑ Ⓒ Ⓓ	112. Ⓐ Ⓑ Ⓒ Ⓓ	150. Ⓐ Ⓑ Ⓒ Ⓓ
37. Ⓐ Ⓑ Ⓒ Ⓓ	75. Ⓐ Ⓑ Ⓒ Ⓓ	113. Ⓐ Ⓑ Ⓒ Ⓓ	
38. Ⓐ Ⓑ Ⓒ Ⓓ	76. Ⓐ Ⓑ Ⓒ Ⓓ	114. Ⓐ Ⓑ Ⓒ Ⓓ	

PRACTICE TEST 2

Practice CCRN Test 2

16

Directions: This is the second of two, 150-question comprehensive practice tests. Do not attempt to complete these tests until you have reviewed each section of the book and have completed the tests related to each section. The pretest questions and the questions that follow each section focus more on "facts." Questions found in each final comprehensive test require application, evaluation, and analysis of knowledge. Master the book contents until you can achieve a score of at least 80% on the comprehensive tests prior to taking the CCRN® exam.

1. The patient develops blood pressure 82/48, heart rate 126/minute, temperature 35°C, hemoglobin 8.9 g/dL, WBC 4,000, bands 22%. A pulmonary artery catheter was inserted and the following measurement obtained: pulmonary artery pressure 22/8 mmHg, central venous pressure 1 mmHg, pulmonary artery occlusive pressure 4 mmHg, cardiac output 7.0 L/minute, systemic vascular resistance of 600 dynes/s/m5.

   The patient needs:

   (A) continued fluids, blood transfusion, pressors.
   (B) discontinue fluids, blood transfusion, warming.
   (C) reduce fluid rate, positive inotropes, preload reducers.
   (D) continued fluids, pressors, antibiotics.

2. The nurse notices that patients receiving PCA therapy have had more adverse effects and safety reports over the past month. She asks the clinical nurse specialist whether anyone else has noted this increase, and the CNS says "No." What would be the ideal strategy to pursue at this point?

   (A) Poll the unit nurses and two noncritical care units about whether an increase of adverse events has been noticed.
   (B) Discuss the finding with the author of the hospital PCA Standing Orders.
   (C) Undertake a chart audit of all patients receiving PCA therapy in the previous six months.
   (D) List all future adverse events for the next 30 days.

3. The physician asks the nurse to call with any sign of increased intracranial pressure. Clinical changes indicative of an increase in ICP for the majority of neurological problems are seen in which order of progression (early to late) of those listed below?

(A) pupillary inequality, change in level of consciousness, vital sign changes
(B) change in level of consciousness, vital sign changes, pupillary inequality
(C) vital sign changes, pupillary inequality, pupils fixed and dilated
(D) change in level of consciousness, pupillary inequality, vital sign changes

4. Which of the following assessments is most important in order to identify a complication for the patient with Guillain-Barré syndrome?

(A) vital capacity
(B) O$_2$ saturation
(C) pupil reaction
(D) temperature

5. Which of the following would the nurse anticipate with the initiation of a nitroprusside (Nipride) infusion?

(A) decrease contractility
(B) increase pulmonary vascular resistance
(C) decrease afterload
(D) increase preload

6. The patient was admitted 12 hours ago with an acute inferior wall MI. Which of the following would be expected on the 12-lead ECG?

(A) ST elevation and deep Q-waves in I, II, aVL
(B) ST depression in I, aVL
(C) ST elevation and deep Q-waves in V2, V3, V4
(D) ST depression in II, III, aVF

7. The patient admitted with bleeding esophageal varices with a known history of alcohol abuse demonstrates tremulousness, mild anxiety, and diaphoresis 48 hours after admission. He is alert and oriented. Which of the following interventions is most effective for this patient?

(A) Continue to monitor mental status closely.
(B) Obtain an order for the CIWA-ar protocol.
(C) Obtain a complete blood count (CBC).
(D) Apply a vest restraint.

8. The patient was admitted status post fall from a 3rd-story roof. Chest X-ray reveals fracture of left ribs 4 through 6, and chest excursion on the left is diminished. Patient vital signs include: B/P 84/54, heart rate 130, respiratory rate 32. Which of the following immediate interventions is indicated?

(A) oxygen, fluid bolus, left chest tube insertion
(B) intubation, pressors, left chest tube insertion
(C) oxygen, fluid bolus, pericardiocentesis
(D) intubation, fluids, emergency surgery

9. The patient with a cerebral arterial embolus most likely has thrombi in which of the following?

(A) femoral artery
(B) left atrium or left ventricle
(C) superior vena cava
(D) right atrium or right ventricle

10. A Type I diabetic is training for a 10K run and develops tachycardia, slurred speech, and confusion. Which of the following does the patient most likely need?

(A) immediate glucose source
(B) insulin
(C) CT of the head
(D) fluids

PRACTICE TEST 2

11. Fluid and electrolyte balance require close monitoring for the patient with acute pancreatitis due to which of the following?

 (A) increased diuresis secondary to pancreatic enzyme release
 (B) increased incidence of hypercalcemia
 (C) increased capillary permeability resulting in fluid loss from the vascular space
 (D) hypoglycemia due to pancreatic cell destruction

12. The patient is status post percutaneous coronary intervention, and labs reveal a PTT of 210 seconds. Which of the following is indicated?

 (A) heparin
 (B) vitamin K
 (C) protamine sulfate
 (D) fresh frozen plasma

13. The nurse notices that the patient admitted with acute pancreatitis demonstrates left hand spasm when inflating the B/P cuff on the patient's left arm. Which of the following is the most likely assessment?

 (A) positive Chvostek sign, hypophosphatemia
 (B) positive Trousseau sign, hypocalcemia
 (C) positive Kernig's sign, hypermagnesemia
 (D) positive Cullen's sign, hypercalcemia

14. The nurse is interested in getting approval for a protocol that he learned from a nationally known expert at a nursing conference he recently attended. Which of the following strategies would be most effective in convincing hospital leadership that the new protocol is financially worthwhile?

 (A) Send copies of the protocol and the conference presentation to the nursing leadership.
 (B) Present to the nursing leadership a summary of research that relates the protocol to decreased length of patient stay.
 (C) Outline favorable patient outcomes that have been demonstrated at other hospitals that adopted the protocol.
 (D) Ask for a meeting with the unit medical director to request adoption of the protocol.

15. A patient develops acute onset of inspiratory and expiratory wheezing throughout the lung fields. Which of the following statements is correct?

 (A) The patient has acute heart failure and requires morphine.
 (B) The patient has an asthma exacerbation and requires bronchodilators.
 (C) The patient has an asthma exacerbation and requires corticosteroids.
 (D) The patient has acute heart failure and requires a diuretic.

16. Which of the following ventilator settings or patient assessments is most likely to predict success with ventilator liberation or weaning?

 (A) FiO_2 70% or less
 (B) negative inspiratory force of < -25 cm H_2O
 (C) minute ventilation 15 L/min
 (D) vital capacity 3–5 L

17. Pressure support ventilation has which of the following positive effects?

    (A) It decreases the oxygen requirements.
    (B) It decreases the work of breathing.
    (C) It decreases the work of muscles.
    (D) It decreases the tidal volume requirements.

18. The patient had a prolonged period of hypotension status postsurgical repair of a leaking AAA. The patient developed ATN. Which of the following are likely to develop?

    (A) acidosis, azotemia, hyperkalemia
    (B) anemia, alkalosis, hypercalcemia
    (C) acidosis, hypotension, hypomagnesemia
    (D) hypertension, azotemia, hypokalemia

19. The patient receiving mechanical ventilation and tube feeding is suspected of having aspirated. Which of the following are most likely to develop if the patient has aspiration?

    (A) decrease in minute ventilation, drop in SaO_2
    (B) decrease in respiratory rate and low-pressure alarm
    (C) increase in negative inspiratory force and bilateral infiltrates on chest film
    (D) increase in peak inspiratory pressure and right-sided infiltrate on chest film

20. The patient presents with methamphetamine overdose. Which of the following initial interventions should the nurse anticipate?

    (A) monitor renal function, protect patient from self-harm
    (B) monitor for rhabdomyolysis, prepare for intubation
    (C) initiate cooling, fluid replacement
    (D) initiate naloxone (Narcan), monitor renal function

21. Which of the following is CORRECT regarding continuous venovenous hemofiltration (CVVH) therapy?

    (A) prevent life-threatening electrolyte imbalance
    (B) remove immunoglobins for those with autoimmune disease
    (C) correct fluid balance
    (D) increase colloid oncotic pressure

22. A man is admitted with a gunshot wound to the head. His right pupil is dilated and nonreactive. This indicates damage to cranial nerve:

    (A) II.
    (B) III.
    (C) V.
    (D) IX.

23. The patient is admitted with fever and nuchal rigidity. A lumbar puncture is performed. Which of the following findings most likely indicates bacterial rather than viral meningitis?

    (A) CSF glucose of 30 mg/dL
    (B) CSF with elevated WBCs and protein
    (C) fever greater than 40°C
    (D) decreased level of consciousness

24. Which of the following assessment findings indicate possible ARDS?

    (A) PaO_2 95 mmHg on FiO_2 1.00
    (B) SvO_2 0.65
    (C) PaO_2 65 on room air
    (D) A-A gradient 8 mmHg

25. Which of the following are NOT a part of the Circle of Willis?

    (A) left and right anterior cerebral
    (B) left and right internal carotid
    (C) posterior cerebral and posterior communicating
    (D) middle cerebral and basilar

26. A patient is admitted with intestinal obstruction. Which of the following assessments would the nurse anticipate for this patient?

 (A) rigid, boardlike abdomen, absent bowel sounds, rebound tenderness, pain worse with movement
 (B) dull, right upper-quadrant pain, rebound tenderness
 (C) tympanic percussion note, cramping pain, abdominal distention, high-pitched tinkling sounds
 (D) boring, epigastric pain, abdominal tenderness, normal bowel sounds

27. The patient was admitted with hypertensive crisis, and a nitroprusside (Nipride) infusion was begun. Which of the following is a priority assessment?

 (A) symptoms of nausea and vomiting
 (B) blood pressure every 1 to 2 minutes until stable
 (C) thiocyanate level
 (D) liver enzymes

28. A patient admitted with systolic heart failure developed hypotension, tachycardia, decreasing urine output, cool and clammy skin, decreasing level of consciousness, and tachypnea. Which of the following medical orders should the nurse anticipate?

 (A) negative inotropes, antiarrhythmics, cardiac glycoside
 (B) positive inotropes, diuretics, vasodilators
 (C) beta blockers, ACE inhibitors, diuretics
 (D) calcium-channel blockers, positive inotropes, amiodarone

29. The patient with status asthmaticus will most likely have which of the following?

 (A) wheezing, atrial fibrillation
 (B) silent chest, diastolic murmur
 (C) wheezing, giant V-waves
 (D) silent chest, pulsus paradoxus

30. Which of the following would be contraindicated in the treatment of SIADH?

 (A) hypertonic saline and diuretics
 (B) vasopressin
 (C) fluid restriction
 (D) phenytoin (Dilantin)

31. The patient was admitted with signs of acute embolic stroke, and fibrinolytic therapy is anticipated. Which of the following is a priority determination?

 (A) home medications
 (B) symptom onset
 (C) allergy history
 (D) risk factor assessment

32. The patient is admitted with community-acquired pneumonia and speaks only Spanish. Which of the following strategies is effective in this situation?

 (A) Get a hospital translator; stand next to the translator while speaking and as close to the patient as possible.
 (B) Allow extra time for the hospital translator to decode medical terms when providing the translation.
 (C) Speak slowly in English, using hands and pictures when indicated.
 (D) Ask the wife to translate, provide all of the information, and then take patient questions through the translator.

33. The patient was admitted with ST elevation and deep Q-waves in V1, V2, V3. The patient suddenly complains of shortness of breath and develops a loud holosystolic murmur that is loudest at the left sternal border, 5th intercostal space. Which of the following has the patient most likely developed?

 (A) ventricular septal defect
 (B) acute ischemia
 (C) cardiac tamponade
 (D) papillary muscle dysfunction

34. Which of the following ABGs (obtained on room air) is most indicative of acute respiratory failure?

   (A) pH 7.18; pCO_2 25; pO_2 64;.HCO_3 11
   (B) pH 7.20; pCO_2 58; pO_2 61; HCO_3 25
   (C) pH 7.35; pCO_2 61; pO_2 62; HCO_3 41
   (D) pH 7.25; pCO_2 45; pO_2 68; HCO_3 18

35. The patient is experiencing alcohol withdrawal and reports bugs crawling on his arms and on the walls. Which of the following nursing interventions is most appropriate for this patient?

   (A) Whisper to colleagues to control the noise.
   (B) Explain the actual circumstances to the patient.
   (C) Provide therapeutic touch to calm the patient.
   (D) Explain to the patient that the hallucinations are not real.

36. Which of the following is most indicative of cardiogenic shock?

   (A) Cardiac index 1.9 $L/min/m^2$
   (B) PAOP 9 mmHg
   (C) SvO_2 70%
   (D) SVR 1000 dynes/s/cm^{-5}

37. The patient is admitted with upper GI bleeding, hypotension, and tachycardia. Which of the following lab results would be expected?

   (A) elevated BUN, elevated serum sodium
   (B) metabolic acidosis, decreased PT
   (C) elevated PTT, decreased sodium
   (D) decreased WBC, elevated platelets

38. A 90 kg male patient with ARDS is receiving mechanical ventilation with the following settings: Assist control mode, rate 18/minute; FiO_2 70%; Vt 450 mL; PEEP 5 cm H_2O. ABGs are obtained and reveal the following: pH 7.36, PCO_2 50, pO_2 49, HCO_3 25. Which of the following interventions should the nurse anticipate?

   (A) increase the FiO_2
   (B) increase the rate
   (C) increase the Vt
   (D) increase PEEP

39. Which of the following is most indicative of distributive shock?

   (A) SVR 490 dynes/s/cm^{-5}
   (B) CVP 1 mmHg
   (C) heart rate 130/minute
   (D) PAOP 7 mmHg

40. Which of the following is TRUE regarding surfactant?

   (A) It is produced by the Type I alveolar cells.
   (B) It prevents atelectasis.
   (C) It increases the work of breathing.
   (D) It decreases lung compliance.

41. Which of the following are related to hypokalemia?

   (A) ACE inhibitors and crush injuries
   (B) diarrhea and hemolysis
   (C) alkalosis and thiazide diuretics
   (D) acidosis and vomiting

42. A research study is being conducted to look at the effectiveness of a newer drug to manage patient agitation. A patient is too ill to make his own decisions. While the nurse is in the patient's room, a family member is approached by one of the research staff and asked to consent to participate in the study. When the family member asks if there are any risks, she is told not to worry of risks and "Here is the form, sign here." How should the patient's nurse respond?

(A) Report what was overheard to the ethics committee.
(B) Contact the primary investigator on the study.
(C) Review the protocol with the patient's surrogate decision maker.
(D) Smile at the family member and leave the room.

43. An 81-year-old patient admitted 4 days ago is experiencing periods of agitation alternating with withdrawal. Which of the following is the most appropriate initial nursing intervention?

(A) Keep the lights on, and put the television on the music station.
(B) Provide a private room, and restrict visiting to family.
(C) Review the medication list, and ensure periods of uninterrupted sleep.
(D) Contact the physician for a benzodiazepine order.

44. The patient has been in the ICU with respiratory failure and hepatic failure secondary to metastatic cancer for 6 days without improvement. The family, who seems to understand the patient's condition, refuses to agree to a do-not-resuscitate order at a family meeting with the multidisciplinary team. The patient's SpO_2 acutely drops to 74%, and the physician orders the FiO_2 to be maintained at 40%. Which of the following should the nurse do at this time?

(A) Ask the physician to provide a rationale for the order.
(B) Continue the FiO_2 at 40%.
(C) Request that the family speak with the physician.
(D) Administer analgesia and sedating medication to avoid discomfort.

45. A 22-year-old patient was admitted to the ED with weakness and history of aching and fever for 2 days. The patient was hypotensive, was not responsive to fluids, and was admitted to the critical care unit with blood pressure 80/60. A pulmonary artery catheter was inserted with the following values obtained: right atrial pressure 14 mmHg; PAOP 16 mmHg; cardiac output 2.0 L/min; SVR 1800^{-5}. Which of the following treatments would you anticipate?

(A) emergent pericardiocentesis
(B) antibiotics
(C) pressors
(D) continue aggressive fluids

46. The patient is in cardiogenic shock and not responsive to positive inotropic drug therapy. The nurse asks the cardiologist if preparation should begin for an intra-aortic balloon insertion, but the physician said the patient has a contraindication to this therapy. The patient most likely has which of the following?

    (A) ventricular septal defect
    (B) aortic valve regurgitation
    (C) mitral valve regurgitation
    (D) aortic valve stenosis

47. The patient is admitted with stage II hepatic encephalopathy. Which of the following assessments is most likely for this patient?

    (A) coma
    (B) respiratory acidosis
    (C) asterixis
    (D) decreased serum ammonia

48. Heart failure is most often associated with which of the following arrhythmias?

    (A) third-degree AV block
    (B) atrial fibrillation
    (C) ventricular bigeminy
    (D) atrial tachycardia

49. While preparing the patient for transfer from the critical care unit, the patient states, "I will probably end up back here tomorrow since they don't know what to do for me on the other unit." Which of the following is the most appropriate response?

    (A) "You seem concerned about going to the other unit."
    (B) "The nurses are very well trained on that unit."
    (C) "The doctors all feel you don't need us anymore."
    (D) "We need your bed for an extremely ill lady in the emergency room."

50. After admitting a 19-year-old trauma patient in critical condition, the nurse enters the family waiting room and is approached by 8 family members with questions. Which of the following INITIAL responses is appropriate?

    (A) Tell the family you will contact the trauma surgeon to come and speak with them.
    (B) Explain to the family you will meet with them when the chaplain arrives.
    (C) Request that the family identify a spokesperson.
    (D) Inform the family that the patient's condition is critical.

51. An obstetrical patient, 1 hour status post abruptio placental delivery, is noted to have pink urine and oozing from the IV insertion site. Which of the following laboratory tests would most likely be ordered at this time?

    (A) D-dimer and PT
    (B) fibrin split products and creatinine
    (C) Pitocin level and magnesium
    (D) factor X and BUN

52. A patient was admitted with a history of several syncopal episodes at home. On arrival, the patient was in normal sinus rhythm with a QTc of 0.50 seconds. The patient suddenly developed a non-sustained episode of polymorphic ventricular tachycardia. Which of the following interventions would be most appropriate at this time?

    (A) defibrillation
    (B) amiodarone IV
    (C) magnesium IV
    (D) synchronized cardioversion

53. A patient with DKA would most likely present with which of the following?

    (A) decreased anion gap
    (B) volume overload
    (C) hypokalemia
    (D) low serum osmolality

54. Which of the following will worsen hepatic encephalopathy?

    (A) normal saline
    (B) carbohydrates
    (C) aldactone
    (D) GI bleeding

55. A patient has a temporary transvenous pacemaker set at 70/min on demand. The nurse notices that the patient's heart rate is 78/min, and pacer spikes are noted in the patient's native beats. Which of the following interventions is indicated at this time?

    (A) Check the pacing connection to the generator.
    (B) Decrease the rate.
    (C) Increase the sensitivity.
    (D) Increase the mA.

56. A patient with aortic regurgitation develops atrial fibrillation with a rate of 92/minute, B/P is 115/78. Which of the following medical orders should the nurse anticipate?

    (A) cardiac glycoside and calcium-channel blocker
    (B) antiarrhythmic and beta agonist
    (C) beta blocker and vasopressor
    (D) beta blocker and calcium-channel blocker

57. The patient with which of the following signs most likely has a tension pneumothorax?

    (A) absent breath sounds on the affected side, hypotension, distended neck veins
    (B) dull to percussion on the affected side, hypertension, flat neck veins
    (C) diminished breath sounds on the affected side, tracheal deviation to the affected side, hypotension
    (D) absent breath sounds on the affected side, tracheal deviation to the opposite side, flat neck veins

58. The patient is 2 days status post head injury, keeps asking for water, and has urine output of 300 mL/hour. Which of the following lab findings and treatment should the nurse expect?

    (A) serum sodium decreased, serum osmolality increased, administer phenytoin
    (B) serum sodium decreased, serum osmolality decreased, administer phenytoin
    (C) serum sodium increased, serum osmolality decreased, administer vasopressin
    (D) serum sodium increased, serum osmolality increased, administer vasopressin

59. The patient is status post craniotomy. Which of the following positions is optimal for the patient?

    (A) the position that prevents postoperative pain
    (B) the position that increases intracranial pressure
    (C) on the side opposite of the surgery
    (D) upright to maximize cerebral venous outflow

60. The patient was admitted with a sudden death arrhythmia and required insertion of an implantable cardiac defibrillator (ICD). The wife is anxious that the patient's ICD will not work and the patient will have another cardiac arrest after discharge. Which of the following would be the most appropriate response of the nurse?

    (A) "Now that he has the ICD, you do not need to worry."
    (B) "Would you be less anxious if you learned how to do CPR?"
    (C) "Your town has an excellent EMS system."
    (D) "I will ask the cardiologist to speak to you and give you more information."

61. Measurement of hemodynamic data is most accurate when obtained:

    (A) at the end of the T-wave.
    (B) every hour.
    (C) at the end of the respiratory cycle, end expiration.
    (D) from the digital readout on the monitor.

62. The patient has acute respiratory failure secondary to a pulmonary embolism. The patient has a respiratory rate of 28/minute, lungs clear, SpO_2 is 88% on 4L/nasal cannula, blood pressure is 88/58. Which of the following is accurate regarding this patient?

    (A) The embolism is massive, and alveolar dead space is increased.
    (B) The patient's D-dimer is negative, and fibrinolytic therapy is indicated.
    (C) The patient requires mechanical ventilation and a norepinephrine infusion.
    (D) The shunting is massive, and PEEP therapy is indicated.

63. The physician orders a bowel regimen for a patient with DIC. What is the rationale for the physician order?

    (A) prevent large bowel obstruction
    (B) decrease risk of GI bleeding
    (C) prevent fluid and electrolyte imbalance
    (D) decrease risk of intracranial hemorrhage

64. Which of the following may cause left ventricular failure?

    (A) pulmonary embolism, aortic stenosis
    (B) mitral stenosis, acute coronary syndrome
    (C) hypertension, aortic regurgitation
    (D) mitral regurgitation, COPD

65. Which of the following hemodynamic profiles is indicative of hypovolemic shock?

    (A) SvO_2 55, PAOP 16, SVR 1,600
    (B) SvO_2 65, PAOP 8, SVR 1,200
    (C) SvO_2 55, PAOP 3, SVR 1,500
    (D) SvO_2 85, PAOP 3, SVR 500

66. Which of the following findings definitively demonstrates hypoventilation?

    (A) pCO_2 46
    (B) pO_2 59
    (C) pH 7.50
    (D) respiratory rate 10/min

67. The patient has acute lung injury (ALI) and septic shock. Which of the following assessments of oxygenation would be most likely for this patient?

    (A) pO_2 50, SvO_2 50
    (B) pO_2 80, SvO_2 80
    (C) pO_2 50, SvO_2 85
    (D) pO_2 55, SvO_2 50

68. The patient was admitted with a carboxyhemoglobin level of 55%. Which of the following is appropriate treatment?

    (A) Provide FiO_2 of 100% until the SpO_2 is > 95%.
    (B) Provide positive pressure ventilation until the patient's level of consciousness is normal.
    (C) Provide FiO_2 of 100% until the carboxyhemoglobin level is < 10%.
    (D) Provide treatment in a hyperbaric oxygen chamber until the patient's level of consciousness is normal.

69. Which of the following would be expected for the patient with renal hypoperfusion?

    (A) urine sodium greater than 20 and serum osmolality greater than urine osmolality
    (B) urine sodium less than 20 and serum osmolality greater than urine osmolality
    (C) urine sodium greater than 20 and urine osmolality greater than serum osmolality
    (D) urine sodium less than 20 and urine osmolality greater than serum osmolality

70. A patient is admitted with middle meningeal artery bleed. Which of the following problems does the patient most likely have?

    (A) subdural hematoma
    (B) subarachnoid hemorrhage
    (C) epidural hematoma
    (D) AV malformation

71. A patient developed confusion and combativeness 2 days post-op. Which of the following would determine that the patient has delirium?

    (A) The patient is speaking incoherently, rambling.
    (B) The family reports this is the patient's usual behavior.
    (C) The patient is attentive when you speak.
    (D) Some days the patient is oriented better than other days.

72. A 55-year-old female is admitted with subarachnoid hemorrhage (SAH). Which of the following interventions is indicated for this patient?

    (A) Provide hypotonic intravenous fluids.
    (B) Secure her airway in the event of respiratory arrest.
    (C) Prevent hypoventilation.
    (D) Administer antibiotics to prevent infection.

73. The patient has ST elevation in V1, V2, and V3. Which of the following is the patient at risk of developing?

    (A) sinus exit block or sinus arrest
    (B) second-degree heart block, Type I
    (C) second-degree heart block, Type II
    (D) third-degree heart block, complete

74. A patient is admitted with ST elevation MI, hypotensive, and heart rate 42/minute, more P-waves than QRS complexes, wide QRS, and PR intervals constant. Which of the following arteries is most likely blocked?

    (A) left anterior descending
    (B) left main
    (C) left circumflex
    (D) right coronary artery

75. The patient presents one month status post gastric bypass bariatric surgery with vomiting, headache, diplopia, and memory loss. The patient most likely needs which of the following?

(A) vitamins
(B) antibiotics
(C) potassium
(D) emergent surgery

76. Which of the following would be goals of therapy for a patient with dilated (congestive) cardiomyopathy?

(A) Decrease the preload, and decrease the afterload.
(B) Increase the preload, and increase the afterload.
(C) Decrease the preload, and increase the afterload.
(D) Increase the preload, and decrease the afterload.

77. A patient was admitted with chest pain and ST elevation in leads II, III, and aVF. Several hours after a PCI, the patient developed a drop in blood pressure to 82/52, bibasilar crackles, and urine output of 25 mL in the past hour. Which of the following hemodynamic profiles would the patient be expected to have?

(A) CO 5.8; SVR 500; PAP 19/6
(B) CO 2.8; SVR 725; PAP 25/14
(C) CO 3.5; SVR 1800; PAP 42/22
(D) CO 4.8; SVR 950; PAP 32/11

78. The patient with acute ST elevation MI is receiving a heparin infusion in order to do which of the following?

(A) prevent platelet aggregation on the clot
(B) prevent conversion of prothrombin to thrombin
(C) promote conversion of plasminogen to plasmin
(D) prevent conversion of thrombin to fibrinogen

79. A patient is admitted with hepatic failure. Which of the following treatments should the nurse anticipate?

(A) Provide higher doses of insulin to treat hyperglycemia.
(B) Provide sedation with benzodiazepines.
(C) Treat dehydration with lactated Ringer's.
(D) Treat ascites with spironolactone (Aldactone).

80. The patient was admitted status post full cardiac arrest on the step-down unit and died prior to his wife's arrival to the hospital. Which of the following should the nurse do in order to prepare for the wife's arrival?

(A) Plan to provide the wife with information about the care that was provided to the patient prior to his death.
(B) Arrange to allow the wife to view the patient in the morgue after she arrives.
(C) Ensure that the physician is available when the wife arrives.
(D) Have the chaplain available to escort the wife to the waiting room when she arrives.

81. A patient has a right-sided chest tube. The nurse notes that during inspiration and expiration, the water in the water seal chamber rises and falls. What does this assessment indicate?

(A) a pleural leak
(B) a tension pneumothorax
(C) normal fluctuation in pleural pressure
(D) intact connection to suction

82. The patient with acute lung injury (ALI) is receiving mechanical ventilation with the following settings: FiO_2 60%, assist control of 12/min, Vt 4 mL/kg, PEEP 15 cm H_2O. Which of the following is an important nursing intervention for this patient?

   (A) Avoid disconnecting the ventilator circuit from the ETT.
   (B) Increase the Vt.
   (C) Ensure that suction passes are greater than 15 seconds.
   (D) Decrease the PEEP and then the FiO_2.

83. Pulmonary assessment reveals bronchial breath sounds and whispered pectoriloquy. Which of the following should the nurse expect?

   (A) partial pneumothorax
   (B) air trapping
   (C) pulmonary consolidation
   (D) pulmonary edema

84. The patient sustained a crush injury at a construction site. Urine is tea colored, 20 mL/hour; creatinine kinase (CK) is 15,000 U/L. The nurse knows the patient is at risk for which of the following?

   (A) heart failure
   (B) hyperkalemia
   (C) alkalosis
   (D) acute liver failure

85. The patient is receiving assist-control ventilation, currently not assisting the ventilator. ABGs reveal the following: pH 7.29; pCO_2 52; pO_2 69; HCO_3 29. Which of the following statements is correct?

   (A) The patient has partially compensated respiratory acidosis; increase the breath rate.
   (B) The patient has uncompensated metabolic acidosis; increase the FiO_2.
   (C) The patient has uncompensated respiratory acidosis; decrease the tidal volume (Vt).
   (D) The patient has partially compensated metabolic acidosis; decrease the peak flow rate.

86. The patient presented with a lower-leg wound with purulent drainage and generalized weakness. Temperature was 39°C, B/P 82/38 mmHg, heart rate 140/minute, hemoglobin 9.1 gm/dL, WBC 3,000, and bands 25%. A total of 1,500 mL isotonic solution was infused, and a central venous catheter was inserted. Currently the CVP is 7 mmHg, B/P 80/40 mmHg, and heart rate 132/minute. Which of the following interventions is appropriate?

   (A) Continue the fluid at 50 mL/hour, start a dopamine infusion, and titrate to a urine output of 30 mL/hour.
   (B) Continue the fluid boluses, start a norepinephrine infusion, and titrate to a mean arterial pressure (MAP) ≥ 65 mmHg.
   (C) Continue the fluid boluses, infuse PRBCs, and titrate to a CVP of 8 mmHg.
   (D) Discontinue the isotonic fluid, begin 0.45 normal saline at 50 mL/hour, and begin a phenylephrine infusion.

87. The patient is receiving an angiotensin-converting inhibitor (ACE). What assessments are important?

(A) heart failure symptoms and hypokalemia
(B) proteinuria and hyperkalemia
(C) thrombocytopenia and hepatotoxicity
(D) dysrhythmias and hyponatremia

88. A 19 year old presents with raccoon eyes and bruising behind the right ear after falling from a one-story roof. You notice clear fluid draining from his nose. The most appropriate intervention would be to:

(A) insert a nasogastric tube to prevent vomiting.
(B) suction the nasopharynx as needed.
(C) insert nasal packing until the physician arrives.
(D) tape rolled sterile gauze under his nose.

89. Which of the following may trigger vasospasm post-aneurysm repair for subarachnoid hemorrhage?

(A) hypokalemia
(B) dehydration
(C) nimodipine
(D) hypertension

90. All of the following are true of obstructive pulmonary disease EXCEPT for:

(A) dynamic hyperinflation occurs due to too much air in lungs.
(B) air trapping and auto-PEEP are common.
(C) expiratory flow rates are high.
(D) asthma, emphysema, and bronchitis are examples.

91. The patient presents with eye deviation to the left, right homonymous hemianopsia, right-sided weakness, and left pupil dilation. The patient most likely has which of the following?

(A) left-sided stroke
(B) right temporal lobe tumor
(C) central herniation
(D) meningitis

92. The patient with chronic liver failure with acute GI bleeding is likely to receive which of the following agents?

(A) octreotide (Sandostatin)
(B) lactulose (sorbitol)
(C) lactated Ringer's
(D) beta blockers

93. The patient is admitted with acute-onset chest pain at rest, ST elevation, and deep Q-waves in leads V5, V6, I, and aVL. Which of the following is the most accurate?

(A) The patient is having an acute posterior wall MI; emergent PCI is indicated.
(B) The patient is having an acute anterior wall MI; fibrinolytic therapy is indicated.
(C) The patient is having an acute inferior wall MI; emergent PCI is indicated.
(D) The patient is having an acute lateral wall MI; fibrinolytic therapy is indicated.

94. The purpose and management of a mediastinal chest tube include which of the following?

(A) promote lung re-expansion, keep drainage system lower than the chest, clamp when transporting patient

(B) improve gas exchange postoperatively, report bubbling in the negative pressure chamber, monitor SpO_2

(C) remove serosanguinous fluid from the operative site, gently milk visible clots to keep patent, report output of greater than 100 mL/hours for 2 consecutive hours

(D) prevent cardiac tamponade postoperatively, prepare to transfuse PRBCs if output greater than 100 mL for the hour, report bubbling in the suction chamber

95. Which of the following is indicative of cor pulmonale?

(A) right ventricular failure secondary to pulmonary hypotension

(B) right ventricular enlargement secondary to pulmonary hypertension

(C) pulmonary edema secondary to right ventricular failure

(D) left ventricular failure secondary to chronic hypoxemia

96. Differentiation of DKA and HHS is best done by examining which of the following?

(A) serum osmolality

(B) serum sodium

(C) serum glucose

(D) serum potassium

97. The patient 1-month status post burr hole and evacuation of a subdural hematoma presents with positive Brudzinski's and positive Kernig's signs. Which of the following is most likely the etiology of these signs?

(A) a recurrence of the subdural hematoma

(B) hydrocephalus

(C) a central nervous system infection

(D) increased intracranial pressure

98. All disciplines (nursing, respiratory, dietitian, and physical and speech therapists) are responsible for documentation of discharge teaching. Which of the following is the best strategy to coordinate teaching provided to the patient?

(A) Discuss patient teaching at daily care conferences.

(B) Review each discipline's flow sheet of documentation at shift change.

(C) The same flow sheet should be used to document patient teaching by all disciplines.

(D) Each discipline documents in the record that the other discipline's flow sheet was reviewed daily.

99. Hypotension, distended neck veins, distant heart sounds, widening mediastinum, clear lungs, narrowing pulse pressure, and pulsus paradoxus are signs of what problem and require which interventions?

(A) hypovolemia, fluid resuscitation, identify and correct underlying cause

(B) diastolic heart failure, control heart rate, calcium-channel blockers, avoid positive inotropes

(C) cardiac tamponade, emergent pericardiocentesis or return to the operating room if post-op cardiac surgical patient

(D) cardiogenic shock, positive inotropes, afterload reduction, IABP therapy

100. Which of the following is correct related to a shift of the oxyhemoglobin dissociation curve to the left?

(A) It may be due to a decrease of arterial pH.
(B) It will cause easier release of oxygen from hemoglobin.
(C) It may drop the SaO_2.
(D) It may be due to hypothermia.

101. The patient is admitted with acute pancreatitis. Which of the following lab profiles will the patient most likely have?

(A) elevated serum calcium, elevated serum amylase, elevated total protein
(B) decreased serum glucose, elevated bilirubin, decreased serum lipase
(C) decreased serum calcium, elevated serum amylase, decreased total protein
(D) elevated serum glucose, decreased alkaline phosphatase, elevated calcium

102. The chest pain due to pericarditis differs from the chest pain due to acute coronary syndrome in that the chest pain with pericarditis:

(A) is a sudden, ripping pain between the shoulder blades.
(B) increases with deep inspiration.
(C) is a squeezing, tight heaviness.
(D) decreases with activity.

103. Which of the following is a primary treatment for the patient with severe sepsis?

(A) vasopressors
(B) antibiotics
(C) steroids
(D) antipyretics

104. Which of the following ABGs reveals severe hypoxemia with respiratory acidosis?

(A) pH 7.56, pCO_2 28, pO_2 38, HCO_3 24
(B) pH 7.19, pCO_2 78, pO_2 40, HCO_3 28
(C) pH 7.34, pCO_2 46, pO_2 60, HCO_3 21
(D) pH 7.21, pCO_2 29, pO_2 48, HCO_3 14

105. The patient has septic shock. Which of the following assessments would the nurse expect?

(A) SVR 1,400, ejection fraction 30%
(B) SVR 525, cardiac output 9 L
(C) SVR 1,200, ejection fraction 60%
(D) SVR 600, cardiac output 3 L

106. Arterial hypoxemia may occur with a pulmonary embolism due to which of the following?

(A) anatomic shunt
(B) diffusion defect
(C) pulmonary hypotension
(D) ventilation/perfusion mismatch

107. The nurse is caring for a patient with rhabdomyolysis secondary to a crush injury. Which of the following orders should the nurse question?

(A) mannitol
(B) monitor serum potassium level
(C) urine for myoglobin
(D) infuse 0.45 normal saline at 100 ml/hour

108. While orienting a new nurse to the unit, the orientee's patient experiences cardiac arrest and requires resuscitation. The preceptor arrives and sees that the orientee has not lowered the head of the bed. Which of the following represents the best response the preceptor could make to instruct this new nurse?

(A) Immediately begin chest compressions.
(B) Reposition the patient supine.
(C) Initiate the unit's code blue response.
(D) Ask the orientee why she did not lower the head of the bed.

109. A patient is admitted with pelvic fracture. Which member of the healthcare team should be consulted first in order to optimize recovery?

  (A) physical therapist
  (B) wound care consultant
  (C) social service
  (D) dietitian

110. Which of the following results in death for the patient with status epilepticus?

  (A) respiratory failure
  (B) pulseless electrical activity
  (C) cerebral hypermetabolism
  (D) intracranial hemorrhage

111. Which of the following nursing interventions is appropriate related to the care of the post-PCI patient?

  (A) Apply a pressure dressing after 5 minutes of direct pressure for acute groin bleeding.
  (B) Administer atropine and dopamine for hypotension secondary to vasovagal response.
  (C) Monitor for ST changes on the bedside monitor in the lead that showed the greatest change.
  (D) Adjust the head of the bed, administer an analgesic, and reposition for acute back pain.

112. A patient presents with complaints of ripping back pain, dizziness, dyspnea, and widening mediastinum on the chest radiograph. Which of the following should the nurse anticipate the patient most likely has?

  (A) a dissecting thoracic aneurysm and requires vasopressors and surgery if the aneurysm is greater than 6 cm in size
  (B) an abdominal aortic aneurysm and requires blood transfusion and surgery if the aneurysm is greater than 5 cm in size
  (C) a dissecting thoracic aneurysm and requires aggressive blood pressure control and emergent surgery
  (D) cardiac tamponade and requires fluids and emergent pericardiocentesis

113. The patient had an arteriogram. Which of the following should the nurse closely assess?

  (A) serum creatinine
  (B) mean arterial pressure
  (C) WBCs
  (D) liver enzymes

114. Which of the following patient histories has the greatest risk of coronary artery disease?

  (A) diabetes, male, age 66
  (B) diabetes, use of beta blockers, obese
  (C) smoking, LDL of 70, age 28
  (D) hypertension, history of alcohol abuse, female

115. The trauma patient, who is a Jehovah's Witness, has 1,500 mL chest tube output in 2 hours and has a hematocrit of 20%. Which of the following interventions is most appropriate for the patient?

  (A) administer donated PRBCs
  (B) administer a non-blood volume expander, such as saline
  (C) obtain an ethics consult
  (D) administer 500 mL of albumin

116. The patient's wife is expressing concern about the meaning of the numbers on the patient monitor. Which of the following is the most appropriate nursing response?

    (A) "Nurses are closely watching the numbers."
    (B) "There is no problem unless an alarm sounds."
    (C) "The trend of the numbers is more important than intermittent changes."
    (D) "What about the numbers concerns you?"

117. Two days after admission for pulmonary embolism, the patient's laboratory report reveals a 55% decrease in the platelet count, no clinical change. Which of the following is indicated FIRST?

    (A) infuse platelets
    (B) discontinue all heparin exposure
    (C) order enzyme-linked immunosorbent assay (ELISA)
    (D) start a direct-thrombin inhibitor

118. Provision of a dobutamine infusion at 10 mcg/kg/min to the patient with cardiogenic shock provides which of the following effects?

    (A) It decreases myocardial oxygen demand.
    (B) It improves myocardial contractility.
    (C) It increases the threshold for ventricular fibrillation.
    (D) It dilates coronary arteries.

119. Which of the following are signs of syndrome of inappropriate ADH excretion (SIADH)?

    (A) low urine output, elevated serum osmolality, hypernatremia, elevated urine sodium
    (B) elevated urine output, elevated serum osmolality, hypernatremia, low urine sodium
    (C) elevated urine output, low serum osmolality, hyponatremia, low urine sodium
    (D) low urine output, low serum osmolality, hyponatremia, and elevated urine sodium

120. The nurse notices during assessment of the patient that the patient has developed Cullen's sign. Which of the following problems has most likely developed?

    (A) acute liver failure
    (B) esophageal varices
    (C) small bowel obstruction
    (D) hemorrhagic pancreatitis

121. The patient admitted with acute respiratory failure is very upset regarding the new diagnosis of lung cancer. The nurse understands that a useful strategy to use for this type of situation is to frame the new diagnosis as a new life challenge for the patient to meet. Which of the following statements would help the patient see the new diagnosis in this light?

    (A) Determine how the patient has met past life challenges.
    (B) Explain the tumor is small and the diagnosis was caught early.
    (C) Assist the patient to prepare for death and call clergy.
    (D) Remind the patient that therapeutic options are now more successful.

122. In which heart block are the PR intervals variable and the R-R intervals regular?

(A) first-degree AV heart block
(B) second-degree AV heart block, Type I
(C) second-degree AV heart block, Type II
(D) third-degree AV heart block

123. Care of the critically ill mechanically ventilated patient includes:

(A) routine instillation of saline down the ETT for suctioning.
(B) use of higher tidal volumes and airway pressure for patients with ARDS.
(C) disconnection of the patient with critical PEEP to transport off the unit.
(D) hyper-oxygenation before, during, and after the suctioning procedure.

124. The patient with Type I diabetes is admitted with DKA, is admitted with stuporous mental status, and responds to shaking with moaning. Which of the following is the most likely cause of the patient's mental status?

(A) acidosis
(B) hypovolemia
(C) hyperkalemia
(D) infection

125. A patient has a right temporal lobe tumor and history of a seizure prior to admission. Which of the following would be the most ominous sign for this patient?

(A) right pupil 5 mm, left pupil 3 mm
(B) left-sided weakness since admission
(C) left-sided headache
(D) right facial bruise

126. The acute and critical care nurse may be required to teach patients and families how to perform care. Which of the following principles of teaching is accurate?

(A) Teaching is best done at the beginning of the day.
(B) A complex procedure is best taught in one session.
(C) Written instruction is the most effective method for adult learners.
(D) Knowledge of the importance of learning is the first step.

127. A magnesium infusion is being administered to a patient after several non-sustained episodes of torsades de pointes ventricular tachycardia. Which of the following clinical findings would indicate the infusion should be discontinued?

(A) hyper-reflexia
(B) hypotension
(C) supraventricular tachycardia
(D) tachypnea

128. The patient receiving mechanical ventilation has a peak inspiratory pressure of 70 cm H_2O and a plateau pressure of 35 cm H_2O. Which assessment and intervention is most likely correct?

(A) The patient has ARDS; decrease the tidal volume.
(B) The patient has a pulmonary embolus; begin anticoagulation.
(C) The patient has pneumonia; increase the FiO_2.
(D) The patient has asthma exacerbation; administer a bronchodilator.

129. Management of acute pancreatitis includes which of the following?

(A) antibiotics for all patients
(B) close lung assessment for all patients
(C) nasogastric tube for all patients
(D) avoid narcotics for all patients

130. The patient developed third-degree AV block, rate 46/minute, and B/P 76/44. Which of the following is the most effective intervention?

(A) atropine 0.5 mg IV
(B) contact physician for pacemaker insertion
(C) fluid bolus
(D) transcutaneous pacing

131. The patient presents with salicylate overdose. Which of the following acid-base disturbances is expected?

(A) metabolic alkalosis, respiratory alkalosis
(B) metabolic acidosis, respiratory acidosis
(C) metabolic alkalosis, respiratory acidosis
(D) metabolic acidosis, respiratory alkalosis

132. Which of the following is indicative of massive pulmonary embolism?

(A) B/P 78/58, SpO_2 88%, increased PAOP
(B) B/P 170/102, SpO_2 86%, decreased mean pulmonary artery pressure
(C) B/P 82/52, SpO_2 85%, increased alveolar dead space
(D) B/P 158/98, SpO_2 89%, decreased pulmonary vascular resistance (PVR)

133. The patient is receiving volume resuscitation. Which of the following would be indicative of successful resuscitation?

(A) Cardiac index 2.3 $L/min/m^2$
(B) CVP 3 mmHg
(C) base deficit 5 mmol/kg
(D) oxygen consumption of 225 $mL/min/m^2$

134. The definitive diagnosis of pulmonary embolism is made with which of the following?

(A) pulmonary angiogram
(B) chest X-ray
(C) ventilation/perfusion scan
(D) arterial blood gas

135. A patient was admitted with multiple trauma and brief hypotension. The following day, the patient is hypertensive, tachycardic, and tachypneic with bilateral lung crackles. BUN is 100 mg/dL, and creatinine is 3.2 mg/dL. Which of the following should be the initial treatment?

(A) hemodialysis
(B) mannitol 25% IV
(C) hemofiltration
(D) fluid bolus

136. The patient had onset of gait disturbance, falling, lack of coordination. The CT demonstrated a tumor. Which of the following areas of the brain is most likely involved?

(A) frontal lobe
(B) cerebellum
(C) parietal lobe
(D) occipital lobe

137. A patient has had a stormy course with numerous complications and is manifesting signs of depression. Which of the following interventions is CONTRAINDICATED for the patient?

(A) Force the patient to make decisions related to his/her care.
(B) Provide a safe environment.
(C) Encourage the patient to express his/ her feelings.
(D) Involve family members and the patient's support system.

138. The patient sustained trauma from a fall down the basement stairs. Which of the following is the highest priority?

(A) stabilize cervical spine
(B) assess blood pressure
(C) identify facial fractures
(D) initiate IV access

139. The patient was admitted with acute anterior wall MI and is now hypotensive, sinus tachycardia, tachypnea with SpO_2 0.89, lung crackles, S3 heart sound, and restlessness. Which of the following interventions is anticipated at this time for this patient?

   (A) negative inotropes, antiarrhythmics, digoxin
   (B) beta blockers, diuretics, aspirin
   (C) positive inotropes, vasodilators, diuretics
   (D) adenosine, ACE inhibitors, calcium-channel blockers

140. What positive hemodynamic effects do nitrates provide for chest pain secondary to coronary artery disease?

   (A) They increase afterload and decrease myocardial oxygen demand.
   (B) They decrease afterload and increase myocardial contractility.
   (C) They increase preload and increase myocardial contractility.
   (D) They decrease preload and decrease myocardial oxygen demand.

141. The patient with chronic alcoholism is at risk for which of the following?

   (A) hyperkalemia
   (B) hypomagnesemia
   (C) hyperphosphatemia
   (D) hyponatremia

142. The patient is admitted with chest pain. ECG shows ST elevation in leads V1, V2, V3. The day after admission, the patient developed a drop in blood pressure and a holosystolic murmur on the left sternal border, 5th intercostal space. The nurse suspects the patient has developed:

   (A) a ventricular septal defect.
   (B) left ventricular failure.
   (C) acute mitral valve regurgitation.
   (D) right ventricular failure.

143. A 72-year-old patient admitted with pneumonia has a known history of Alzheimer's disease and is cared for by his daughter. The patient keeps trying to pull out his intravenous lines and get out of the bed. Which of the following interventions is most effective for maintaining the patient's safety?

   (A) Maintain wrist restraints around the clock.
   (B) Involve family members as many hours as possible with the patient's care.
   (C) Request and order a psychotropic medication.
   (D) Reorient the patient frequently and remind him of the need for the intravenous lines.

144. A patient has a blood pressure of 150/96, heart rate 110/minute, respiratory rate of 32/minute, and SpO_2 of 0.89. Auscultation reveals diminished breath sounds over the right lung fields, and tracheal deviation to the right is present. Which of the following interventions is the definitive treatment?

   (A) initiate oxygen and observe response
   (B) right-sided needle thoracostomy
   (C) endotracheal intubation
   (D) right-sided chest tube insertion

145. Which of the following is a major effect of acute lung injury (ALI) or acute respiratory distress syndrome (ARDS)?

   (A) decreased compliance
   (B) increased alveolar surface area
   (C) decreased capillary permeability
   (D) increased oxygen delivery

146. A patient with a 3-year history of intermittent claudication is now complaining of left foot pain at rest. Which of the following assessment findings is likely and which of the interventions is indicated?

(A) absent pulses, cool toes, edema; apply TED hose and SCDs
(B) ankle-brachial index of 1.2, edema, pallor; elevate left leg above level of heart
(C) positive venous Doppler, reddish color; warm compresses
(D) ankle-brachial index of 0.8, minimal edema, cool toes; reverse Trendelenburg

147. The patient is 3 hours status post percutaneous coronary intervention (PCI) with successful deployment of a stent to the LAD coronary artery. The patient suddenly complains of low back pain and vital sign assessment reveals: B/P 82/58, heart sinus tachycardia 122/minute, and respiratory rate 28/minute; no bleeding is seen at the femoral insertion site. Which of the following has most likely occurred?

(A) retroperitoneal bleed
(B) cardiac tamponade
(C) thoracic aneurysm dissection
(D) stent re-occlusion

148. A patient with a transvenous temporary pacemaker in place has been 100% paced at a rate of 72/minute. The pacemaker now demonstrates pacing spikes without a QRS, and the patient's heart rate is 40/minute. Which of the following is the most appropriate initial intervention?

(A) Increase the pacemaker rate.
(B) Decrease the mA.
(C) Pull back the pacing wire.
(D) Reposition the patient.

149. The patient with known alcohol abuse is admitted 2 weeks status post tendon repair due to hand laceration. The patient is lethargic. The skin is warm and flushed. The surgical site is red, hard, and tender to touch. Vital signs are temperature of 102.5°F, B/P 82/38, heart rate 130, respiratory rate 24. The nurse should anticipate initial treatment to include which of the following?

(A) stat CBC, antipyretics, rapid fluid administration
(B) dopamine administration, CT of head, monitor for alcohol withdrawal
(C) rapid administration of isotonic fluids, antipyretics, vitamin administration
(D) blood cultures, antibiotics, rapid administration of isotonic fluids

150. The patient is admitted with ST elevation in leads II, III, aVF and an S4 heart sound at the apex. The patient developed hypotension; lungs are clear. Which of the following is accurate related to this patient?

(A) The patient most likely has an anterior infarction and requires pressors.
(B) The patient most likely has a right ventricular infarction and requires fluids.
(C) The patient most likely has an anterior infarction and requires positive inotropes.
(D) The patient most likely has an inferior infarction and requires afterload reduction.

ANSWER KEY
Practice Test 2

1.	D	39.	A	77.	C	115.	B
2.	C	40.	B	78.	D	116.	D
3.	D	41.	C	79.	D	117.	B
4.	A	42.	C	80.	A	118.	B
5.	C	43.	C	81.	C	119.	D
6.	D	44.	A	82.	A	120.	D
7.	B	45.	A	83.	C	121.	A
8.	A	46.	B	84.	B	122.	D
9.	B	47.	C	85.	A	123.	D
10.	A	48.	B	86.	B	124.	B
11.	C	49.	A	87.	B	125.	A
12.	C	50.	C	88.	D	126.	D
13.	B	51.	A	89.	B	127.	B
14.	B	52.	C	90.	C	128.	D
15.	B	53.	C	91.	A	129.	B
16.	D	54.	D	92.	B	130.	D
17.	B	55.	C	93.	D	131.	D
18.	A	56.	A	94.	C	132.	C
19.	D	57.	A	95.	B	133.	D
20.	C	58.	D	96.	A	134.	A
21.	C	59.	D	97.	C	135.	B
22.	B	60.	B	98.	C	136.	B
23.	A	61.	C	99.	C	137.	A
24.	A	62.	A	100.	D	138.	A
25.	D	63.	D	101.	C	139.	C
26.	C	64.	C	102.	B	140.	D
27.	B	65.	C	103.	B	141.	B
28.	B	66.	A	104.	B	142.	A
29.	D	67.	C	105.	B	143.	B
30.	B	68.	C	106.	D	144.	D
31.	B	69.	D	107.	D	145.	A
32.	A	70.	C	108.	B	146.	D
33.	A	71.	A	109.	D	147.	A
34.	B	72.	C	110.	C	148.	D
35.	B	73.	C	111.	C	149.	D
36.	A	74.	A	112.	C	150.	B
37.	A	75.	A	113.	A		
38.	D	76.	A	114.	A		

ANSWERS EXPLAINED

1. **(D)** The clinical picture is one of septic shock. The patient needs continued fluids but also vasopressors to restore vascular tone. The patient does not require blood transfusion as transfusion is not indicated unless there is active bleeding or the hemoglobin is < 7.0 g/dL. Neither reduction of fluid rate nor preload reducers are indicated as the right and left ventricular preload is already low.

2. **(C)** Taking the initiative to collect accurate data will determine the scope of the problem, if there actually is one, and is the first step in getting additional support from key stakeholders. Choices (A) and (B) do not produce evidence of the problem. Choice (D), although an attempt to produce data, will not produce data as powerful as a 6-month retrospective analysis.

3. **(D)** Changes occur from "higher" to "lower" centers of the brain, cerebrum to brain stem. Change in level of consciousness (LOC) is representative of higher (cerebrum) centers. Pupillary change is at the level of the transtentorial notch. Vital sign changes are the last and are representative of brain stem compression. The remaining 3 choices do not represent typical anatomical sites of ICP increase.

4. **(A)** Guillain-Barré syndrome (GBS) results in ascending bilateral paralysis, and monitoring vital capacity will identify diaphragmatic involvement. O_2 saturation decrease is a late sign of hypoventilation. Pupil monitoring is done for a change in ICP, which is not typical of GBS. Temperature change is not typical of GBS.

5. **(C)** Nitroprusside (Nipride) is a potent dilator drug that decreases preload and afterload. The drug does not affect contractility and does not increase either PVR or preload.

6. **(D)** The leads that represent the inferior wall of the LV are II, III, and aVF. Therefore, acute changes would occur in 2 or more of these 3 leads. ST depression and positive troponin would be found in an NSTEMI of the inferior wall. Leads I, aVL represents the high lateral wall of the left ventricle; V2, V3, V4 represent the anterior wall of the LV.

7. **(B)** The patient is demonstrating early signs of alcohol withdrawal. A symptom-triggered protocol for administration of benzodiazepines is effective in preventing advanced delirium tremens (DTs). Simple monitoring of mental status will not prevent progression of withdrawal symptoms. The patient is not exhibiting signs of alteration of blood count. A restraint should not be used unless other strategies have failed and the patient is in danger of harming himself or others. Additionally, restraints have been shown to exacerbate delirium.

8. **(A)** If O_2, fluids, and chest tube are rapidly initiated, intubation may not be needed, and pressors should not be used for this type of traumatic injury. There are no signs of cardiac tamponade. Although surgery may be needed later, the immediate need is not surgery based on the information provided.

9. **(B)** Emboli in the left side of the heart are most likely to migrate to the brain. Lower-extremity or right-sided emboli are more likely to migrate to the lungs and cause a PE.

10. **(A)** The physical exertion increases glucose utilization and decreases insulin requirements, which results in hypoglycemia. Hypoglycemia increases adrenaline production (tachycardia) and affects brain cells, resulting in mental status change.

11. **(C)** The massive fluid shifts may result in hypovolemic shock. Pancreatic enzyme release does not result in diuresis. Acute pancreatitis results in hypocalcemia, not hypercalcemia. Pancreatitis results in hyperglycemia, not hypoglycemia.

12. **(C)** The patient received heparin during the procedure, had inadequate heparin reversal, and needs the agent that reverses heparin. Heparin will further prolong the PTT. Vitamin K is the reversal agent for warfarin. There is no evidence that the patient's prolonged PTT is due to a deficiency of clotting factors and requires FFP.

13. **(B)** Chvostek sign causes twitching of facial muscles. Kernig's sign due to meningeal irritation results in hamstring pain when the leg is straightened. Cullen's sign is discoloration around the umbilicus, a sign of retroperitoneal bleeding.

14. **(B)** Information that demonstrates decreased length of stay will reduce costs. Knowledge of the protocol does not demonstrate financial benefit. Although outlining favorable patient outcomes is an important selling point, it does not demonstrate financial benefit. Ensuring support of unit key stakeholders is important but does not address financial benefit.

15. **(B)** Although the pulmonary edema of heart failure may trigger bronchospasm resulting in wheezing, there would also be pulmonary crackles. Although steroids are used for an asthma exacerbation, bronchodilators are a higher priority. Diuretics are not used for bronchospasm but, rather, for pulmonary edema and fluid overload.

16. **(D)** A vital capacity of at least 3 L/min indicates the strength to support independent ventilation. The remaining 3 choices are not predictive of successful weaning.

17. **(B)** Pressure support (PS) assists inspiratory phase of spontaneous breaths (the degree of support dependent on the PS setting) and decreases the work of breathing. It does not decrease oxygen requirements or tidal volume requirements. Pressure support may prevent tiring of the diaphragm, but choice (C) does not specify this muscle.

18. **(A)** Acute renal failure does not result in alkalosis, and anemia is usually seen in chronic renal failure. Blood pressure may be high or low with acute renal failure, therefore B/P is not a definitive sign of acute renal failure. ARF generally results in high electrolyte levels, not low magnesium and calcium levels.

19. **(D)** Lung aspiration will result in increased airway secretions that will cause an increase in peak inspiratory pressure. Due to the shorter, straighter right mainstem bronchus, most aspirations occur to the right lung, not bilaterally. Minute ventilation would be expected to increase (not decrease) due to an increase (not a decrease) in respiratory rate. Negative inspiratory force would most likely drop, not increase.

20. **(C)** Although renal function should be monitored, it is not an initial intervention. Respiratory depression is not a common effect of methamphetamine overdose, and naloxone is not an antidote.

21. **(C)** CVVH does remove some body waste products (although it is not as efficient as hemodialysis). However, CVVH is mainly used for the critically ill unstable patient who may not tolerate hemodialysis. CVVH provides for replacement of fluids as needed to the vasculature. It may indirectly prevent life-threatening electrolyte imbalance, although close electrolyte monitoring during CVVH is needed in order to prevent severe

imbalance. Choice (B) describes plasmapheresis. The purpose of CVVH is not to restore oncotic pressure.

22. **(B)** Pupillary changes are due to compression of the oculomotor nerve, CN III. Cranial nerve (CN) II is the optic nerve, responsible for vision, i.e., affected with some strokes and results in homonymous hemianopsia. CN V is the trigeminal nerve (corneal reflex), and CN IX is the glossopharyngeal nerve (gag reflex).

23. **(A)** Viral meningitis will not lower the CSF glucose, but bacterial meningitis will. The remaining 3 choices may be seen with both bacterial and viral meningitis.

24. **(A)** The PaO_2 to FiO_2 ratio is < 200 for the patient with ARDS, as choice (A) demonstrates. (Additionally the patient would need to meet the other criteria for ARDS.) The ARDS patient would not have normal mixed venous oxygen. The oxygen would be low. The PaO_2 to FiO_2 ratio for choice (C) is 310, which is too high for ARDS. An A-A gradient of 8 mmHg is normal and would not be seen in ARDS.

25. **(D)** The basilar and middle cerebral vessels are not part of the Circle of Willis; the remaining choices are included in the Circle of Willis.

26. **(C)** Choice (A) describes peritonitis. Choice (B) describes appendicitis. Choice (D) describes acute pancreatitis.

27. **(B)** Nitroprusside is a potent preload and afterload reducer. Close B/P monitoring is required, especially when the agent is initiated in order to detect too great of a drop in the pressure. The remaining 3 options may be adverse effects of nitroprusside but would not occur immediately or would not be life-threatening.

28. **(B)** The clinical picture is one of cardiogenic shock. A positive inotrope (dopamine 5 to 10 mcg/kg/min, not a high dose) will increase contractility. A diuretic (usually given after the positive inotrope) will decrease LV preload. A vasodilator will decrease LV afterload. All of these will increase coronary artery perfusion and cardiac output. The remaining choices include negative inotropic agents that may make the shock worse. Antiarrhythmics are not needed.

29. **(D)** Atrial fibrillation, diastolic murmur, and giant V-waves are not clinical signs of status asthmaticus.

30. **(B)** Vasopressin is ADH, and there is excessive ADH production in SIADH. Therefore, vasopressin administration is contraindicated. Hypertonic saline and diuretics may be indicated in order to treat the hyponatremia and fluid overload. Fluid restriction, especially free water, is indicated. Phenytoin may be ordered as it decreases production of ADH.

31. **(B)** Fibrinolytic therapy is indicated if the patient presents within 4.5 hours of symptom onset. Once this is established, contraindications for fibrinolytic therapy are identified.

32. **(A)** When using a translator, the patient needs to know the information is coming from the nurse through the translator and the nurse needs to stay physically present. Refrain from using medical jargon when communicating with patients, directly or through a translator, in order to avoid creating a misunderstanding. If the patient does not know English, there is no point in speaking English. Although touching and using gestures may be helpful when the translator is not present, it is not adequate for

providing an overview of the plan of care and important point. It is **not** advisable to use a family member as a translator as subjectivity may enter the translation. Additionally, when using a translator, give small bits of information, stop and allow the translation, and then resume with more information in order to prevent translator omission of information.

33. **(A)** The patient has an acute anterior wall MI, usually caused by a LAD plaque rupture. LAD occlusion may lead to intraventricular septum ischemia/necrosis and a VSD. Acute anterior wall MI does not cause cardiac tamponade or papillary muscle dysfunction. The patient has ST elevation, and deep Q-waves, signs of a myocardial infarction; acute ischemia results in ST depression or T-wave inversion not ST elevation.

34. **(B)** This ABG demonstrates acute, uncompensated respiratory acidosis, hypercapneic respiratory failure with a $PCO_2 > 50$, and pH < 7.30. Choice (A) demonstrates acute metabolic acidosis with partial compensation. Choice (C) demonstrates fully compensated respiratory acidosis (therefore a chronic condition). Choice (D) demonstrates uncompensated metabolic acidosis. None of the ABGs demonstrates acute hypoxemic respiratory failure as none has $pO_2 < 60$.

35. **(B)** Whispering may trigger paranoia. Touch may aggravate the symptoms. Logical explanations are not especially useful for the patient with DTs.

36. **(A)** In addition to the low CI, cardiogenic shock will cause an elevation of the left heart pressures (PAOP), arterial constriction (elevated SVR), and low mixed venous oxygenation.

37. **(A)** The volume depletion associated with hemorrhage results in factitious dehydration (high BUN and sodium). As volume is restored, the BUN and sodium will normalize.

38. **(D)** The PEEP setting of 5 cm H_2O is too low for treatment of ARDS, so there is opportunity to adjust this setting. Since PEEP is still quite low, there would not be a need to increase an already high FiO_2 setting. Permissive hypercapnea is expected and tolerated quite well for the patient with ARDS as tidal volumes need to be kept low (permissive hypercapnea). Therefore, choices (B) and (C) would not be good alternatives.

39. **(A)** The chief characteristic of distributive shock (septic, anaphylactic) is massive vasodilation that results in a low SVR. Although the other choices are associated with distributive shock, they may also be seen in hypovolemic shock.

40. **(B)** Surfactant prevents alveolar collapse. Surfactant is produced by the Type II alveolar cells, not the Type I cells. Surfactant decreases the work of breathing, not increases it. Surfactant increases lung compliance, thereby decreasing the work of breathing. It does not decrease compliance.

41. **(C)** There is increased loss of potassium with the use of thiazide diuretics. Additionally, chloride is lost. When chloride is lost, renal tubules reabsorb bicarbonate, which may lead to metabolic alkalosis. Vomiting and diarrhea may cause hypokalemia. However, use of ACE inhibitors, crush injury, hemolysis, and acidosis (metabolic) may all lead to hyperkalemia.

42. **(C)** Immediate nurse engagement to correct the staff researcher's omission of providing information to the patient will be most effective for all sides. Eventually, a discussion will need to occur with the primary investigator. Right now, though, engagement

is the best strategy. Involvement of the ethics committee may also be needed at a later time. Choice (D) is passive and is not best for the patient.

43. **(C)** Medications and sleep deprivation may cause the signs the patient is experiencing. Environmental stimulation, isolation, and benzodiazepines increase the incidence of delirium in the elderly. Benzodiazepines may be used for this population if other strategies are not effective or if immediate patient safety is an issue.

44. **(A)** The family still desires full therapy, and the patient now requires an increase in FiO_2 in order to maintain oxygenation. The nurse needs to advocate for the family's wishes, and discussion with the physician is the first step. Keeping the FiO_2 at 40% would not be honest. Advising the family to speak to the physician is a passive approach. Choice (D) is palliative care, but this is not the family's choice at this time.

45. **(A)** The patient has cardiac tamponade as evidenced by equilibration of right and left heart pressures and narrowing pulse pressure. The question is more challenging in that the usual signs of cardiac tamponade (bulging neck veins, distant heart sounds, widening mediastinum, pulsus paradoxus) are not provided. The history of fever might indicate antibiotics are needed. However, severe sepsis/septic shock usually has low RA, PAOP, and low SVR. Pressors would increase an already high SVR (afterload) and increase the work of the heart. Fluids are not indicated for a patient with elevated RA and PAOP. The etiology of cardiac tamponade may be a viral infection that led to a pericardial effusion, resulting in tamponade.

46. **(B)** If the aortic valve is unable to close completely, when the IAB inflates during diastole, blood will go backward into the left ventricle, which would not provide the desired hemodynamic benefits. IAB therapy may be done with any of the other conditions.

47. **(C)** Elevated NH_3 may cause hands to tremor, "flap" when hands are extended. Coma is found in stage 4 liver failure. Respiratory alkalosis is typical of liver failure, not respiratory acidosis. Serum ammonia increases, not decreases.

48. **(B)** Due to increased left heart pressures, the left atrium often enlarges and predisposes the patient to atrial fibrillation. Heart failure is also associated with ventricular tachycardia (but not ventricular bigeminy). However, VT is not a choice. Because of the predisposition to VT, the patient may qualify for an ICD device. Third-degree block or atrial tachycardia are not specifically associated with heart failure.

49. **(A)** It is best to explore with the patient the source of the point of view expressed and then address this. The remaining choices are not as effective.

50. **(C)** Communication through one designated person is most efficient for the nursing staff, and this family decision can be passed on from shift to shift. It is not best practice for the nurse to defer family communication to other healthcare team members. Choice (D) does not provide the family with sufficient information and is open to many interpretations.

51. **(A)** The patient, who most likely had excessive bleeding during the complicated delivery with resultant consumption of clotting factors, has signs of early DIC. A prolonged PT and positive D-dimer would help confirm the diagnosis. Although elevated FSP is the most definitive lab test for DIC, creatinine would not be helpful. Pitocin, magnesium, BUN, and factor X levels are not definitive tests for DIC.

52. **(C)** The patient is having episodes of torsades de pointes VT, a polymorphic VT secondary to prolonged QT interval. Magnesium is indicated in order to decrease the QT. Lidocaine and amiodarone will increase the QT and exacerbate torsades VT (as will procainamide and any other drug that prolongs QT). Since the arrhythmia is not sustained, synchronized cardioversion is not indicated.

53. **(C)** Although acidosis results in an elevated serum potassium, the total body potassium is low in DKA due to fluid loss. This becomes evident as the acidosis is corrected. Therefore, potassium replacement needs to begin as soon as the serum potassium reaches "normal."

54. **(D)** The blood in the intestine results in the breakdown of protein, which will raise the serum NH_3, and the NH_3 further irritates the brain. The remaining 3 choices do not increase NH_3 or worsen encephalopathy.

55. **(C)** The pacemaker is not effectively sensing the patient's own beats, and an increase in the sensitivity is needed. To increase the sensitivity, the sensitivity dial on the device is **decreased** (so that it will sense "smaller," the patient's own ECG waves). The remaining 3 choices would not be helpful.

56. **(A)** Although the patient seems stable, the cardiac glycoside, i.e., digoxin, which is a mild positive inotrope, will improve contractility needed with the loss of cardiac output secondary to atrial fibrillation. The calcium-channel blocker will help keep the rate controlled. "Antiarrhythmic" is too vague, and beta agonist will have no benefit. A beta blocker would help control rate; however, a vasopressor would not be indicated. Providing either a beta blocker **or** a calcium blocker is indicated but not both.

57. **(A)** Hypertension, flat neck veins, and tracheal deviation to the affected side are not signs of a tension pneumothorax.

58. **(D)** The patient has signs of diabetes insipidus (DI). There is a deficiency of antidiuretic hormone (ADH) with large volume fluid loss, resulting in dehydration and potential hypovolemic shock. Water loss will increase serum sodium and serum osmolality. The treatment is to provide what the patient is not able to produce—vasopressin. Additionally, the urine specific gravity will be very low. Phenytoin (Dilantin) may cause DI. Choice (C) is not correct.

59. **(D)** Elevation of the head of the bed will allow venous outflow and help decrease ICP. None of the other positions will prevent elevated ICP.

60. **(B)** The literature has demonstrated learning CPR has been beneficial to families of sudden cardiac death (SCD) survivors, provides a sense of empowerment, and at times, has saved the patient's life. Choice (A) may not be true. Choice (C) does not provide a sense of empowerment. Even if the family knows how and when to access the EMS system, early, effective CPR improves outcome. Choice (D) is deferring nurse accountability.

61. **(C)** During end expiration, there is no interference by thoracic pressure changes seen during inspiration. There is no evidence that the end of the T-wave or every hour affects the accuracy of measurements. The digital readout on the monitor may not always be accurate, especially in the presence of respiratory artifact. The printed waveform strip

or analysis of the waveform on the monitor using the scale is the most accurate method to determine hemodynamic readings.

62. **(A)** The patient has hypotension and hypoxemia, which are evidence of massive PE. A pulmonary embolus prevents pulmonary perfusion, which results in dead space. The larger the PE is, the greater the degree of dead space. The D-dimer would be positive, not negative, since a clot is present. There are possible options other than mechanical ventilation and pressor infusion, such as fibrinolytic therapy if the patient does not have contraindications. PE results in increased dead space, not shunting. PEEP is not indicated.

63. **(D)** Straining may suddenly increase intracranial pressure and result in hemorrhage. Constipation will not suddenly result in the remaining 3 problems.

64. **(C)** Elevated systemic pressure or back flow of blood into the LV may increase left heart pressures to the point where ejection will be impeded, leading to LV failure. Pulmonary embolism will result in right heart failure. Acute coronary syndrome does not necessarily cause LV failure. COPD may result in RV failure.

65. **(C)** The mixed venous O_2 will drop in hypovolemic shock due to a drop in oxygen delivery. The left heart pressure will drop due to decreased venous return (left ventricular preload). The SVR will increase due to compensatory vasoconstriction.

66. **(A)** The pCO_2 is the best indicator of ventilation, and anything greater than 45 mmHg is considered outside normal range. Hypoxemia is a late indicator of hypoventilation. Choice (C) is an indicator of hyperventilation. Respiratory rate needs to be monitored. Because depth of respiration and factors that affect diffusion at the alveolar-capillary interface also impact ventilation, the respiratory rate is not as reliable an indicator as is the pCO_2 (or waveform capnography).

67. **(C)** Refractory hypoxemia is seen with ALI/ARDS and poor oxygen utilization (VO_2), which results in an elevated mixed venous O_2 typical of septic shock.

68. **(C)** Do not use SpO_2 to monitor oxygenation status for the patient with CO poisoning. Positive pressure ventilation (PPV) will not achieve the goal of therapy (CO level return to normal), and LOC alone is not the endpoint of therapy.

69. **(D)** Initially, renal hypoperfusion results in prerenal renal failure. The renal tubules are not yet destroyed. Therefore, they will hold onto sodium (resulting in decreased urine sodium) and concentrate urine in an attempt to counteract the effects of decreased perfusion. After the renal tubule basement membrane is damaged (intrarenal renal failure), the tubules can no longer do the above. Urine sodium will be high and urine osmolality will be low.

70. **(C)** The middle meningeal artery lies above the dura, tough covering of the brain right under the temporal bone that, if traumatized, results in an arterial epidural bleed. The remaining choices are due to problems other than middle meningeal artery disruption.

71. **(A)** Incoherent speech and rambling are signs of disorganized thinking, which is a component of delirium. Delirium is an acute problem, not chronic. Inattentiveness, not attentiveness, is a component of delirium. Although fluctuation of mental status is a component of delirium, the fluctuation occurs within a 24-hour period, not over days.

72. **(C)** Acidosis secondary to hypoventilation will result in vasodilation that, in turn, will increase ICP. Hypotonic fluids should be avoided due to their propensity to leave vascular space and increase ICP. Respiratory arrest should be avoided. Antibiotics are not given prophylactically for SAH.

73. **(C)** The patient is having an anterior-septal myocardial infarction, most often due to occlusion of the left anterior descending (LAD) artery. This problem may affect perfusion to the common bundle of HIS of the conduction system, which may result in a second-degree heart block Type II. (If the patient is symptomatic, he/she will most likely require transcutaneous pacing as atropine is not generally effective.) The remaining 3 choices are more often associated with an acute inferior MI, which is due to a right coronary artery occlusion, and decreases perfusion to the SA and AV nodes.

74. **(A)** The patient has bradycardia secondary to high-grade second-degree AV block, Type II, which often occurs due to a conduction defect of the bundle of HIS (not the AV node). The bundle of HIS is supplied by the LAD. Occlusion of the arteries described in the remaining 3 choices would not usually lead to a second-degree AV block, Type II.

75. **(A)** Bariatric surgical patients may have alteration in absorption, which results in vitamin deficiency. There is no indication for any of the other 3 choices.

76. **(A)** The patient with dilated cardiomyopathy has signs of systolic heart failure that would benefit from a reduction of LV preload (PAOP) and a decrease in afterload (decrease SVR). The other choices would either not benefit this patient population or may actually cause harm.

77. **(C)** The patient seems to have developed acute heart failure severe enough to drop the B/P; therefore, the CO will drop. Afterload will increase in attempt to compensate. The left heart pressure will be elevated due to the inability of the LV to empty, which will result in an elevated PAD pressure.

78. **(D)** By preventing conversion of thrombin to fibrinogen, heparin, which is an anticoagulant, prevents the existing thrombus from getting larger and prevents future formation of thrombi. Choice (A) describes the effects of platelet inhibitors such as clopidogrel. Choice (B) describes the effects of the anticoagulant warfarin. Choice (C) describes the effects of the thrombolytic, clot-dissolving drug tissue plasminogen activator (tPa).

79. **(D)** Aldactone is a potassium-sparing diuretic that is used to prevent the hypokalemia associated with a thiazide diuretic. It is important to prevent hypokalemia in the presence of liver failure as a secondary acidosis may result. Liver failure patients tend to develop hypoglycemia, not elevated blood glucose. Sedation should be avoided as it may mask encephalopathy. Lactated Ringer's may result in acidosis if the liver cannot metabolize the lactate, therefore 0.9 saline is the preferred isotonic solution.

80. **(A)** Although the wife will be grief stricken, the knowledge that everything possible was done offers some comfort. (Do not say, "We did everything we could," without providing a few details.) Choice (B) may not meet the wife's needs (although it could be arranged if specifically requested). Although having the physician or chaplain present may provide support to the nurse, they may not be as effective strategies as choice (A) in meeting the wife's needs.

81. **(C)** A pleural leak or tension pneumothorax would result in bubbling in the negative water seal chamber. Intact connection to suction would be assessed by evaluating the suction chamber or suction indicator, not the negative-pressure water seal chamber.

82. **(A)** PEEP enables alveolar recruitment. Disconnection will result in massive derecruitment and hypoxemia. Even with immediate reconnection, time will be needed for the hypoxemia to resolve. The remaining 3 choices are not beneficial strategies and may be harmful for the patient with ALI/ARDS.

83. **(C)** The remaining 3 choices do not typically present with bronchial breath sounds or whispered pectoriloquy.

84. **(B)** The patient has signs of rhabdomyolysis, a result of massive destruction of skeletal muscle cells. When these cells lyse, they release CK and intracellular potassium. None of the other choices is a typical result of rhabdomyolysis.

85. **(A)** An increase in the rate (or in Vt) would decrease the pCO_2. The remaining choices have incorrect acid-base interpretations.

86. **(B)** The patient has septic shock. There is SIRS, organ dysfunction (hypotension), and incomplete response to fluids. Since the CVP is still slightly less than 8 mmHg, fluids should be continued. However, norepinephrine needs to be initiated. Dopamine is not a first-line agent for septic shock. Blood administration is not indicated for a patient not actively bleeding and with a hemoglobin of 9.1 gm/dL. A hypotonic solution such as 0.45 saline and the pressor phenylephrine are not indicated in septic shock.

87. **(B)** The ACEI drugs may affect renal function as evidenced by proteinuria and/or hyperkalemia (or elevated serum creatinine). The clinical signs listed in choices (A), (C), and (D) are not caused by ACEI drugs.

88. **(D)** The clinical signs seem to be that of a basilar skull fracture. Clear drainage from the nose is most likely CSF, which should be allowed to drain. Nasogastric tube insertion may be dangerous in the presence of a skull fracture as the tube may get displaced to the brain. Suctioning or nasal packing may result in infection of meninges.

89. **(B)** Hypovolemia needs to be avoided as it has been associated with cerebral vasospasm post-SAH repair. The remaining 3 choices are not associated with vasospasm.

90. **(C)** In obstructive pulmonary disease, expiratory flow rates are LOW. The remaining choices are **true** of obstructive pulmonary disease.

91. **(A)** A left-sided problem will result in ipsilateral pupil change, eye deviation toward the problem, and contralateral vision and motor changes.

92. **(B)** It is important to increase transit time of blood through the gut in order to prevent the breakdown of protein, which will increase serum NH_3 and increase chance of encephalopathy. Although octreotide may be used for GI bleeding, it is used for all types of GI bleeding, not only for those with liver failure. Lactated Ringer's may cause acidosis. Beta blockers have no special role in the treatment of GI bleeding or liver failure.

93. **(D)** Leads V5 and V6 represent the lower LV lateral wall, and leads I and aVL represent the high lateral wall of the LV. The remaining 3 choices are not correct.

94. **(C)** The mediastinal tube does **not** promote lung re-expansion and should not be clamped during patient transport as lung re-collapse may occur. A mediastinal tube does not improve gas exchange. Transfusion would not be anticipated for output of > 100 mL in 1 hour but more likely for two consecutive hours.

95. **(B)** Pulmonary hypotension and left ventricular failure are not signs of cor pulmonale. There may be pulmonary edema if there is concomitant LV failure. However, the pulmonary edema would not be due to RV failure but to LV failure.

96. **(A)** Although HHS generally has higher serum glucose than DKA, there may be some crossover. However, the serum osmolality is always elevated in HHS due to the higher fluid loss, whereas serum osmolality in DKA may be normal or only slightly elevated. This is due to the fact that DKA develops more rapidly and fluid loss occurs over a shorter period of time.

97. **(C)** A positive Brudzinski's sign and Kernig's sign (along with nuchal rigidity) indicate meningeal irritation/infection. These signs are not typical of the remaining 3 choices.

98. **(C)** When all team members document on the same flow sheet, effective communication is more likely to occur. Choice (A) does not ensure all members of the interdisciplinary team have access to the daily discussions. Choices (B) and (D) are less efficient and foster a "silo" mentality in planning patient care.

99. **(C)** These are signs of cardiac tamponade. Treatment for the medical patient would be emergent pericardiocentesis. Treatment for the post-op cardiac surgical patient would be emergent return to the OR. The clinical picture described would not be seen with hypovolemia, diastolic heart failure, or cardiogenic shock.

100. **(D)** A **left** shift of the oxyhemoglobin dissociation curve will occur with alkalosis, low pCO_2, low temp, low 2,3-DPG. Each of these prevents release of O_2 from hemoglobin, which may slightly raise the SaO_2.

101. **(C)** Calcium is used in the autodigestive process in acute pancreatitis, which will decrease serum calcium; amylase is produced in the pancreas and increases with pancreatic inflammation; protein may decrease due to increased capillary permeability caused by inflammation. Additionally, the serum glucose may increase due to beta 2 cell damage, serum lipase increases, and alkaline phosphatase rises, which make the other 3 choices incorrect.

102. **(B)** Sudden ripping pain between the shoulder blades is most likely a thoracic aneurysm dissection. A squeezing, tight heaviness is most likely angina. Pericarditis does not necessarily decrease with activity.

103. **(B)** Early initiation of antibiotics decreases mortality of severe sepsis/septic shock. Vasopressors are indicated for severe sepsis refractory to fluid resuscitation (septic shock). Steroids are not a primary intervention for sepsis. Antipyretics are provided for fever, when present, but are not considered life-saving.

104. **(B)** Choice (A) demonstrates severe hypoxemia, and uncompensated respiratory alkalosis. Choice (C) demonstrates moderate hypoxemia with respiratory and metabolic acidosis. Choice (D) demonstrates metabolic acidosis with partial compensation.

105. **(B)** The patient in septic shock has massive vasodilation (low SVR). Due to low arterial resistance, the CO is initially high.

106. **(D)** Complete occlusion of a pulmonary vessel obstructs blood flow past ventilated alveoli. It results in a mismatch of ventilation and perfusion. Gas exchange cannot occur. A PE is not an anatomic defect. Diffusion is not impeded. Pulmonary pressure increases, not decreases.

107. **(D)** The patient with rhabdomyolysis requires large volumes of 0.9 normal saline (an isotonic solution) and bicarbonate in some of the IV fluid in order to flush and buffer the renal tubules. The 0.45 normal saline is a hypotonic solution and will not adequately flush the renal tubules. Instead, it will rapidly leave the vascular compartment and get displaced intracellularly. The remaining 3 choices are appropriate interventions for this patient.

108. **(B)** The preceptor needs to do what is best for the patient in this emergency situation. Beginning chest compressions with the head of the bed elevated would not be the best intervention for the patient. Choice (C) is avoidance behavior. Discussing the situation at that moment with the orientee is not correct. This needs to be done later, after the emergency.

109. **(D)** The most immediate need of the patient with pelvic fractures is adequate nutrition and prevention of malnutrition, which will delay recovery. Physical therapy and social service consults may be needed at a future time but are not immediate priorities. No information indicates that the patient presented with a wound, therefore a wound care consultant is not indicated. Preventative measure should be instituted by nurses for all trauma patients.

110. **(C)** The continual firing of neurons in the brain tissue consumes a great deal of O_2. The brain does not store O_2. Therefore, the hypermetabolism results in massive brain cell death. Although ventilation is not normal during generalized tonic-clonic seizure, respiratory failure is addressed with intubation and would not be fatal. Although skeletal muscle breakdown may lead to hyperkalemia that may in turn result in PEA, the continuous muscle activity can be controlled with clinical paralysis. Status epilepticus does not cause intracranial hemorrhage.

111. **(C)** Monitoring the patient in his/her "fingerprint" lead will detect artery re-occlusion. If acute groin bleeding occurs, it would require more than 5 minutes of manual pressure. Vasovagal response generally occurs during sheath removal. Acute back pain is a sign of possible retroperitoneal bleeding, which may occur post-PCI. However, interventions include a stat CT scan and fluids, not the interventions described.

112. **(C)** The symptoms are typical of a dissecting thoracic aneurysm, which requires both emergent surgery regardless of size and B/P control. Signs and symptoms are different for abdominal aortic aneurysm and cardiac tamponade.

113. **(A)** Any patient who has been exposed to contrast medium is at risk for nephropathy. Renal function should be closely monitored, especially for those at high risk for contrast-induced nephropathy. The remaining 3 problems are not usual complications after an arteriogram.

114. **(A)** Diabetes, male sex, and age greater than 65 are all CAD risk factors. Use of beta blocker, LDL of 70, age of 23, history of alcohol abuse, and female sex are not CAD risks.

115. **(B)** Auto-transfusion is within the accepted practice of Jehovah's Witnesses and a good alternative. Choices A and D are not acceptable to Jehovah's Witnesses. An ethics consult (choice C) is not necessary as auto-transfusion is an acceptable alternative. If the patient's blood loss was not able to be auto-transfused, the patient/family would need to be given an explanation of the consequences of their decisions related to refusal of transfusion and the hospital legal department may need to be contacted as to how to best proceed.

116. **(D)** It is best to determine what specifically is causing anxiety rather than begin an explanation that may further confuse the family and increase anxiety. Choice (A) is too vague and will most likely not reduce anxiety. Choice (B) will be problematic as many times, alarms are false and are not a sign of patient deterioration. Although choice (C) is an attempt to reassure, it might not directly relate to the family's concerns.

117. **(B)** The patient, who would have had heparin for the PE, has signs of heparin-induced thrombocytopenia (HIT). The first intervention is to stop all heparin to prevent progression of the problem. Infusion of platelets is indicated for only active bleeding or extremely low platelets (platelet count of ~ 10,000). Although the ELISA test may be ordered, the decision to discontinue heparin is not delayed until the ELISA results are available. A direct thrombin inhibitor will be needed, but first heparin is stopped.

118. **(B)** Dobutamine stimulates beta-1 receptors of the cardiac muscle. This results in a positive inotropic effect, which is beneficial (although beta-1 stimulation will increase myocardial oxygen demand/work). Dobutamine does not cause the clinical effects described in the other 3 choices.

119. **(D)** There is increased production of antidiuretic hormone with SIADH, resulting in a drop in urine output. As a result, there is a dilutional hyponatremia, sodium loss in urine, and drop in serum osmolality due to fluid retention.

120. **(D)** Hemorrhagic pancreatitis may result in retroperitoneal bleeding. Cullen's sign is not typical of the other 3 problems.

121. **(A)** Exploring how the patient has met past life challenges will assist the patient identify coping mechanisms. Choices (B) and (D) may give the patient hope, but not assist in identification of coping strategies. Choice (C) may not be warranted at this time.

122. **(D)** First-degree AV heart block has constant (but long) PRI. Second-degree AV heart block, Type I, more often has irregular R-R intervals due to grouped beating (unless it is a 2:1 Wenckebach, which is not always able to be determined). Second-degree AV heart block, Type II, may have irregular R-R intervals.

123. **(D)** Hyperoxygenation will prevent potential adverse effects of hypoxemia during the suctioning procedure. The remaining 3 choices are contraindicated for the situations described.

124. **(B)** The total body fluid loss results in intracellular dehydration of brain cells, which results in mental status change. The other 3 choices have little or no effect on mental status change. They affect other organ systems.

125. **(A)** The patient has a right-sided brain abnormality. An acute increase in ICP will cause a sudden pupil change on the side of the problem. Weakness since admission is not a sign of an acute change. Unilateral headache is not an ominous sign for the patient with brain tumor. Lethargy for 24 hours is not an acute change.

126. **(D)** Adults learn best when they understand the importance and reason for the need to learn. Choice (A) is not a proven fact. Choice (B) is not true. A complex procedure should be broken down into several sessions in order to prevent sensory overload, which impedes learning. Adults (as well as children) have various preferred learning styles (written, auditory, kinesthetic). Therefore, the same approach cannot be used for all individuals. The combination of written, auditory, and kinesthetic (hands-on) may be best.

127. **(B)** Hypermagnesemia may result in hypotension. It may also cause depressed reflexes, not hyper-reflexia, and may cause bradyarrhythmias, not SVT. Hypermagnesemia may result in hypoventilation, not tachypnea.

128. **(D)** The extremely elevated peak inspiratory pressure reflects bronchospasm. The relatively normal plateau pressure reflects that the problem is not at the lung level.

129. **(B)** The inflamed pancreas may result in elevation of the diaphragm, left lower lobe atelectasis, bilateral crackles, and even ARDS. The patient needs close lung assessment. Antibiotics and gastric decompression are not needed for most patients. The patient does need opiate drugs for the severe pain even though all opiates may constrict the sphincter of Oddi. This constriction is not going to worsen the pain as thought in years past.

130. **(D)** The patient with complete heart block will not generally respond to atropine. The patient is clinically unstable. Therefore, the patient cannot wait for insertion of a transvenous pacemaker. The hypotension is due to the low heart rate (which needs to be increased), not hypovolemia. Therefore, fluid bolus is not the treatment of choice.

131. **(D)** Hyperventilation results from direct stimulation of the respiratory center by salicylic acid. Increased bicarbonate excretion results in metabolic acidosis.

132. **(C)** There is increased dead space ventilation with pulmonary embolism (PE) since there is ventilation without perfusion. Additionally with massive PE, hypotension and hypoxemia are present due to the severity of the pulmonary hypertension and degree of V/Q mismatch. The PAOP is a left heart pressure and does not increase with PE. The mean PA pressure increases with massive PE. It does not decrease. The PVR increases (not decreases). Hypertension is not a clinical indicator of a massive PE.

133. **(D)** Successful volume resuscitation would result in normal oxygen consumption/utilization. The remaining 3 choices would not indicate the target has been reached during volume resuscitation.

134. **(A)** Although not often done due to its invasiveness, only an angiogram allows visualization of the occluded vessel. A PE does not alter the chest X-ray in any specific, unique manner. A V/Q scan demonstrates a perfusion defect. However, COPD may also cause perfusion defects due to alveolar destruction. Although the ABG may be altered, there is no finding specific for a PE.

135. **(B)** Administration of diuretics in order to "challenge" the kidneys is an initial treatment for acute renal failure (as long as obstruction and hypotension are not present). An isotonic fluid bolus may also be initially given as long as there are no signs of fluid overload. In this case, the patient does have signs of fluid overload. Hemodialysis may be needed if initial interventions are not effective. Hemofiltration may be used if initial treatment is not effective for the patient with hypotension.

136. **(B)** The cerebellum (or hind brain) is responsible for balance and equilibrium. The remaining 3 areas of the brain control different functions.

137. **(A)** The patient with signs and symptoms of clinical depression has trouble making decisions. Forcing the patient to make decisions may increase anxiety and anger and is not therapeutic. The remaining 3 choices have been shown to be effective interventions with depression and are indicated.

138. **(A)** If a patient sustained any injury at all to the cervical spine, any movement will worsen the injury and may lead to respiratory arrest secondary to paralysis. All other choices will need to be dealt with but are not as important as cervical spine stabilization.

139. **(C)** The clinical picture is one of extreme heart failure, cardiogenic shock. The patient needs an increase in contractility (positive inotrope), a decrease in preload (diuretics), and a decrease in afterload (vasodilators). Providing a positive inotrope first (perhaps dopamine) will help increase the B/P, and then the other 2 agents can be given. Negative inotropes and antiarrhythmics are not indicated and may even be harmful. Aspirin is not an agent used for cardiogenic shock. Beta blockers and calcium-channel blockers are negative inotropes and are not indicated.

140. **(D)** Nitrates dilate the venous bed, which decreases left ventricular preload. In turn, this decreases myocardial workload. Nitrates do not increase afterload. They mildly decrease afterload at higher doses but do not directly affect contractility either positively or negatively. Nitrates do not increase preload; vasoconstriction or fluids have this effect.

141. **(B)** The chronic alcohol abuser is at risk for low magnesium due to poor nutritional status and due to the effect of alcohol on proximal renal tubules, which prevents reabsorption of magnesium. There is also a risk for low phosphate, calcium, and potassium.

142. **(A)** VSD is associated with antero-septal MI, hypotension due to a drop in cardiac output, and the murmur as described. LV failure generally results in an S3 heart sound and lung crackles. Mitral valve regurgitation results in a systolic murmur at the apex. RV failure will not result in the murmur as described.

143. **(B)** The patient with dementia needs familiarity to minimize agitated behavior and to feel safe. So family involvement is highly recommended. Restraints will increase anxiety and fear. Non-pharmacological solutions are always preferable to pharmacological ones. Reorientation is more effective for delirium, whereas it is not very effective for dementia.

144. **(D)** The patient has a right pneumothorax. Initiation of oxygen will resolve the hypoxemia, but it is not the definitive treatment. A needle thoracostomy is not indicated for this patient; it is indicated for a tension pneumothorax. However, this patient does not

have signs of a tension pneumothorax (hypotension, tracheal deviation away from the side of lung collapse). Endotracheal intubation will not resolve the patient's problem.

145. **(A)** In ARDS or ALI, the Type II alveolar cells no longer produce surfactant that is needed to prevent alveolar collapse. With massive atelectasis, lung compliance and functional residual capacity drop. The alveolar surface area decreases (not increases). Capillary permeability increases (not decreases), which results in pulmonary edema. In addition, O_2 delivery decreases due to severe hypoxemia. It does not increase.

146. **(D)** The patient's peripheral arterial disease (PAD) is worsening. The ankle-brachial index is abnormal (it should be > 1), and perfusion of the foot may be aided by keeping the extremity down. Each of the remaining choices have clinical signs not typical of PAD or interventions that are not beneficial.

147. **(A)** The low back pain associated with hypotension after the PCI procedure that involved puncture of the femoral artery is indicative of retroperitoneal bleeding. The remaining problems would not present with the same signs and symptoms.

148. **(D)** If the pacing electrode gets dislodged from the RV wall, there may be loss of capture. By repositioning the patient, the pacing electrode may regain contact with the RV wall. None of the other choices will restore capture.

149. **(D)** The patient has signs of severe sepsis. Interventions included in the other 3 choices are not indicated for severe sepsis.

150. **(B)** The ECG changes are indicative of an acute inferior wall MI, which has a higher probability for an RV infarction than any other type of STEMI. When the RV infarct is large, it results in RV failure with decreased perfusion to the left heart. This, in turn, causes hypotension with clear lungs and is treated with fluids and pressors if fluids alone are not effective. The patient is not having an anterior MI. Afterload reduction would exacerbate the patient's symptoms and is not indicated.

References

AACN Practice Alert, Verification of Feeding Tube Placement (Blind Insertion), 12/2009.

AACN Practice Alert: Delirium Assessment and Management, 2011, *http://www.aacn.org/WD/ practice/docs/practicealerts/delirium-practice-alert-2011.pdf*, accessed March 27, 2014.

AACN Synergy Model for Patient Care. American Association of Critical Care Nurses website. *http://www.aacn.org/wd/certifications/content/synmodel.pcms?pid=1&=&menu=certification*. Accessed June 2, 2014.

American Association of Blood Banks, Standards for Blood Banks and Transfusion Services, 2012, 28th edition.

American Association of Critical Care Nurses practice alert: pulmonary artery pressure measurement. 2009. Available at: *http://www.aacn.org/AACN/practiceAlert.nsf/vwdoc/Practice AlertMain*. Accessed December 2011.

American Heart Association/American College of Cardiology 2011 Guidelines.

Balas M, Vasilevskis EE, Olsen KM, et al. Effectiveness and safety of the awakening and breathing coordination, delirium monitoring/management, and early exercise/mobility bundle (abstract). *Crit Care Med*, 2014, Jan 3 [epub ahead of print], *http://www.ncbi.nlm.nih.gov/ pubmed/24394627*, accessed March 28, 2014.

Bankhead, R., et al. "Enteral Nutrition Practice Recommendations," *Journal of Parenteral and Enteral Nutrition* 33(2):122–67, March–April 2009.

Barr J, Fraser GL, Puntillo K, Ely EW, Gelinas C, Dasta JF, et al. Clinical practice guidelines for the management of pain, agitation, and delirium in adult patients in the intensive care unit. *Crit Care Med* 2013; 41:263–306.

Bellomo R, Ronco C, Kellum JA, et al. Acute renal failure-definition, outcome measures, animal models, fluid therapy and information technology needs: the Second International Consensus Conference of the Acute Dialysis Quality Initiative (ADQI) Group. *Crit Care* 2004; 8:B204.

Burns S. (ed). *AACN Essentials of Critical Care Nursing*, 3rd ed, 2014. McGraw-Hill, New York, New York.

Carlson KK, *Advanced Critical Care Nursing*, 2009, Saunders Elsevier, St. Louis, MO.

Chulay M, Burns SM. A*ACN Essentials of Critical Care Nursing*. 2nd ed. New York, NY: McGraw Hill; 2010.

Correa de Sa, DD, Hodge, DO, Slusser, JP, Redfield, MM, Simari, RD, Burnett, JC & Chen, HH (2010). Progression of preclinical diastolic dysfunction to the development of symptoms. *Heart*, 96 (7), 528–532.

Dellinger RP, Levy MM, Rhodes A, et al. Surviving sepsis campaign: International guidelines for management of severe sepsis and septic shock: 2012, *Crit Care Med* 2013;41:580–637.

Deutschman CS, Neligan PJ. *Evidence-Based Practice of Critical Care*, 2010, Elsevier, Saunders, Philadelphia PA.

Deutschman CS, Neligan PJ. *Evidence-Based Practice of Critical Care*, 2010, Elsevier, Saunders, Philadelphia PA.

Duh SH, Cook JD. Laboratory Reference Range Values. Stedman's Online. Available at *http://www.stedmansonline.com/webFiles/Dict-Stedmans28/APP17.pdf*. Accessed June 17, 2014.

Ely EW, Truman B, Speroff T, et al. Delirium as a predictor of mortality in mechanically ventilated patients in the intensive care unit. *JAMA*, 2004 Apr 14;291(14):1753–1762.

Enteral Nutrition Practice Recommendations Task Force: Bankhead R, Boullata J, Brantley S, et al. Enteral nutrition practice recommendations. *Journal of Parenteral and Enteral Nutrition* 2009;10, 1–46.

Grams ME, Estrella MM, Coresh J, Brower RG, Liu KD, the NHLBI. 2011. Fluid balance, diuretic use, and mortality in acute kidney injury. *Clin J Am Soc Nephrol.* 6(5):966–73.

Guérin C, Girard R, Selli JM, Ayzac L. Intermittent versus continuous renal replacement therapy for acute renal failure in intensive care units: results from a multicenter prospective epidemiological survey. *Intensive Care Med.* 2002;28(10):1411.

Hanlon-Pena, H & Quaal, S. (2011). CE Article: Intra-aortic Balloon Pump Timing: Review of Evidence Supporting Current Practice. *Am J Crit Care* 20, 323–334.

Howard P, Steinmann R, editors. *Sheehy's Emergency Nursing Principles and Practice.* 2010; Mosby/Elsevier, 6th ed., St. Louis, MO.

Jauch EC, Saver JL, Adams HP Jr, et al. Guidelines for the early management of patients with acute ischemic stroke: a guideline for healthcare professionals from the American Heart Association/American Stroke Association. Stroke. 2013: published online before print January 31, 2013, 10.1161/STR.0b013e318284056a, *http://stroke.ahajournals.org/lookup/doi/10.1161/STR.0b013e318284056a*.

Kellum JA, Bellomo R, Ronco C. Kidney attack, *JAMA*, 2012, 307, 21:2265–2266.

Kidney Disease: Improving Global Outcomes (KDIGO). Clinical practice guideline for acute kidney injury. *Kidney Int Suppl.* 2012;2:89–115.

Kirkwood, P. (2002). Ask the Experts. *Critical Care Nurse.* 22, 70–72.

Kushner FG, Hand M, Smith SC Jr, King SB 3rd, 2009 focused updates: ACC/AHA guidelines for the management of patients with ST-elevation myocardial infarction (updating the 2004 guideline and 2007 focused update) and ACC/AHA/SCAI guidelines on percutaneous coronary intervention (updating the 2005 guideline and 2007 focused update): a report of the American College of Cardiology Foundation/American Heart Association Task Force on Practice Guidelines. *J Am Coll Cardiol.* 2009;54:2205–41.

Lameire N, Vanholder R, Van Biesen W. Loop diuretics for patients with acute renal failure: helpful or harmful? *JAMA* 2002; 288:2599.

Lee, Rosemary Koehl. "Intra-Abdominal Hypertension and Abdominal Compartment Syndrome: A Comprehensive Overview," *Critical Care Nurse,* 32(1):19–31, February 2012.

Lewis BE, Wallis DE, Berkowitz SD, et al. Argatroban anticoagulant therapy in patients with heparin-induced thrombocytopenia, *Circulation.* 2001; 103:1838–1843.

Lewis BE, Wallis DE, Berkowitz SD, et al. Argatroban anticoagulant therapy in patients with heparin-induced thrombocytopenia, *Circulation.* 2001; 103:1838–1843.

Longo DL, Fauci AS, Kasper DL, et al. *Harrison's Principles of Internal Medicine,* 18th ed., 2008.

Lynn-McHale Wiegand, D., ed. (2011) *AACN Procedure Manual for Critical Care,* 6th ed. St. Louis, MO: Saunders.

Martindale R, McClave S, Vanek V, et al. Guidelines for the provision and assessment of nutrition support therapy in the adult critically ill patient: Society of Critical Care Medicine and American Society of Parenteral and Enteral Nutrition: Executive Summary. *Crit Care Med* 2009;37(5):1757–1761.

McClave, Snyder (2002) Clinical use of gastric residual volumes as a monitor for patients on enteral tube feeding. *JPEN,* 26(6):S43–S50.

McLean B, Zimmerman JL (editors). *Fundamental Critical Care Support Course,* 4th ed, 2005, SCCM, Mt. Prospect, IL.

Morgan TJ, Acid-base disorders. In Albert RK, Slutsky A, Ranieri M, et al. *Clinical Critical Care Medicine.* 2006, Mosby, Philadelphia PA.

Muller-Plathe O. A nomogram for the interpretation of acid-base data. *J Clin Chem Clin Biochem,* 1987, (25):795–798.

Murray and Nadel's Textbook of Respiratory Medicine. 5th ed. / editors, Robert J. Mason ... [et al.]. Philadelphia, PA : Saunders/Elsevier, c2010.

Nair, PP; Kalita, J, Misra, UK (Jul–Sep 2011). "Status epilepticus: why, what, and how." *Journal of Postgraduate Medicine* 57(3):242–52.

O'Meara, D, et al. (2008). Evaluation of delivery of enteral nutrition in critically ill patients receiving mechanical ventilation. *AJCC,* 17:1, 53–61.

Reddan D, Laville M, Garovic VD. Contrast-induced nephropathy and its prevention: what do we really know from evidence-based findings? *J Nephrol.* 2009;22(3):333–351.

Rice KL, Bennett M, Gomez M, et al. Nurses' recognition of delirium in the hospitalized older adult, *Clin Nurse Spec,* 2011, *www.cns-journal.com,* accessed March 21, 2014.

Standard 66. Transfusion Therapy. "Infusion Nursing Standards of Practice," *Journal of Infusion Nursing* 34(1S):S93–94, January–February 2011. (Level I)

Toto KH, Complex acid-base disorders and associated electrolyte imbalances. In Carlson KK, *Advanced Critical Care Nursing*, 2009, Saunders Elsevier, St. Louis, MO.

Urden L, Stacy K, Lough M. 6th edition (2009) *Critical Care Nursing Diagnosis and Management*. 6th ed. Mosby, St. Louis.

Wright RS, Anderson JL, Adams CD, et al. 2011 ACCF/AHA focused update of the guidelines for the management of patients with unstable angina/non–ST-elevation myocardial infarction (updating the 2007 guideline): a report of the American College of Cardiology Foundation/American Heart Association Task Force on Practice Guidelines. *J Am Coll Cardiol* 2011;57:1920–59.

Improved grades in anatomy and physiology courses start with this selection of BARRON'S titles

Anatomy & Bodybuilding: A Complete Visual Guide
Flexbinding, 978-1-4380-0548-5, $18.99, *Can$21.99*

The Anatomy Student's Self-Test Visual Dictionary
Paperback: 978-0-7641-4724-1, $29.99, *Can$34.50*

The Anatomy Student's Self-Test Coloring Book
Paperback: 978-0-7641-3777-8, $24.99, *Can$29.99*

Barron's Anatomy Flash Cards, 2nd Ed.
Boxed Set, 978-0-7641-6159-9, $26.99, *Can$32.50*

Essential Atlas of Anatomy
Paperback, 978-0-7641-1833-3, $13.99, *Can$16.99*

Essential Atlas of Physiology
Paperback, 978-0-7641-3093-9, $14.99, *Can$16.99*

Dictionary of Medical Terms, 6th Ed.
Paperback, 978-0-7641-4758-6, $14.99, *Can$16.99*

E-Z Anatomy and Physiology, 3rd Ed.
Paperback, 978-0-7641-4468-4, $16.99, *Can$19.99*

The Student's Anatomy of Exercise Manual
Paperback, 978-1-4380-0113-5, $24.99, *Can$28.50*

The Student's Anatomy of Stretching Manual
Paperback, 978-1-4380-0391-7, $24.99, *Can$28.50*

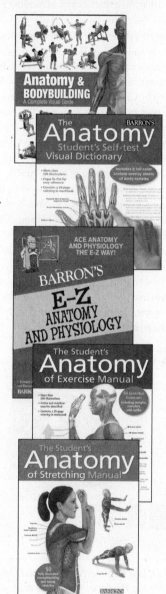

Available at your local book store
or visit **www.barronseduc.com**

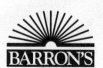

Barron's Educational Series, Inc.
250 Wireless Blvd.
Hauppauge, N.Y. 11788
Call toll-free: 1-800-645-3476

Prices subject to change without notice.

In Canada:
Georgetown Book Warehouse
34 Armstrong Ave.
Georgetown, Ontario L7G 4R9
Call toll-free: 1-800-247-7160

(191a) R 11/14

WE SALUTE THEIR HISTORICAL ACHIEVEMENTS!
From Nightingale to Nursing in the Twenty-first Century

Celebrating Nurses
A Visual History

Dr. Christine Hallett; U.S. Consultant Joan E. Lynaugh, R.N., M.S.N., Ph.D., F.A.A.N.

This refreshing narrative history of nursing marks an exception to standard, often dry academic descriptions of the nursing profession. It presents dramatic, highly readable illustrated stories of nursing's pioneering, often heroic leaders. Following an account of early nineteenth-century nursing practice during the Napoleonic Wars, the book goes on to highlight the life and work of Florence Nightingale who, in the 1850s, elevated nursing to a respected branch of medicine when she served on the Crimean War's battlefields. Also chronicled are the contributions to nursing by Clara Barton, founder of the American Red Cross, and the poet Walt Whitman during the American Civil War. Surgical nursing first became important in the late nineteenth century, following discoveries by Robert Koch in Germany and Louis Pasteur in France of germ theory and infection control. Early twentieth-century accounts chronicle the origin of public health services, and include the story of Adelaide Nutting, the world's first professor of nursing at Columbia Teacher's College in New York. Here too is the story of Edith Cavell, who was executed for helping Allied soldiers escape from German-occupied Belgium during World War I. Nursing's contributions during World War II, as well as in the Korean and Vietnam wars are also described in several vivid accounts. A concluding chapter explains how twenty-first-century nursing has expanded to cover many duties that were once the responsibility of junior doctors. The book's absorbing text is complemented with approximately 200 illustrations and photos.

Hardcover w/jacket, 192 pp., 8 ¹/₂" x 10 ¹/₂"
ISBN-13: 978-0-7641-6286-2, ISBN-10: 0-7641-6286-1
$24.99, Can$29.99

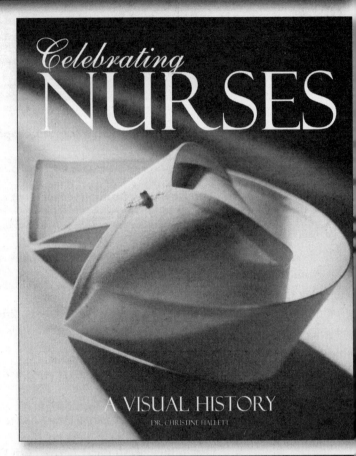

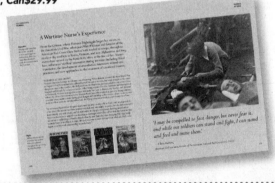

....

Dr. Christine Hallett, Ph.D. is a Registered Nurse and the Director of the Center for the History of Nursing and Midwifery at the University of Manchester, U.K. She also holds fellowships with the Royal Society of Medicine and the Royal Society for the Arts, U.K.

Joan E. Lynaugh, Ph.D., R.N., is Professor Emerita of the School of Nursing at the University of Pennsylvania and the Barbara Bates Center for the Study of the History of Nursing.

....

Highlights from Celebrating Nurses
- Early Military Nursing in the Napoleonic wars and Florence Nightingale in the Crimean War
- What is a Nurse? How the nursing vocation evolved into a highly respected profession
- Surgical Nursing and the emergence of nurses in the operating room
- The Establishment of Nursing Schools, starting in 1907 when Adelaide Nutting at Columbia Teachers College in New York became the world's first nursing professor

Barron's Celebrates National Nurses Week
National Nurses Week is celebrated annually from May 6th, also known as National Nurses Day, through May 12th, the birthday of Florence Nightingale, the founder of modern nursing.

Barron's Educational Series, Inc.
250 Wireless Blvd.
Hauppauge, N.Y. 11788
Call toll-free: 1-800-645-3476

In Canada:
Georgetown Book Warehouse
34 Armstrong Ave.
Georgetown, Ontario L7G 4R9
Call toll-free: 1-800-247-7160

(#190) R 4/10

Prices subject to change without notice.

To order visit us at
www.barronseduc.co
or your local book sto

Barron's puts you on the fast track to success as you prepare for the **NCLEX-RN**

STUDENTS' **#1** CHOICE

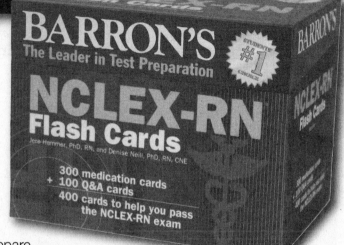

With completion of your nurse training program, you have just one final hurdle to surmount on your career path as a licensed registered nurse—certification by the National Council of State Boards of Nursing. To get certification, you must pass the National Council Licensure Examination for Registered Nurses (NCLEX-RN)—*and Barron's has exactly the help you need for success on that very important exam*.

Flash cards are an effective, time-proven way to prepare for tests of all kinds, and *Barron's NCLEX-RN Flash Cards* have been designed to familiarize you with the questions you'll face on the exam, along with the answers you need to know. The cards are divided into two categories:

BARRON'S

- **300 cards identify medications and their uses**
  Each of these 300 cards names a medication on its front side. It lists its uses, the ways in which it is administered, and its side effects on the back.

- **100 cards present questions like those found on the NCLEX-RN**
  The 100 test question cards closely reflect questions that have appeared on recent actual exams. The questions cover topics that include safe care and environment, safety and infection control, health promotion and maintenance, and related subjects that students are certain to encounter when they take the exam. Answers are printed on each card's reverse side. Easy to use and designed to produce results, *Barron's NCLEX-RN Flash Cards* are your ticket to success as you prepare to take that essential licensure exam.

NCLEX-RN Flash Cards
Jere Hammer, Ph.D., and Denise Neill, Ph.D., R.N., C.N.E.
400 Flash Cards boxed w/enclosed ring,
5 13/16" W x 4 7/16" H x 3 5/8" D
Card size: 5 3/8" x 4"
ISBN 978-1-4380-7085-8
$24.99, *Can$28.50*

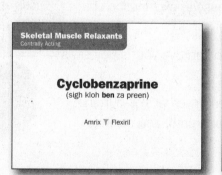

Prices subject to change without notice.

Available at your local book store or visit **www.barronseduc.com**

Barron's Educational Series, Inc.
250 Wireless Blvd.
Hauppauge, NY 11788
Order toll-free: 1-800-645-3476
Order by fax: 1-631-434-3217

In Canada:
Georgetown Book Warehouse
34 Armstrong Ave.
Georgetown, Ont. L7G 4R9
Canadian orders: 1-800-247-7160
Order by fax: 1-800-877-1594

(#215) R7/14

Your first important step on the journey to nursing school

CARROLL COUNTY
JUN 2015
PUBLIC LIBRARY

Barron's Nursing School Entrance Exams 4th Edition

Corinne Grimes, R.N., Ph.D.,
Sandra Swick, R.N., B.C., Ed.D., C.M.S.R.N.,
and Rita Callahan, R.N., B.S.N., M.A., Ph.D.

Does the nursing school program you've applied to require an entrance exam. If yes, then here's the resource that contains all the information and strategies you'll need to get a great score.

Nursing school entrance exams provide nursing programs with specific information relating to an applicant's abilities in content areas that provide the foundation for nursing courses. This includes verbal ability, reading comprehension, numerical or mathematical ability, and life and/or physical sciences.

Inside you'll find: WITHDRAWN FROM LIBRARY

- A multi-part exam that reflects the standards of the most widely given nursing entrance exams, with all questions answered and explained

- Review quizzes with answer explanations in every chapter

- Strategies designed to improve your study skills and test-taking ability

- A subject review covering verbal skill-building, reading comprehension, math, and science

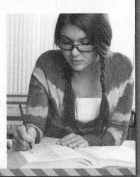

BARRON'S
The Leader in Test Preparation
#1 STUDENTS' CHOICE

NURSING SCHOOL ENTRANCE EXAMS

PREPARATION FOR:
NLN PAX-RN • NET
TEAS • PSB-RN • C-NET-RN

4TH EDITION
Corinne Grimes, R.N., Ph.D.,
Sandra Swick, R.N., B.C., Ed.D., C.M.S.R.N., and
Rita R. Callahan, R.N., B.S.N., M.A., Ph.D.

- A multi-part exam that reflects the standards of the most widely given nursing school entrance exams, with all questions answered and explained
- Review quizzes with answer explanations in every chapter
- Strategies designed to improve your study skills and test-taking ability
- A subject review covering verbal skill-building, reading comprehension, math, and science

Paperback, 312 pp., 8 3/8" x 10 7/8"

ISBN 978-0-7641-4668-8

$18.99, *Can$22.99*

Available at your local book store
or visit **www.barronseduc.com**

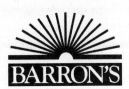

BARRON'S

(#290) R7/14

Barron's Educational Series, Inc.
250 Wireless Blvd.
Hauppauge, NY 11788
Order toll-free: 1-800-645-3476
Order by fax: 1-631-434-3217

In Canada:
Georgetown Book Warehouse
34 Armstrong Ave.
Georgetown, Ont. L7G 4R9
Canadian orders: 1-800-247-7160
Order by fax: 1-800-877-1594

Prices subject to change without notice.